Atlas of 3D Transesophageal Echocardiography in Structural Heart Disease Interventions

Ming-Chon Hsiung • Wei-Hsian Yin
Fang-Chieh Lee • Wei-Hsuan Chiang

Atlas of 3D Transesophageal Echocardiography in Structural Heart Disease Interventions

Cases and Videos

Springer

Ming-Chon Hsiung
Division of Cardiology
Cheng Hsin General Hospital
Taipei, Taiwan

Wei-Hsian Yin
Division of Cardiology
Cheng Hsin General Hospital
Taipei, Taiwan

Fang-Chieh Lee
Division of Cardiology
Cheng Hsin General Hospital
Taipei, Taiwan

Wei-Hsuan Chiang
Division of Cardiology
Cheng Hsin General Hospital
Taipei, Taiwan

ISBN 978-981-10-6936-9 ISBN 978-981-10-6937-6 (eBook)
https://doi.org/10.1007/978-981-10-6937-6

Library of Congress Control Number: 2018931379

Printed on acid-free paper

This Springer imprint is published by the registered company Springer Nature Singapore Pte Ltd. part of Springer Nature
The registered company address is: 152 Beach Road, #21-01/04 Gateway East, Singapore 189721, Singapore

Preface

Interventional cardiology has recently progressed from coronary and noncoronary vascular interventions to interventions for structural heart disease. The procedures have been developed to treat conditions that have been traditionally managed by surgeries and medical therapies. Moreover, the success of interventional therapies depends highly on the skills of transesophageal echocardiographic imaging, especially three dimensional, which allows visualizing the entire scenario in which interventions take place in a single view.

The field is young and worthy of investigations. While the knowledge, principles, and techniques have been well established by numerous previous publications, we share in this book our clinical experiences mainly by introducing classic and unique cases we have dealt with. We have collected a series of over 35 interesting cases. In each of them, background information, clinical presentations, and diagnostic findings are followed by step-by-step approaches of interventional therapies and outcomes after the procedures. The highlight of the book is that we utilize a large number of illustrations, over 700, to demonstrate various cardiovascular pathologies. Most of the figures are three-dimensional transesophageal echocardiograms; they are cooperated with two-dimensional transesophageal echocardiograms, X-rays, fluoroscopies, computed tomograms, etc. Since the echo images we obtained in clinical practice are moving images, we have also included over 450 videos, which serve as a supplement to the static illustrations in the casebook.

The atlas is composed of five chapters. In chapter one, cases received transcatheter aortic valve implantation are described. Valve-in-valve therapy is discussed in chapter two. Chapter three details the MitraClip procedure. Chapter four covers closure of congenital and acquired cardiac defects. Cases suffered from complications after interventional procedures are provided in the last chapter. It is our hope of this volume to offer readers an insider's view of three-dimensional transesophageal echocardiography in structural heart disease interventions and to refresh your clinical training.

Growing from conception to completion, this casebook mirrored many of the experiences of parenting, especially wise from the rearing of our previous book, *Atlas of Perioperative 3D Transesophageal Echocardiography*. Thankfully, Cheng Hsin General Hospital, Taipei, Taiwan, provided us full clinical support.

We also appreciate the Division of Cardiovascular and Heart Center for facilitating transesophageal echocardiography in structural heart disease interventions. Lastly, the entire Echocardiography Laboratory is thanked for compiling the cases and delivering the new book to the public.

Taipei, Taiwan Ming-Chon Hsiung
Taipei, Taiwan Wei-Hsian Yin
Taipei, Taiwan Fang-Chieh Lee
Taipei, Taiwan Wei-Hsuan Chiang

Contents

Brief Introduction of Three-Dimensional Transesophageal Echocardiography in Structural Heart Disease Interventions

Modern technological developments have contributed to the progress of new devices and procedures, which have significantly improved the opportunity to effectively treat structural heart diseases. Interventional cardiology has been receiving rapid and wide execution as a practical alternative treatment to surgery for several congenital and acquired diseases. The advent of transcatheter valve implantation and repair techniques set up one of the main revolutions of the last decades. Such development is also thoroughly related to a continuous progress in cardiac imaging. Certainly, multimodality cardiac imaging, such as X-ray, echocardiography, and computed tomography, has become indispensible in providing precise patient selection and in monitoring the interventional procedures in order to elevate the success rate and minimize the incidence of complications. Additionally, the role of transesophageal echocardiography, which requires a careful and noninvasive imaging instrument, has evolved to support the procedures from the initial planning and intraoperative monitoring to the assessment of the acute result and follow-up.

Transesophageal echocardiography is generally regarded as a fundamental imaging tool for guidance of percutaneous procedure. Coupled with fluoroscopy, it provides detailed and dependable information to the operators, enabling measurement of the annulus diameter, origin of the regurgitation, defects and their rims, visualization of devices, and evaluation of the results. However, conventional two-dimensional transesophageal echocardiography has some intrinsic limitations. Locating guiding wires and catheters and assessing device position, particularly when multiple devices are used, can often be challenging with two-dimensional imaging. Three-dimensional transesophageal echocardiography enables accurate localization of guiding wires and catheters during the procedure. It also provides a surgical view to clearly demonstrate the mitral anatomy. In cases where multiple devices are used, three-dimensional transesophageal echocardiography provides information on their arrangement and relationship with surrounding structures. An innovative echocardiographic imaging tool, real-time three-dimensional transesophageal echocardiography, which is based on miniaturized matrix array transducers, allows three-dimensional imaging in real time without the requirement of multiple-beat acquisition and is especially useful for guidance of every phase of percutaneous procedures.

Even if transesophageal echocardiography has been confirmed to be an essential tool for planning and execution of cardiac interventions, the helpfulness of three-dimensional echo is becoming more and more evident along with the developing skills of operators.

Transcatheter Aortic Valve Implantation

1

1.1 Introduction

Transcatheter aortic valve implantation provides an alternative to surgical aortic valve replacement in patients who have severe aortic stenosis or regurgitation but are poor candidates for surgery. Thus far, two different transcatheter aortic valve implantation systems have dominated the market: the self-expanding Medtronic CoreValve, suitable for a transfemoral or subclavian approach; and the balloon expandable Edwards SAPIEN valve, suitable for a transfemoral or transapical approach.

Prior to the transcatheter aortic valve implantation, a careful evaluation of the aortic valvular complex is required, most often with transthoracic echocardiography and computed tomography. During the procedure, angiography and transesophageal echocardiography play crucial roles monitoring every single process: introduction, delivery, alignment, deployment and releasing of the transcatheter aortic valve. Also, the position of the device and cardiac hemodynamic condition should be confirmed to prevent any possible complication.

This chapter lists several patients who have undergone transcatheter aortic valve implantation with the Medtronic CoreValve and the Edwards SAPIEN valve system with delicate illustrations of transesophageal echocardiography cooperating with computed tomography and angiography demonstrating lesions diagnoses, interventional processes, and clinical outcomes.

Electronic supplementary material The online version of this chapter (https://doi.org/10.1007/978-981-10-6937-6_1) contains supplementary material, which is available to authorized users.

M.-C. Hsiung et al., *Atlas of 3D Transesophageal Echocardiography in Structural Heart Disease Interventions*, https://doi.org/10.1007/978-981-10-6937-6_1

1.2 Transapical SAPIEN Valve Implantation

A 62-year-old female patient had surgical mitral valve replacement seven years ago. She suffered from exertional dyspnea that worsened recently. Auscultation showed irregular rhythm with a grade 3/6 systolic murmur over apex region. Electrocardiogram showed atrial fibrillation and left ventricular hypertrophy. Echocardiogram revealed severe aortic stenosis with moderate regurgitation. Therefore, the heart team decided transcatheter aortic valve implantation (Figs. 1.1, 1.2, 1.3, 1.4, 1.5, 1.6, 1.7, 1.8, and 1.9 ; Videos 1.1a, 1.1b, 1.2, 1.3a, 1.3b, 1.4a, 1.4b, 1.5, 1.6, 1.7, 1.8, and 1.9).

Transapical and transarterial approaches are both available for a SAPINE valve implantation. In this patient who had undergone a surgical mitral valve replacement, which increases the difficulty of crossing the native stenotic valve, transapical approach might be a better option.

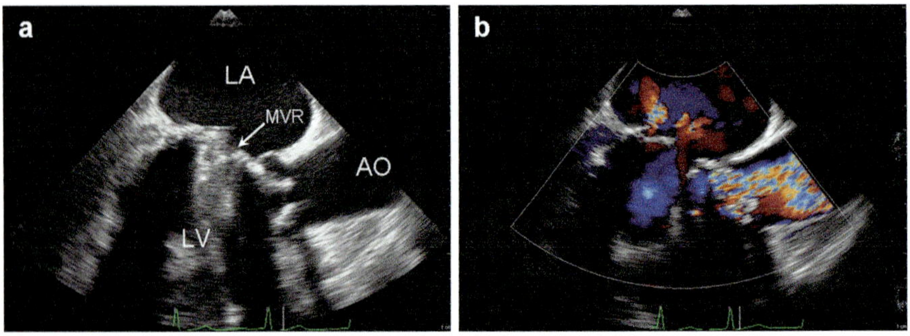

Fig. 1.1 In transesophageal echocardiographic mid-esophageal long-axis view, the patient had received mitral valve replacement (MVR, **a**) with mechanical prothesis before. Calcified aortic valve reduced cusp separation and caused turbulent left ventricular outflow (**b**)

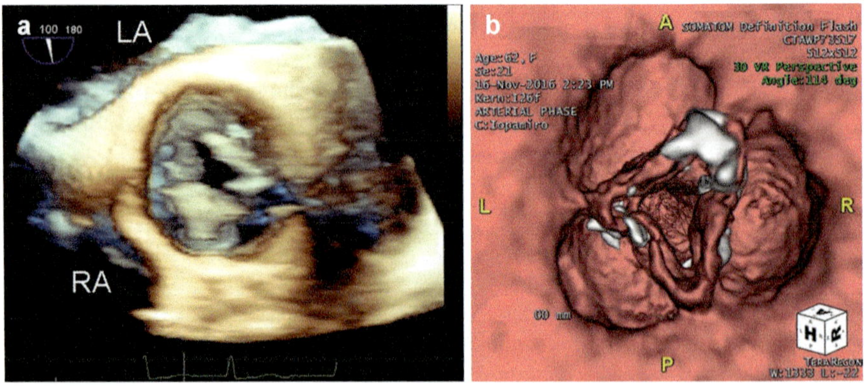

Fig. 1.2 Three dimensional echocardiogram (**a**) and reconstructive computed tomogram (**b**) of aortic valve showed severe calcification of RCC and NCC commissural which reduced the aortic orifice

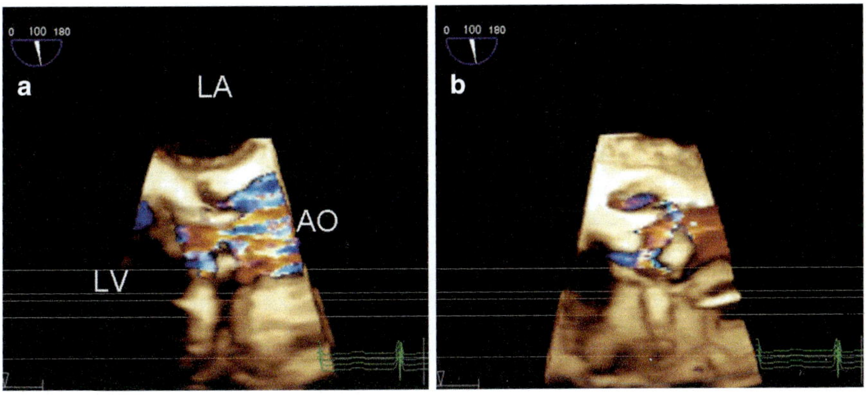

Fig. 1.3 Three dimensional color Doppler showed turbulent outflow across calcified aortic valve in systole (**a**) and moderate aortic regurgitation in diastole (**b**)

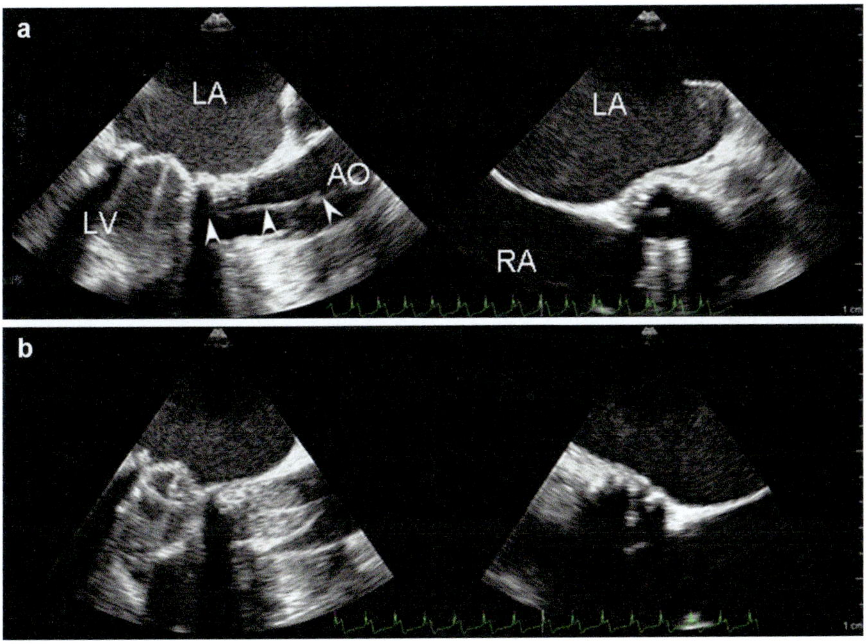

Fig. 1.4 In x-plane views during the transcatheter aortic valve implantation, *rapid pacing (180BPM) was started*, a delivery sheath (arrow heads, **a**) advanced through the stenotic native aortic valve, then the SAPIEN valve was delivered by it and expanded by balloon (**b**)

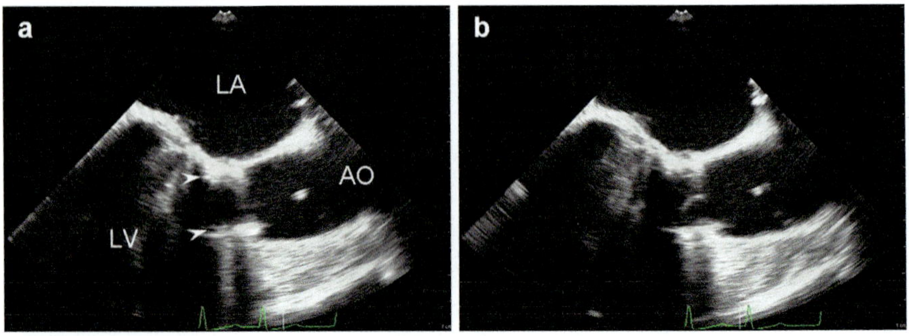

Fig. 1.5 After the transcatheter aortic valve implantation, the SAPIEN valve (arrow heads) presented normal function in systole (**a**) and diastole (**b**)

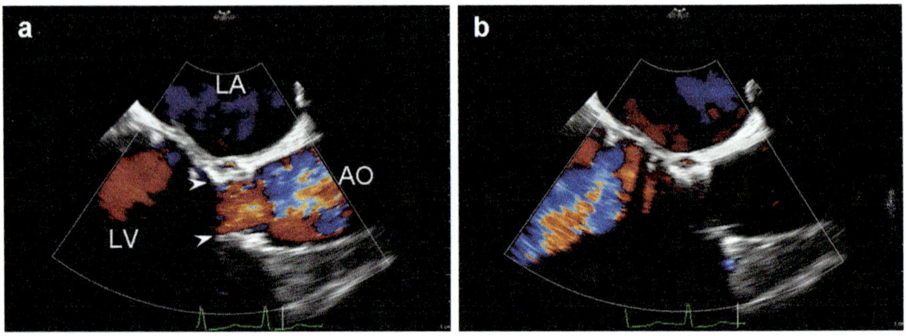

Fig. 1.6 Color Doppler long-axis view after the transcatheter aortic valve implantation. There was no turbulent flow across the SAPIEN valve (arrow heads, **a**), and only trivial paravalvular leakage was present (**b**)

Fig. 1.7 In three dimensional view after the implantation, the SAPIEN valve (arrow heads) was well positioned

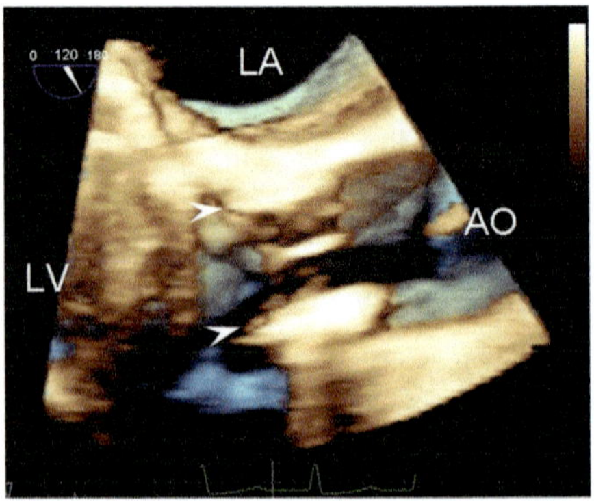

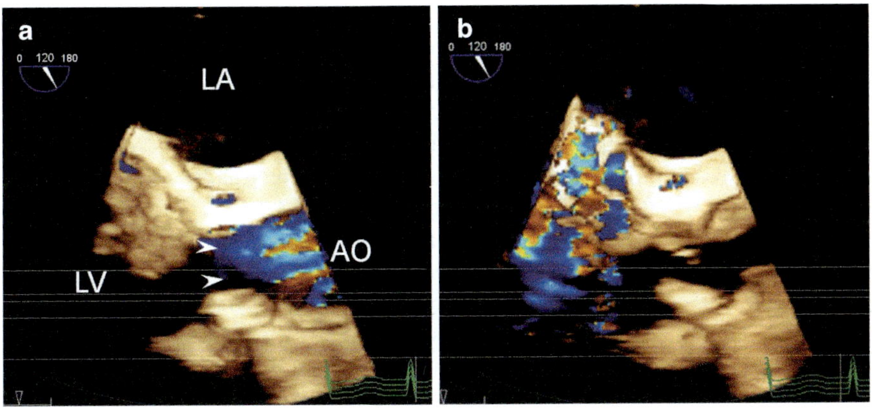

Fig. 1.8 Color Doppler long-axis view after the transcatheter aortic valve implantation. There was no turbulent flow across the SAPIEN valve (arrow heads, **a**), and only trivial paravalvular leakage was present (**b**)

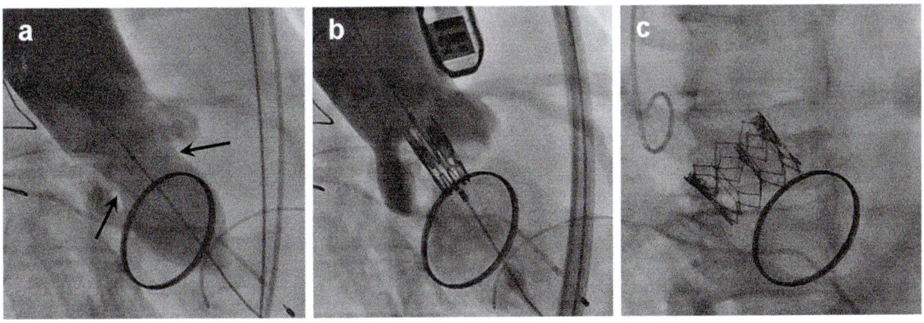

Fig. 1.9 Aortic root angiography during implantation of the SAPIEN valve. (**a**) The contrast injection showed the position of the cusps (arrows) which were unlikely to obstruct the left main artery while being replaced. (**b**) The SAPIEN valve was advanced onto the balloon and aligned between the two radiopaque markers. (**c**) After the procedure, the SAPEIN valve was well expanded

1.3 Transapical SAPIEN Valve Implantation for Lower Limbs Arteries Atherosclerotic Calcifications

A 70-year-old female patient had a history of three-vessel coronary artery bypass graft, type two diabetes mellitus, hypertension and hyperlipidemia. She was found conscious lost then admitted to our emergency department, where tarry stool, shortness of breath and desaturation were noted. Auscultation showed a grade 3/4 murmur over aortic region. Echocardiography revealed critical aortic valve stenosis with the mean and peak gradient are 40 and 60 mmHg respectively. Therefore, due to high risk for open heart surgery, transcatheter aortic valve implantation was indicated (Figs. 1.10, 1.11, 1.12, 1.13, 1.14, 1.15, 1.16, and 1.17; Videos 1.10, 1.11, 1.12a, 1.12b, 1.13a, 1.13b, 1.13c, 1.14, 1.15, 1.16, and 1.17).

Transapical access is a technique entering the left ventricular apex through a small anterolateral intercostal thoracotomy, following by left ventricular puncture and sheath advancement into the ventricular cavity. At the end of the procedure, the apex and thoracotomy are surgically closed.

This approach may reduce danger of iliofemoral injury, arch atheroembolism, and movement during deployment in comparison with transarterial approach. However, the disadvantages include greater risk of ventricular injury, recurrent bleeding, and late apical pseudoaneurysm formation. Most patients receive transapical approach in the presence of severe iliofemoral disease to raise the outcomes.

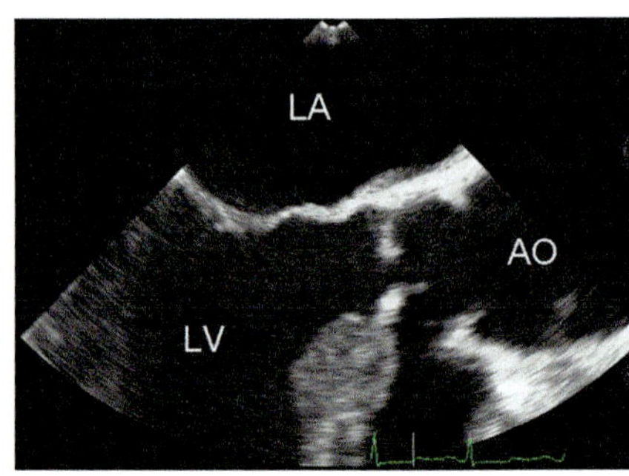

Fig. 1.10 In transesophageal echocardiographic midesophageal long-axis approach, thickened aortic valve restricted cusp mobility and reduced cusp separation

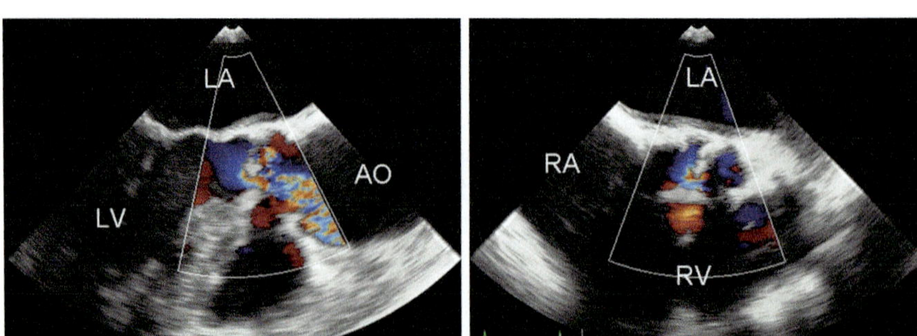

Fig. 1.11 X-plane view with color Doppler showed turbulent flow across the thickened aortic valve

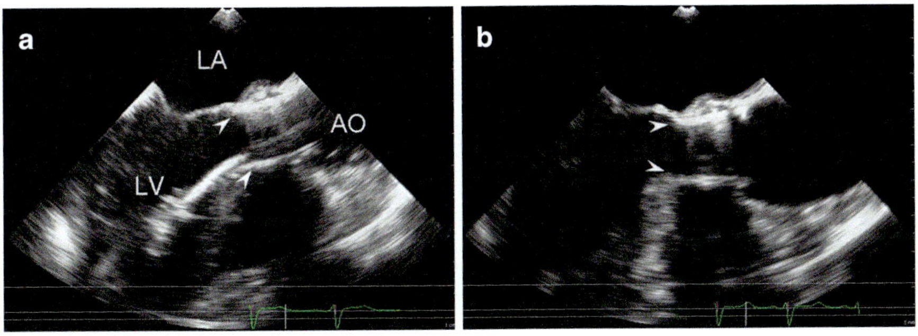

Fig. 1.12 During the transcatheter aortic valve implantation, the SAPIEN valve (arrow heads) was delivered and expanded by the delivery system (**a**), and then released (**b**)

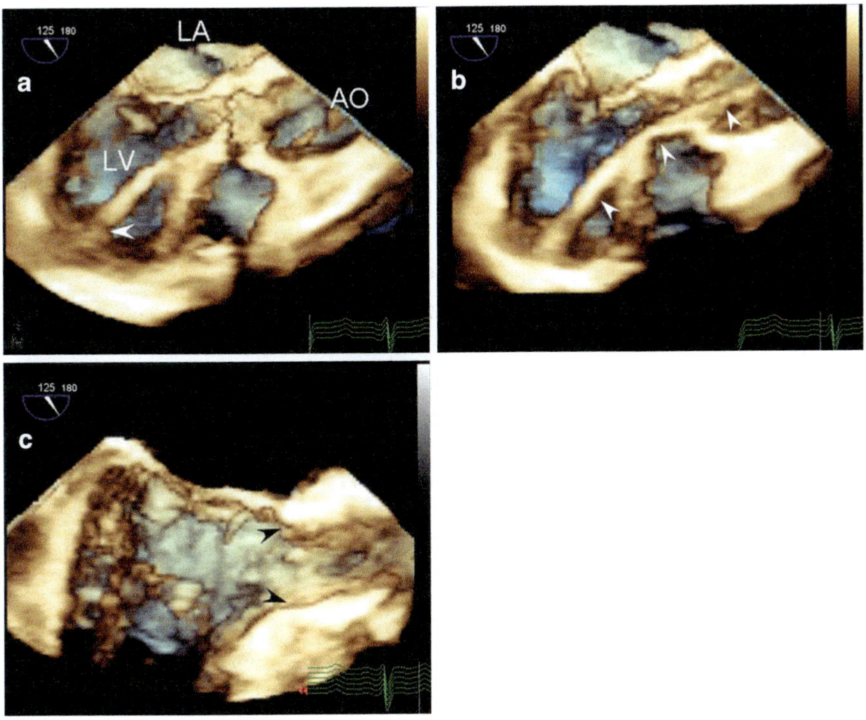

Fig. 1.13 Three dimensional mid-esophageal long- axis views during the transcatheter aortic valve implantation. (**a**) The sheath was advanced into the left ventricular cavity from the apical potion (arrow head). Then the sheath (arrow heads, **b**) crossed the aortic valve for the SAPIEN valve delivery and deployment. (**c**) After the implantation, the SAPIEN valve (arrow heads) was well positioned and expanded

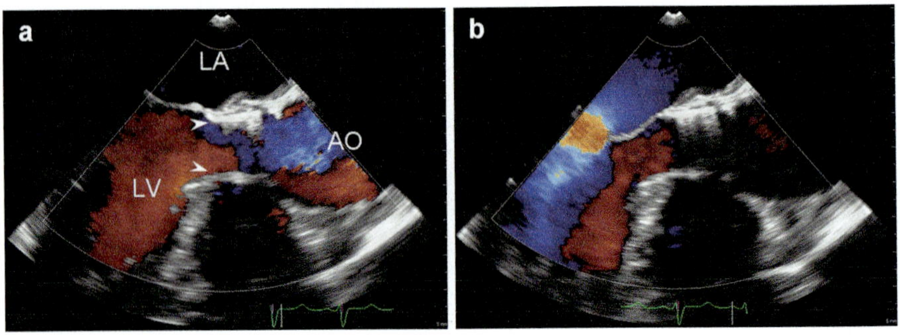

Fig. 1.14 Long-axis views with color Doppler after the transcatheter aortic valve implantation. There was no turbulent flow across the SAPIEN valve (**a**, arrow heads), and only trivial paravalvular leakage was present (**b**)

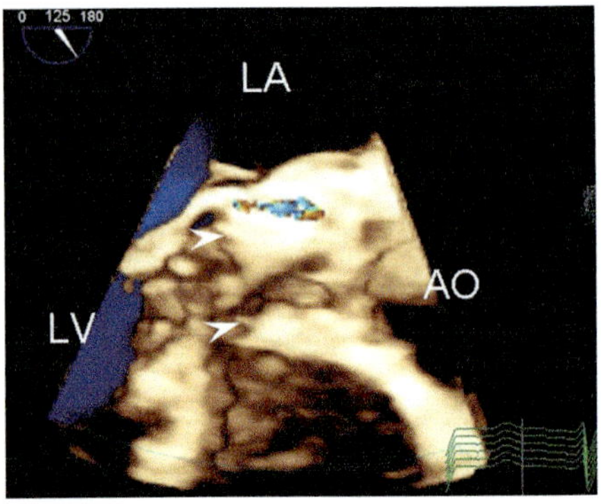

Fig. 1.15 In three dimensional color Doppler after the implantation, the SAPIEN valve (arrow heads) was well positioned with trivial paravalvular leakage present

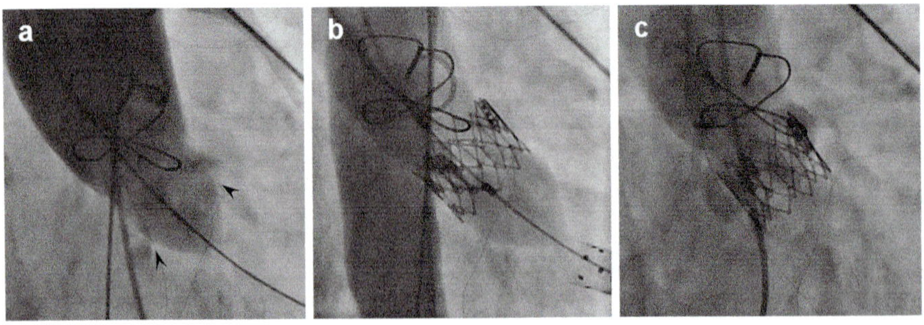

Fig. 1.16 Aortic root angiography during the procedure. (**a**) Contrast injection during valvuloplasty shows the position of cusps (arrow heads). (**b**) The SAPIEN valve was expanded by the balloon. (**c**) After implantation, approximately one half of the valve was below the basal sinus border

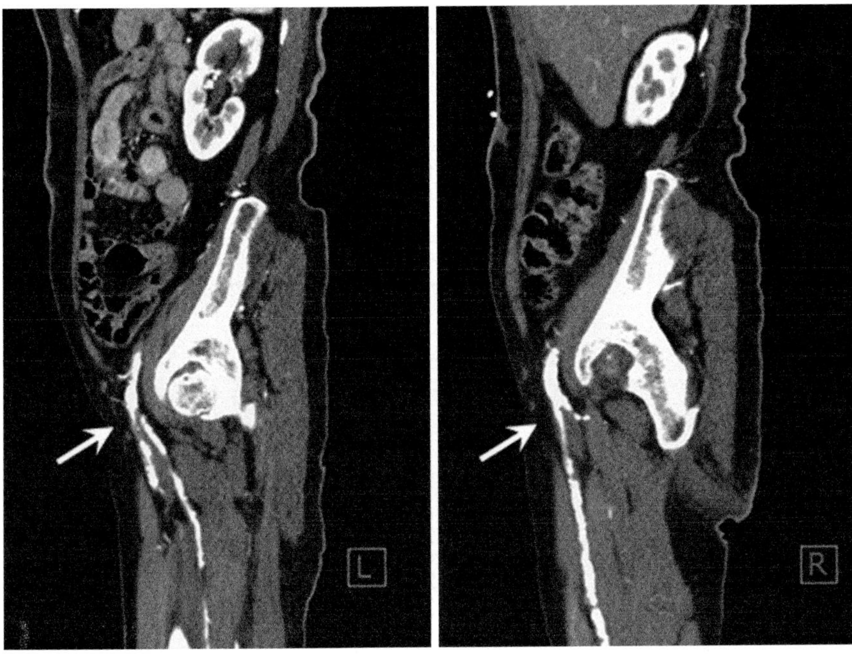

Fig. 1.17 CT showed atherosclerotic calcifications of bilateral iliac arteries and lower limbs arteries (arrows)

1.4 SAPIEN Valve Implantation of Bicuspid Aortic Valve

A 70-year-old male patient had a known history of valvular heart disease with aortic stenosis and hypertension under medical therapy for years. Recently, he suffered from shortness of breath on exertion. Under the impression of his symptoms, transcatheter aortic valve implantation was arranged by the heart team (Figs. 1.18, 1.19, 1.20, 1.21, 1.22, 1.23, 1.24, 1.25, 1.26, 1.27, and 1.28; Videos 1.18, 1.19, 1.20, 1.21a, 1.21b, 1.22, 1.23, 1.24, 1.25, 1.26, 1.27, and 1.28).

Transcatheter aortic valve implantation is not a common treatment to congenital bicuspid aortic valve stenosis because stenotic bicuspid annuli are usually larger and more eccentric than stenotic tricuspid valves. As such, three dimensional imaging is strongly advised for aortic valve size measurement.

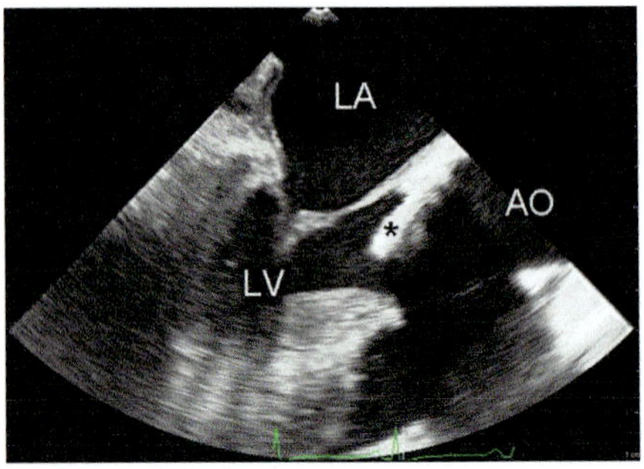

Fig. 1.18 In transesophageal echocardiographic mid-esophageal long-axis view, a giant calcification (asterisk) attached to aortic valve protruded into the left ventricular outflow tract

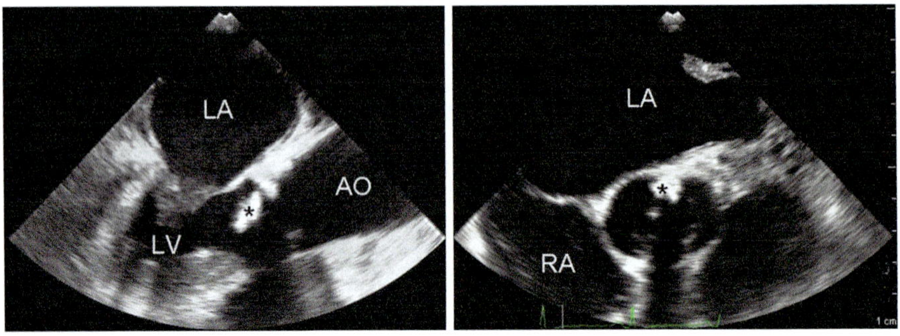

Fig. 1.19 In x-plane view, bicuspid aortic valve with a small elliptical orifice was revealed. There was a giant calcification (asterisk) attached to commissure and protruded into the left ventricular outflow tract

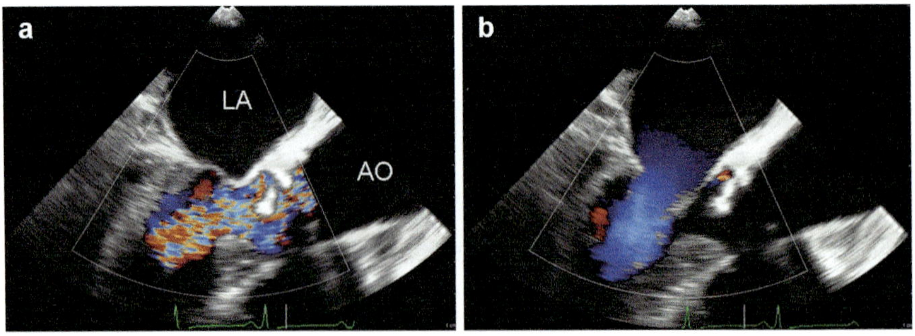

Fig. 1.20 With color Doppler, the thickened aortic valve induced turbulent left ventricular outflow in systole (**a**) and mild regurgitation in diastole (**b**)

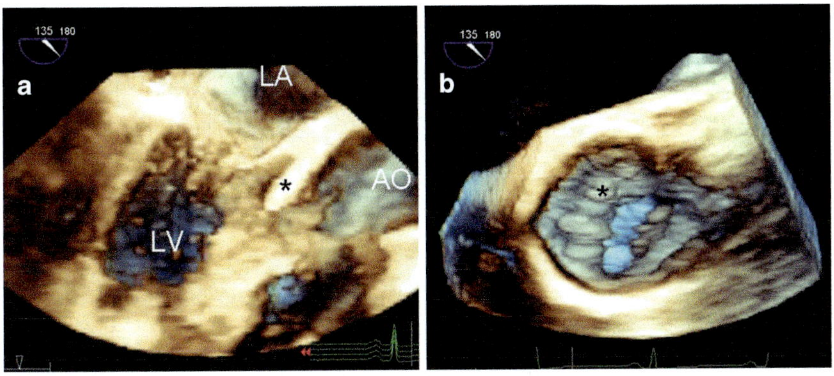

Fig. 1.21 Three dimensional long-axis (**a**) and short-axis (**b**) views of aorta showed bicuspid aortic valve with a giant calcification (asterisk) attached to commissure and protruded into the left ventricular outflow tract

Fig. 1.22 Three dimensional color Doppler showed turbulent left ventricular outflow across the calcified bicuspid aortic valve

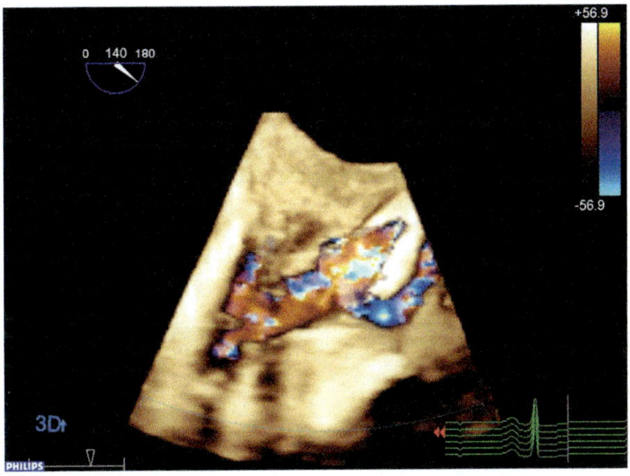

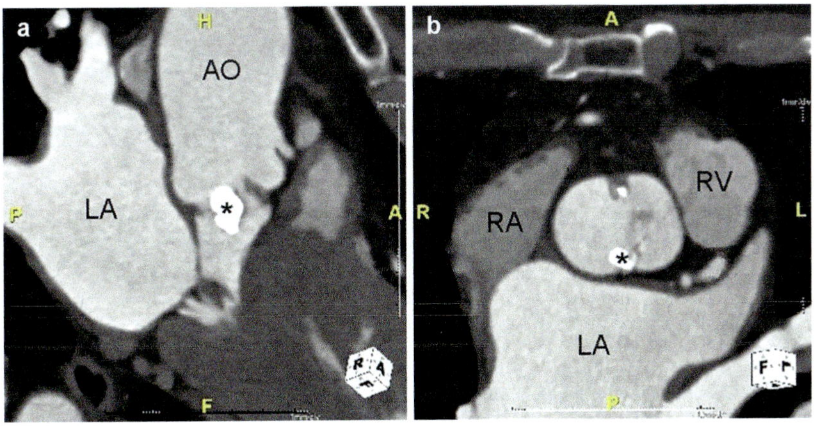

Fig. 1.23 Computed tomographic horizontal plane (**a**) and cross section (**b**) of sinus of Valsalva. Bicuspid aortic valve with a giant calcification (asterisk) attached to commissure and protruded into the left ventricular outflow tract was revealed

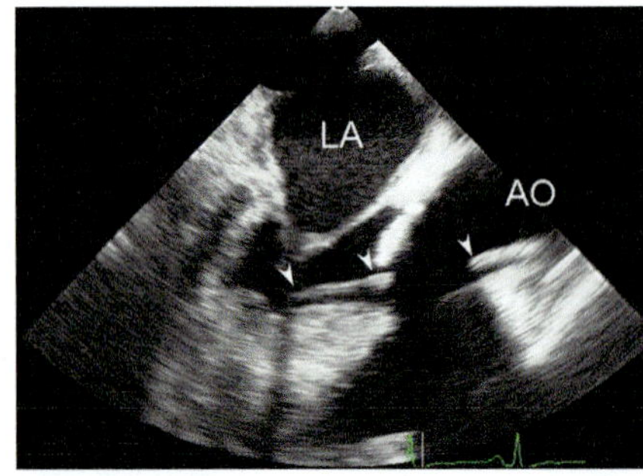

Fig. 1.24 During the transcatheter aortic valve implantation, the guiding sheath (arrow heads) advanced cross the aortic valve

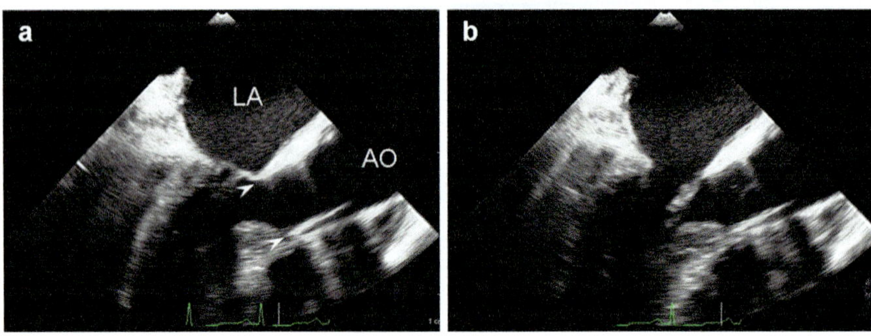

Fig. 1.25 After the transcatheter aortic valve implantation, the SAPIEN valve (26 mm, arrow heads) presented normal function in systole (**a**) and diastole (**b**)

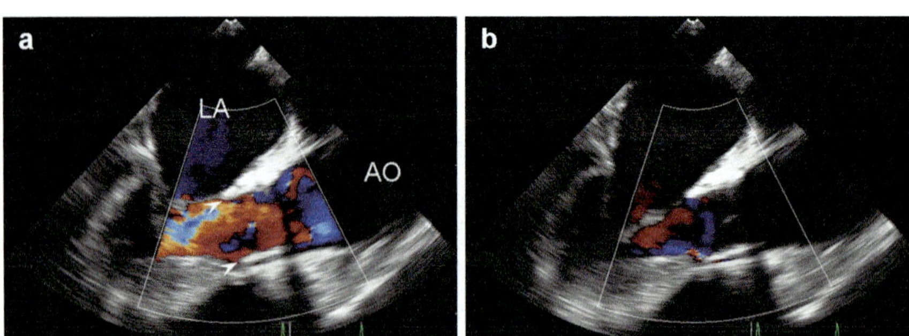

Fig. 1.26 Color Doppler long-axis view after the transcatheter aortic valve implantation. There was no turbulent flow across the SAPIEN valve (arrow heads, **a**), and only trivial paravalvular leakage was present (**b**)

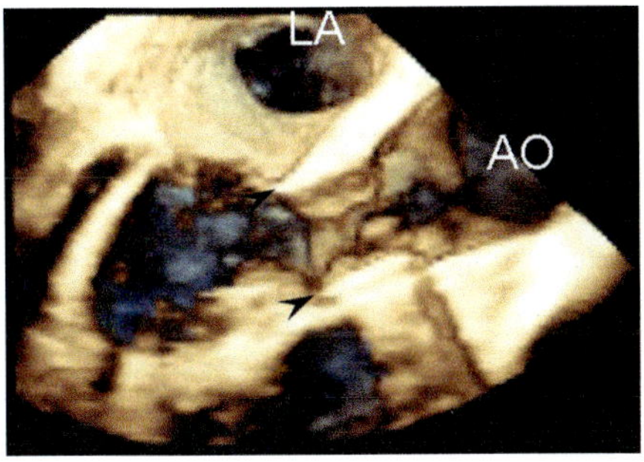

Fig. 1.27 In three dimensional view after the implantation, the SAPIEN valve (arrow heads) was well positioned

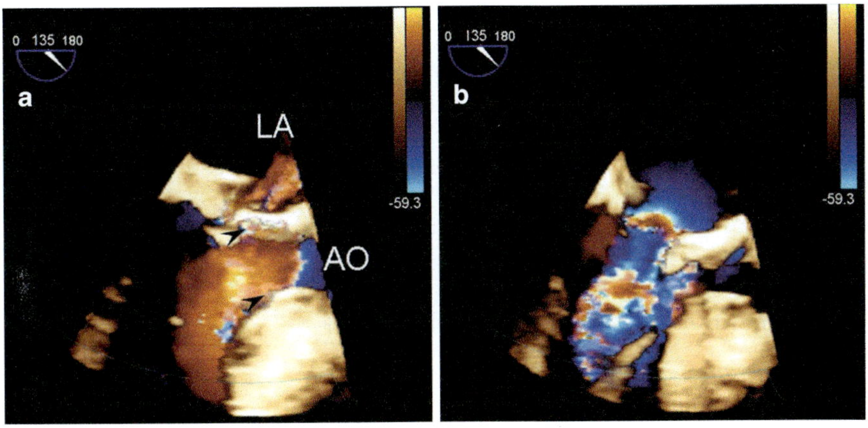

Fig. 1.28 Three dimensional color Doppler long-axis view after the transcatheter aortic valve implantation. There was no turbulent flow across the SAPIEN valve (arrow heads, **a**), and only trivial paravalvular leakage was present (**b**)

1.5 Paravalvular Leakage After CoreValve Implantation Decreased with Time

A 68-year-old female patient suffered from anorexia and shortness of breath. Auscultation showed irregular rhythm with a grade 3/6 diastolic murmur. Chest X-ray showed right side pleural effusion with decreased lung volume. Echocardiogram revealed severe aortic stenosis with moderate regurgitation. Therefore, transcatheter aortic valve implantation was indicated by the heart team (Figs. 1.29, 1.30, 1.31, 1.32, 1.33, 1.34, 1.35, and 1.36; Videos 1.29, 1.30a, 1.30b, 1.31, 1.32a, 1.32b, 1.33, 1.34, 1.35a, 1.35b, and 1.36).

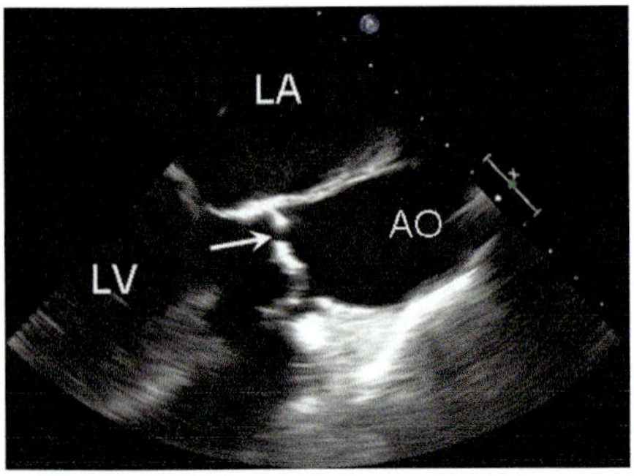

Fig. 1.29 In transesophageal echocardiographic mid-esophageal long-axis view, calcified aortic valve (arrow) reduced cusp mobility

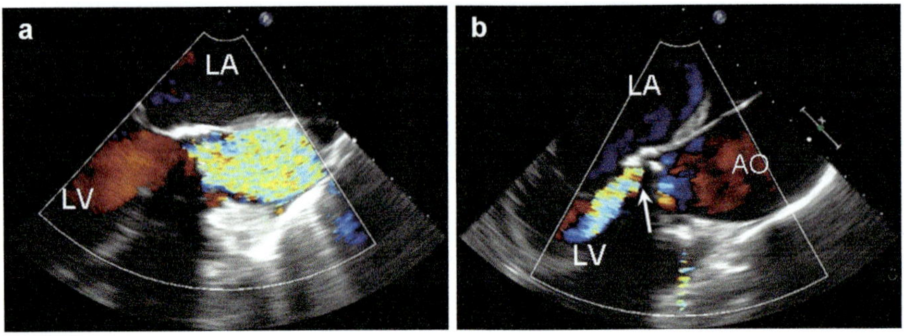

Fig. 1.30 In color Doppler, calcified aortic valve caused turbulent left ventricular outflow in systole (**a**) and moderate regurgitation (arrow, **b**) in diastole

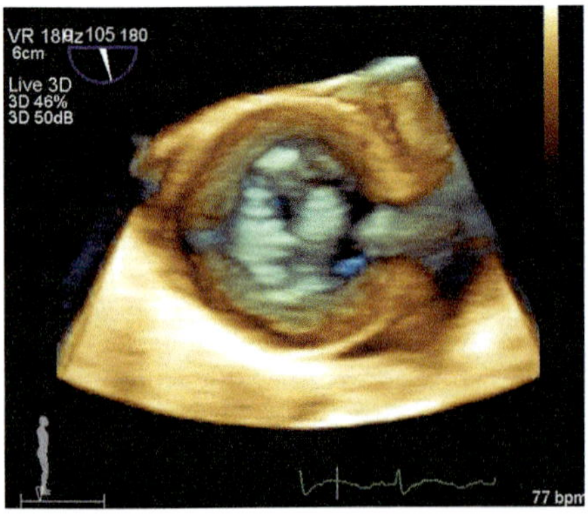

Fig. 1.31 Three dimensional echocardiogram of aortic valve showed severe calcification reducing the aortic orifice

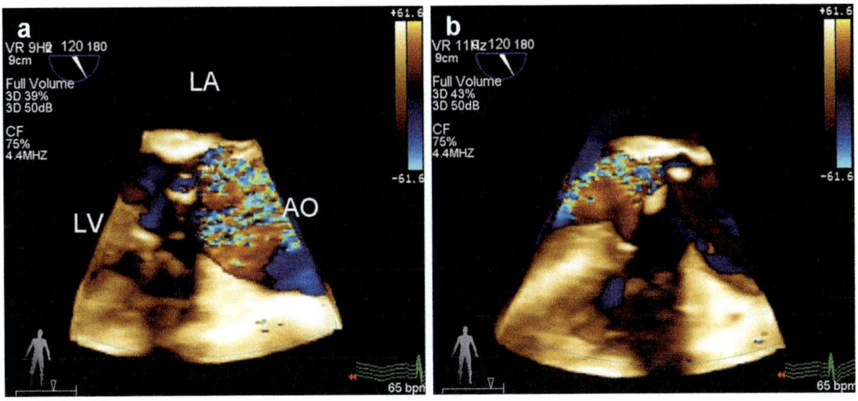

Fig. 1.32 Three dimensional color Doppler showed turbulent outflow across calcified aortic valve in systole (**a**) and moderate aortic regurgitation in diastole (**b**)

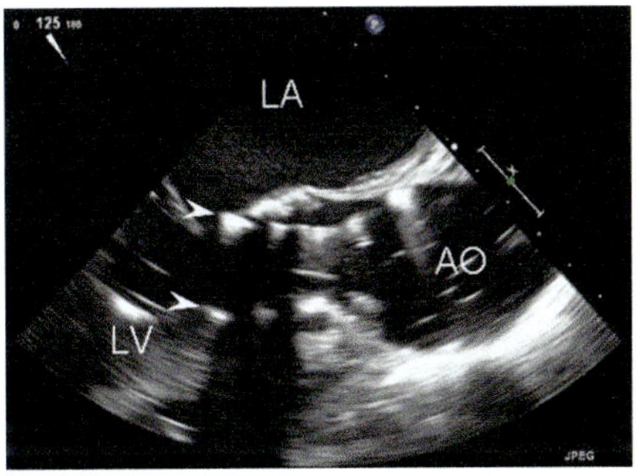

Fig. 1.33 During the transcatheter aortic valve implantation, the CoreValve (arrow heads) was delivered a guiding catheter and deployed

The Metronic CoreValve is a self-expandable transcatrher heart valve. The frame will keep expanding itself even after released till the device fit the aortic annulus thoroughly. Therefore, optimal oversizing of the bioprosthesis can lead to continuous outward expansion of the CoreValve and consequently reduse paravalvular leakage without further postdeployment balloon valvuloplasty.

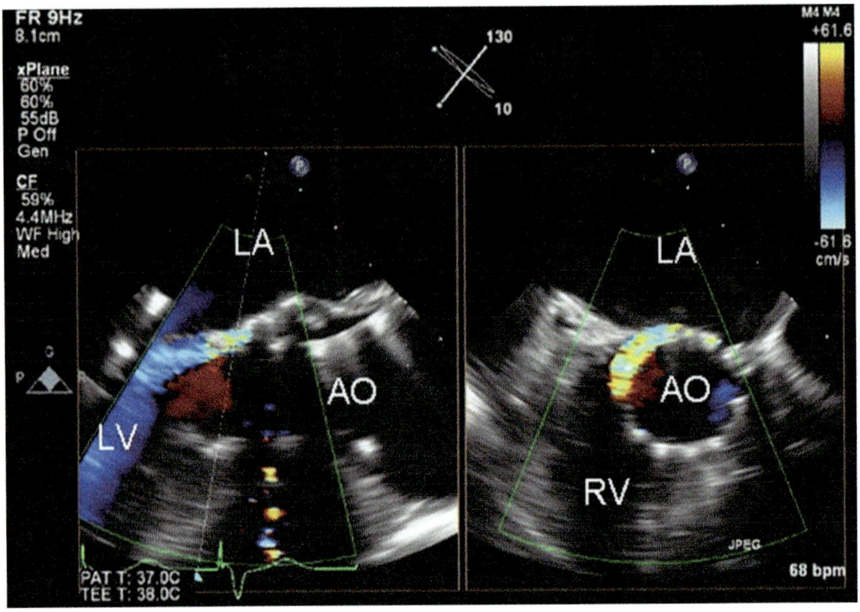

Fig. 1.34 X-plane color Doppler after the transcatheter aortic valve implantation. There was moderate paravalvular leakage from nine o'clock to twelve o'clock position in short-axis view

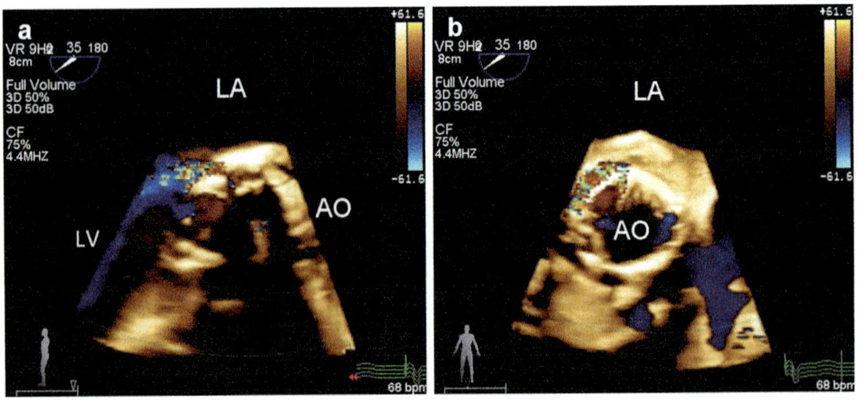

Fig. 1.35 Three dimensional color Doppler of long- (**a**) and short-axis views (**b**) after the implantation. In short-axis view, the origin of the paravalvular leakage accounted for approximately 25% of aortic valve annulus

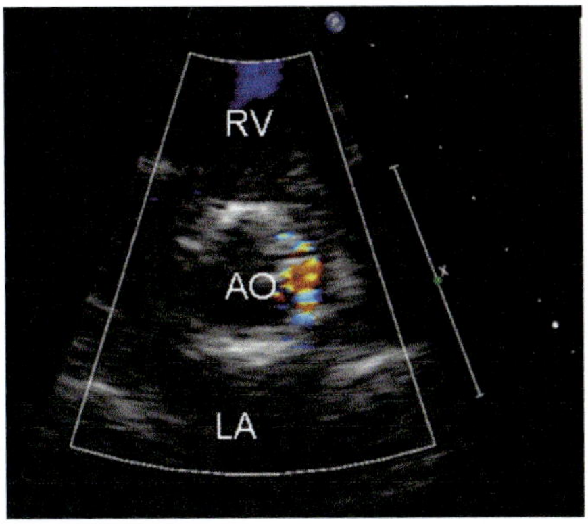

Fig. 1.36 In a transthoracic parasternal short-axis view of a one month follow-up, reduced paravalvular leakage was presented

1.6 CoreValve Implantation After David Operation

A 70-year-old male patient had a history of dilation of aortic root and ascending aorta and had received a David operation a year ago. He suffered from dyspnea recently. Auscultation showed regular rhythm with a grade 3/6 diastolic murmur over right sternal border. Electrocardiogram showed sinus rhythm with left ventricular hypertrophy. Echocardiography revealed severe aortic regurgitation. Therefore, transcatheter aortic valve implantation was indicated by the heart team (Figs. 1.37, 1.38, 1.39, 1.40, 1.41, 1.42, 1.43, 1.44, and 1.45; Videos 1.37a, 1.37b, 1.38, 1.39a, 1.39b, 1.40, 1.41a, 1.41b, 1.42, 1.43, 1.44, and 1.45).

As a result of the high rate of complications associated with the previous David operation, further surgical procedures are increasingly avoided. Owing to calculated preoperative risk, transcatheter aortic valve implantation was considered to be the treatment of choice. During the procedure, the implantation of the CoreValve did not interfere with the graft in the ascending aortic position. Therefore, we can conclude that transcatheter aortic valve implantation can be done in patients with a history of complex thoracic aortic operations.

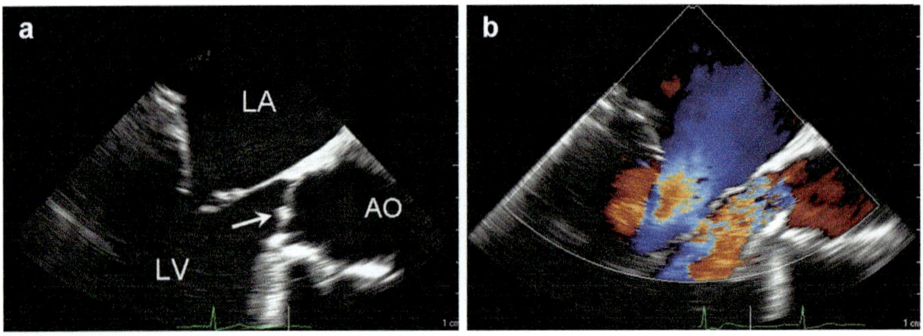

Fig. 1.37 In transesophageal echocardiographic midesophageal long-axis approach, prolapse of aortic right coronary cusp (arrow, **a**) was demonstrated and severe aortic regurgitation was seen by color Doppler (**b**)

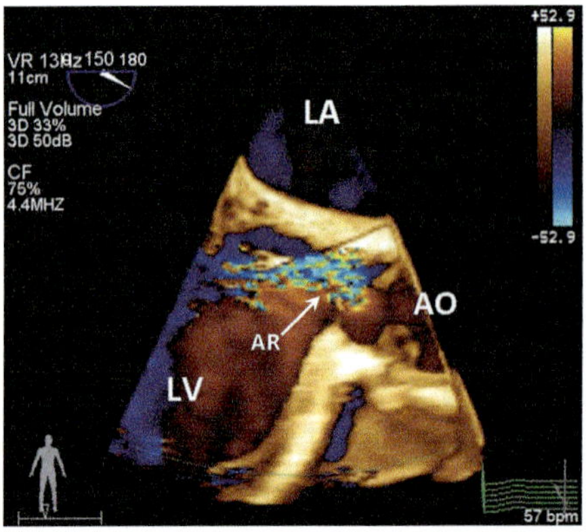

Fig. 1.38 Three dimensional color Doppler showed severe aortic regurgitation (arrow) in diastole

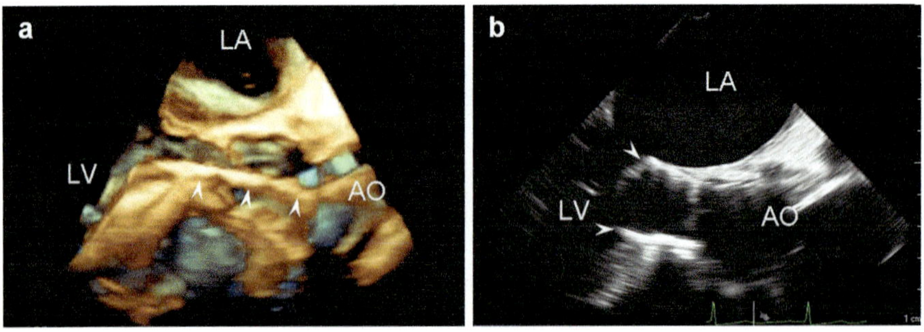

Fig. 1.39 During the transcatheter aortic valve implantation, the guiding catheter (arrow heads, **a**) advanced across the native aortic valve. Afterward, the CoreValve (arrow heads, **b**) was delivered and deployed

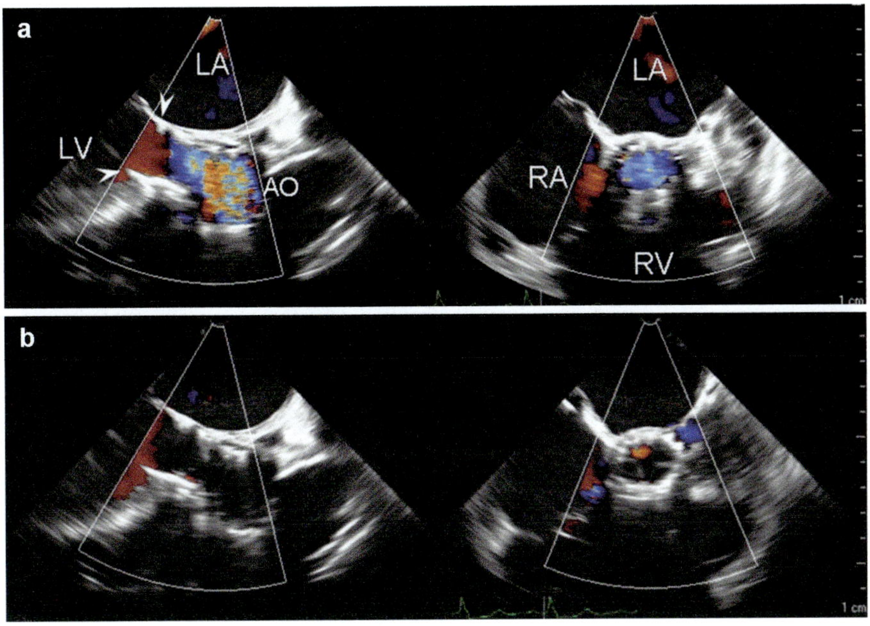

Fig. 1.40 X-plane views with color Doppler after the transcatheter aortic valve implantation. There was no turbulent flow across the CoreValve (arrow heads, **a**) in systole, and only trivial leakage was present in diastole (**b**)

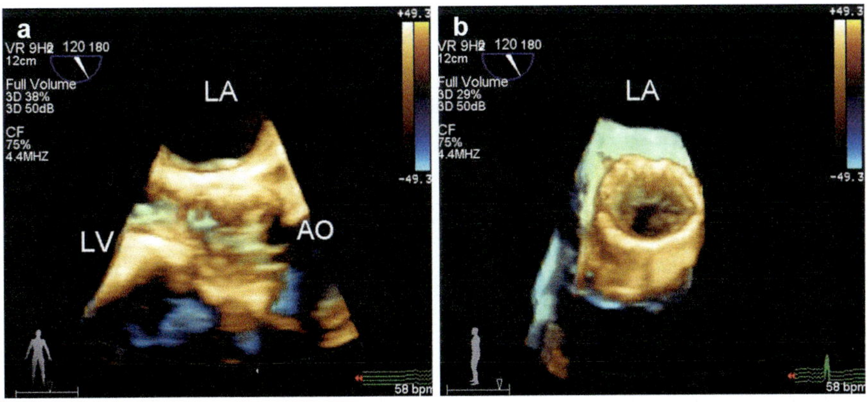

Fig. 1.41 In three dimensional long- (**a**) and short-axis views (**b**) after the implantation, the CoreValve was well positioned

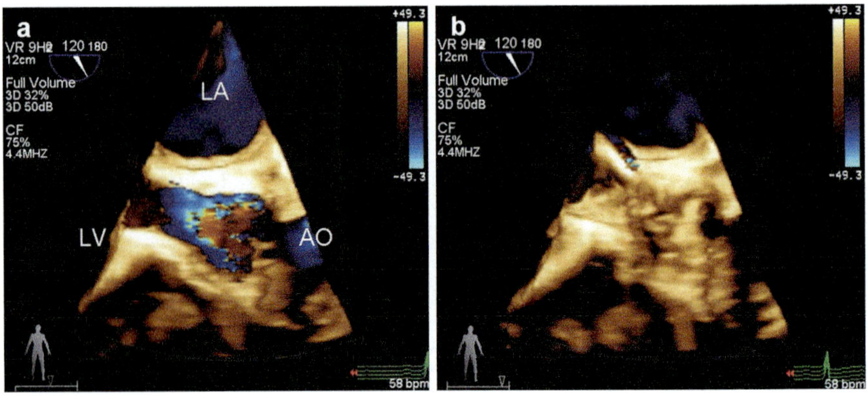

Fig. 1.42 In three dimensional color Doppler after the implantation, there was no turbulent flow across the CoreValve in systole (**a**) and only trivial leakage was present in diastole (**b**)

Fig. 1.43 The one month trans-thoracic follow-up showed normal prosthetic function in apical five-chamber view

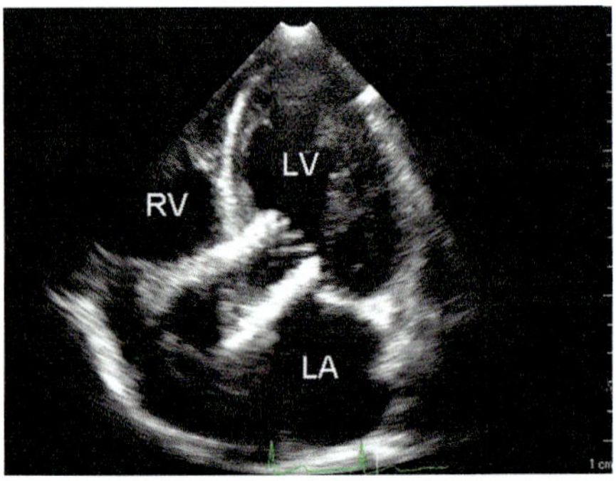

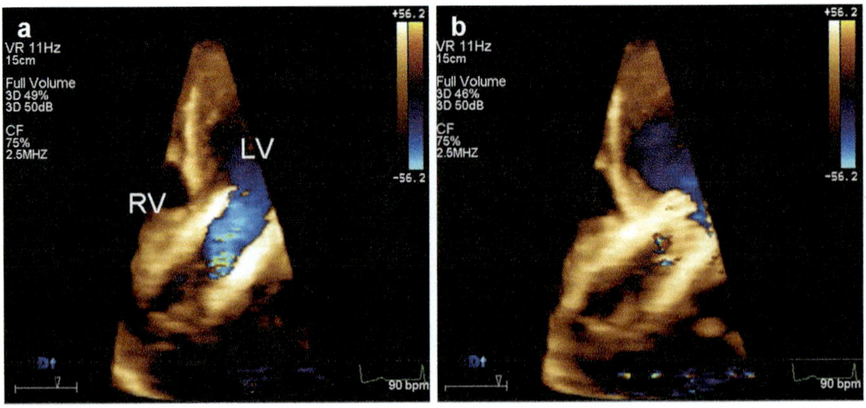

Fig. 1.44 Mild aortic regurgitation was presented by trans-thoracic three dimensional color Doppler in the one month follow-up in systole (**a**) and diastole (**b**)

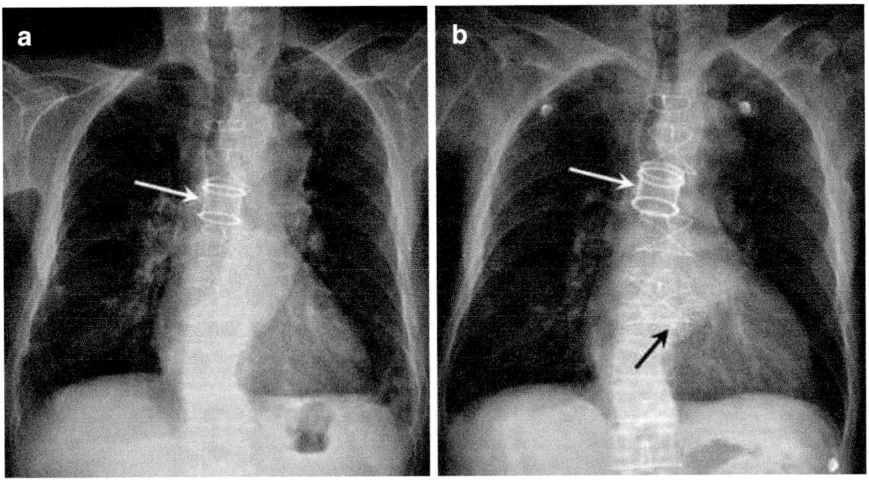

Fig. 1.45 Chest X-rays after the David operation (**a**) and the subsequent transcatheter aortic valve implantation (**b**). Retained surgical wires of median sternotomy, graft in ascending aorta (white arrow), and CoreValve within aortic root (black arrow) were demonstrated

1.7 Valve-In-Valve Implantation of CoreValve for Malposition

A 74-year-old male patient had a known history of critical aortic stenosis. Recently, he suffered from intermittent dyspnea of exertion. Therefore he was admitted and scheduled for a transcatheter aortic valve implantation (Figs. 1.46, 1.47, 1.48, 1.49, 1.50, 1.51, 1.52, 1.53, 1.54, 1.55, 1.56, 1.57, and 1.58; Videos 1.46, 1.47, 1.48, 1.49, 1.50, 1.51, 1.52, 1.53, 1.54, 1.55, 1.56a, 1.56b, 1.57a, 1.57b, and 1.58).

Device malpositioning causing severe paravalvular leakage after transcatheter aortic valve implantation is not a rare finding. It occurs after release of the prosthesis, leading to hemodynamic compromise. It can be managed successfully in selected cases with implantation of a second device inside the malpositioned primary prosthesis. The clinical and echocardiographic outcomes are favorable. The valve-in-valve technique offers a viable therapeutic option in patients with acute significant paravalvular leakage without recourse to emergent surgery.

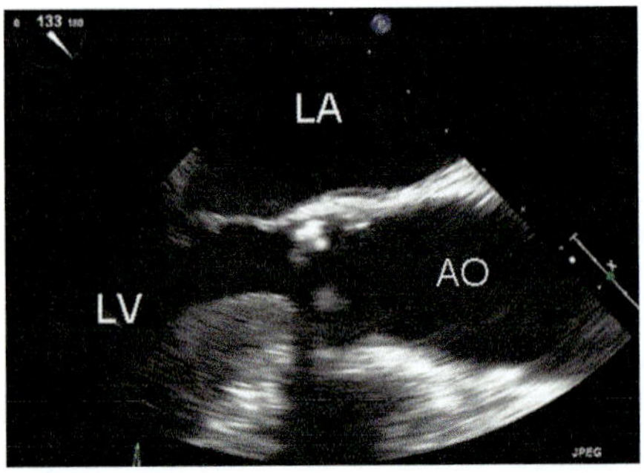

Fig. 1.46 In transesophageal echocardiographic midesophageal long-axis approach, localized calcification of aortic valve was demonstrated

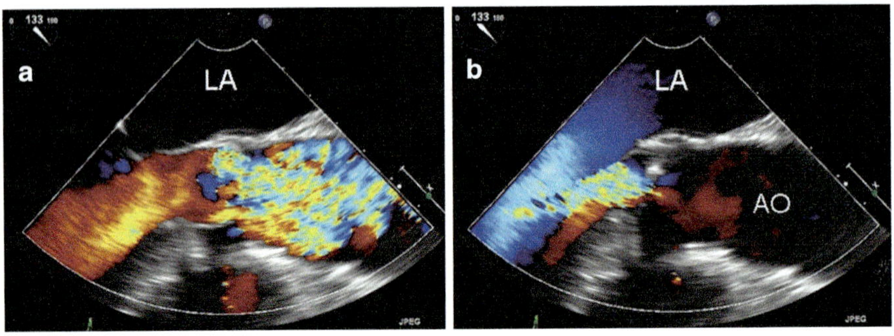

Fig. 1.47 Color Doppler showed turbulence at the level of the calcified aortic valve in systole (**a**) and moderate regurgitation in diastole (**b**)

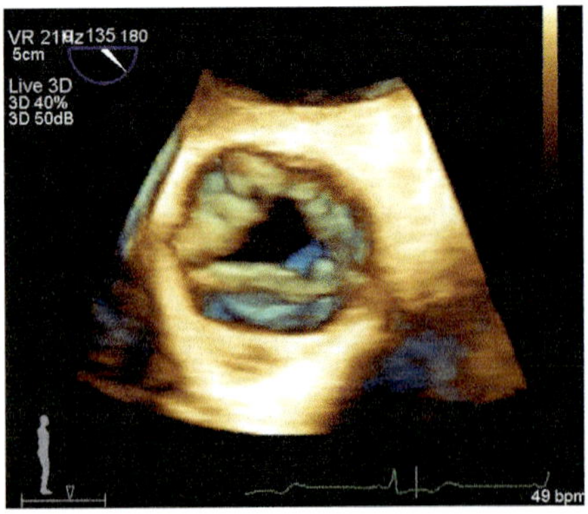

Fig. 1.48 Three dimensional short-axis view of aortic valve showed restrictive valvular morbidity and reduced orifice

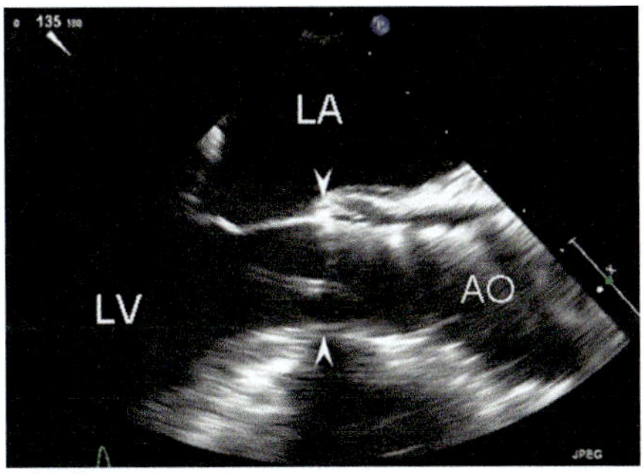

Fig. 1.49 During the transcatheter CoreValve implantation, the position of the device (arrow heads) was below the basal sinus border, which may potentially lead to devise dislocalization

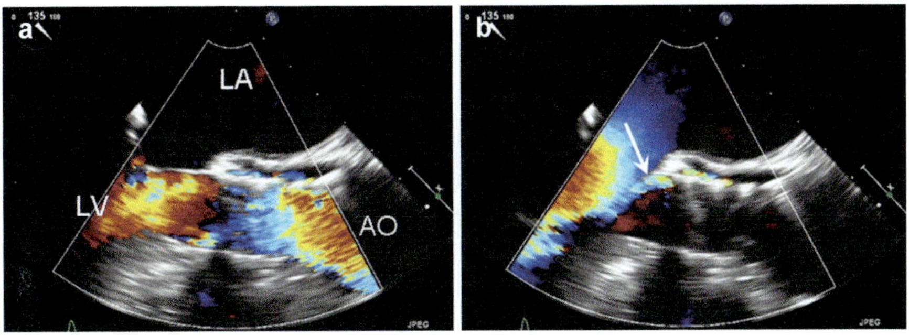

Fig. 1.50 Color Doppler showed smooth flow crossing the CoreValve in systole (**a**) and mild paravalvular leakage was present in diastole (arrow, **b**)

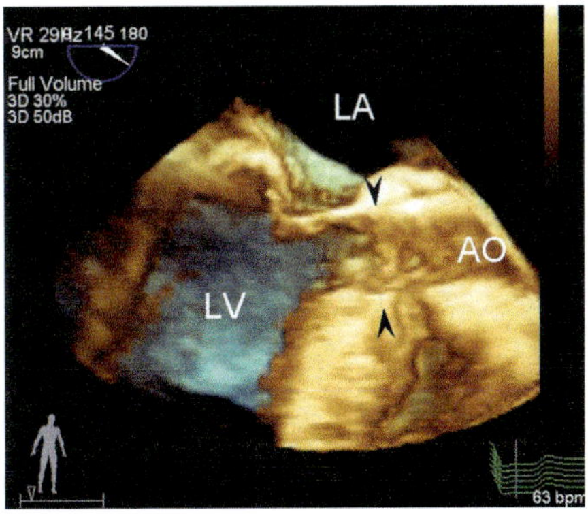

Fig. 1.51 In a three dimensional image, the CoreValve (arrow heads) was implanted lower than the basal sinus border

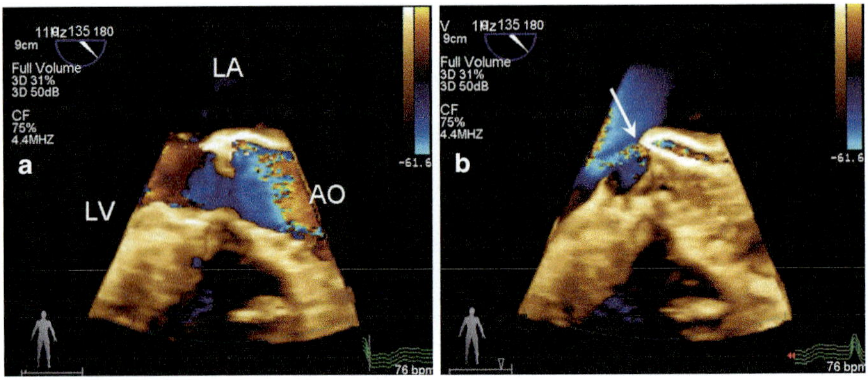

Fig. 1.52 Three dimensional color Doppler showed smooth flow crossing the CoreValve in systole (**a**) and mild paravalvular leakage was present in diastole (arrow, **b**)

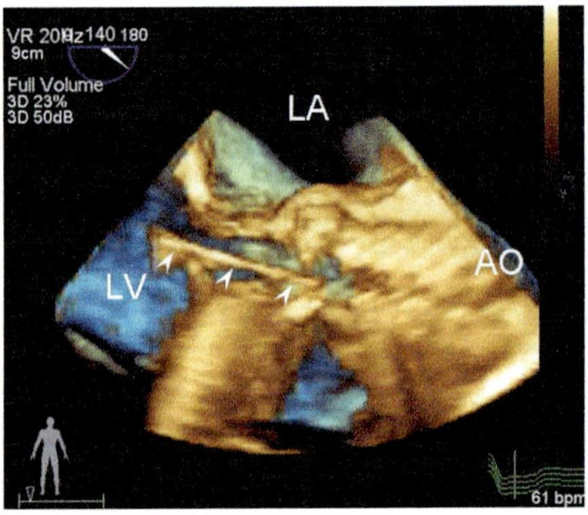

Fig. 1.53 To prevent complications, redo valve-in-valve implacement was indicated right after the preceding procedure. The guiding catheter (arrow heads) was demonstrated within the previous CoreValve

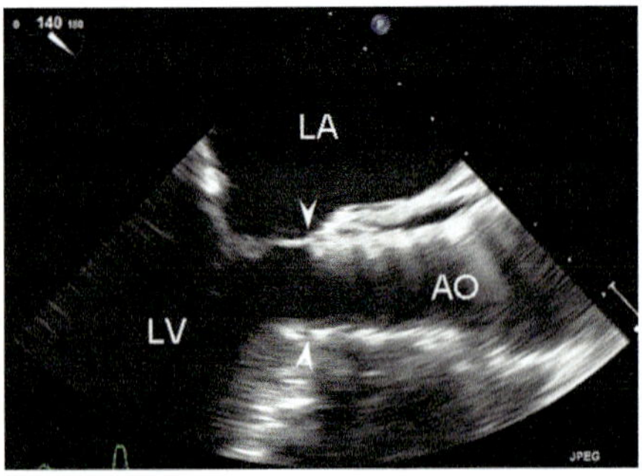

Fig. 1.54 After the redo valve-in-valve procedure, the position of the CoreValve (arrow heads) was revealed beyond the basal sinus border

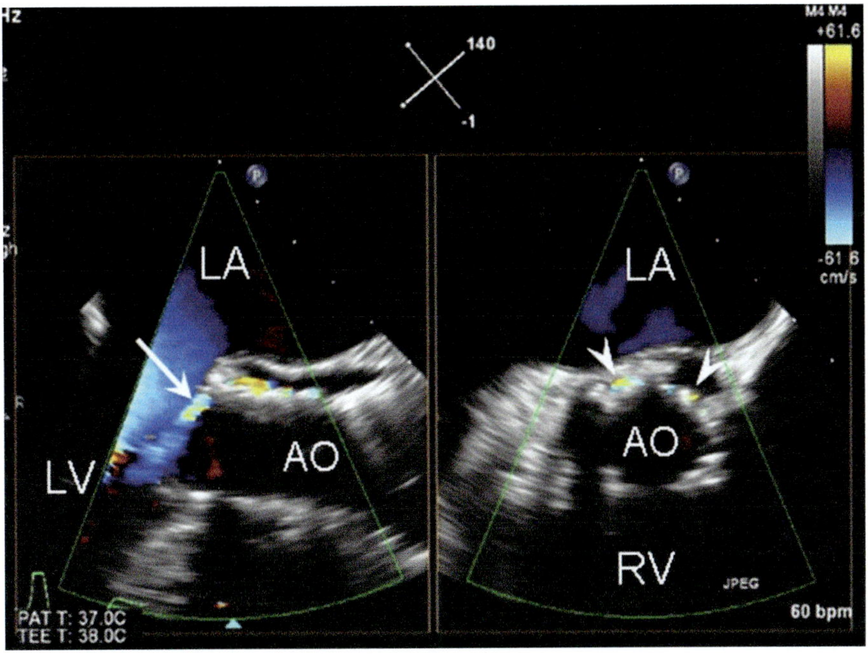

Fig. 1.55 In x-plane color Doppler minimal paravalvular regurgitation (arrows) was present

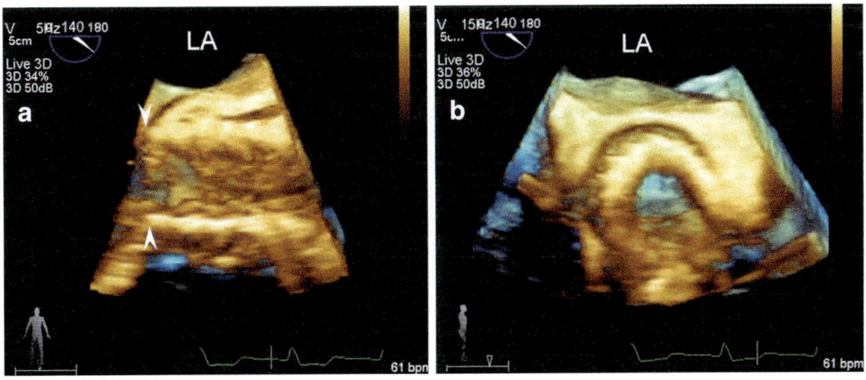

Fig. 1.56 Three dimensional long- (**a**) and short-axis views (**b**) showed the CoreValve (arrows) was implanted beyond the basal sinus border which was a proper position

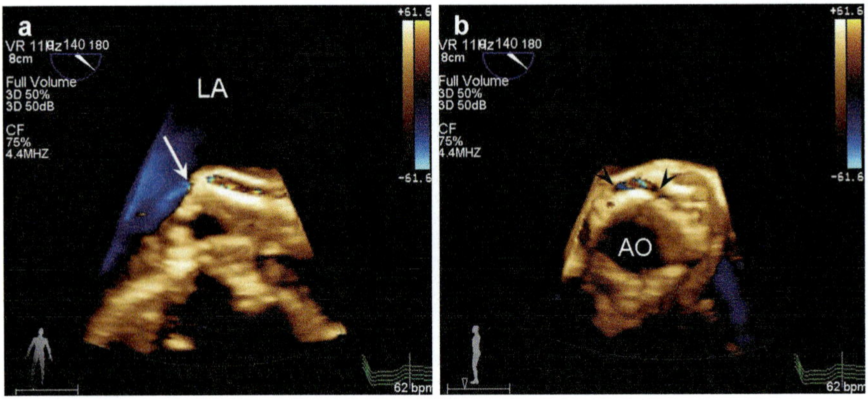

Fig. 1.57 Minimal paravalvular aortic regurgitation (arrows) was demonstrated in three dimensional color Doppler in long- (**a**) and short- (**b**) axis views

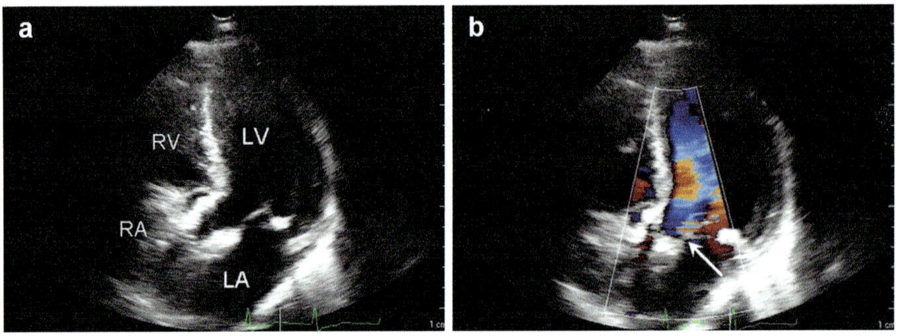

Fig. 1.58 A three-month transthoracic follow-up showed normal prosthetic function in apical five-chamber view (**a**) and reduced paravalvular regurgitation (arrow, **b**) was demonstrated by color Doppler

1.8 Implantation of SAPIEN Valve in CoreValve After David Operation

A 32-year-old male patient had received David operation, repair of right- and non-coronary aortic cusps, reconstruction of ascending aorta, re-implantation of right and left coronary artery, and ligation of coronary fistula. He also had history of infective endocarditis treated by antibiotic for months. This time, he presented with dyspnea and cold sweating as a result of recurrent severe aortic regurgitation (Figs. 1.59, 1.60, 1.61, 1.62, 1.63, 1.64, 1.65, 1.66, 1.67, 1.68, 1.69, 1.70, and 1.71; Videos 1.59a, 1.59b, 1.60a, 1.60b, 1.61, 1.62a, 1.62b, 1.63, 1.64, 1.65, 1.66, 1.67, 1.68a, 1.68b, 1.69a, 1.69b, 1.70, and 1.71).

A valve-in-valve procedure may be necessary in some cases with low implantation level of CoreValve and paravalvular leakage. A CoreValve-in-CoreValve strategy could preclude future engagement of coronary orifice once coronary intervention is needed. Therefore, we strongly recommend the SAPIEN-in-CoreValve approach, leaving only one layer of metal at the level of coronary orifices. On the other hand, the CoreValve served as a rigid frame against non-calcified native aortic valve and the annulus for the SAPIEN valve to settle. This approach may be considered for pure aortic regurgitation in similar patients.

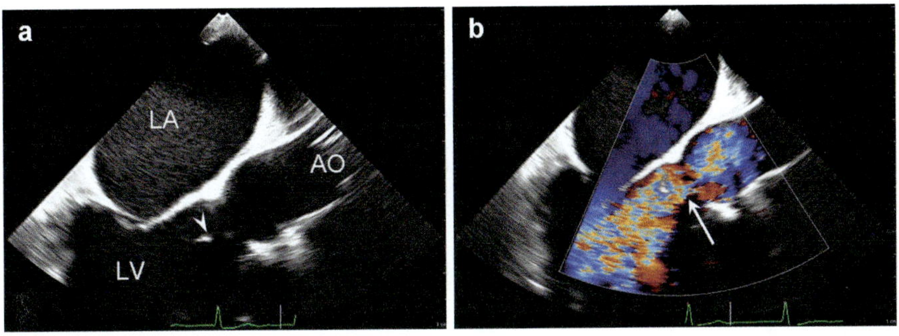

Fig. 1.59 In transesophageal echocardiographic midesophageal long-axis approach, the aortic cusp flailed into the left ventricular outflow tract (arrow heads, **a**). Severe aortic regurgitation was demonstrated by color Doppler (arrow, **b**)

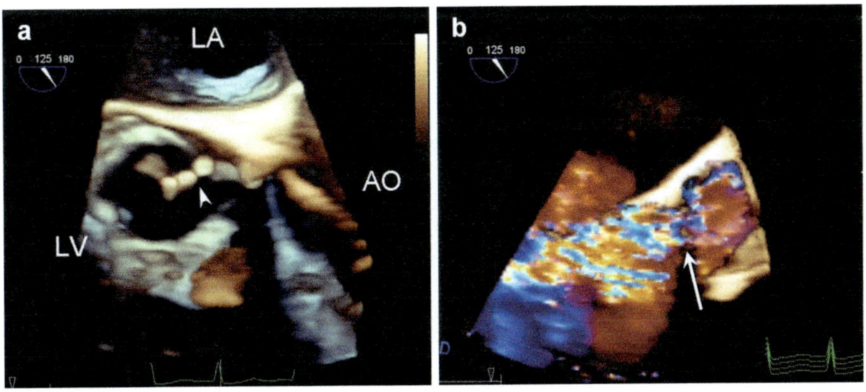

Fig. 1.60 In three dimensional long-axis view, the aortic cusp flailed into the left ventricular outflow tract (arrow heads, **a**). Severe aortic regurgitation was demonstrated by color Doppler (arrow, **b**)

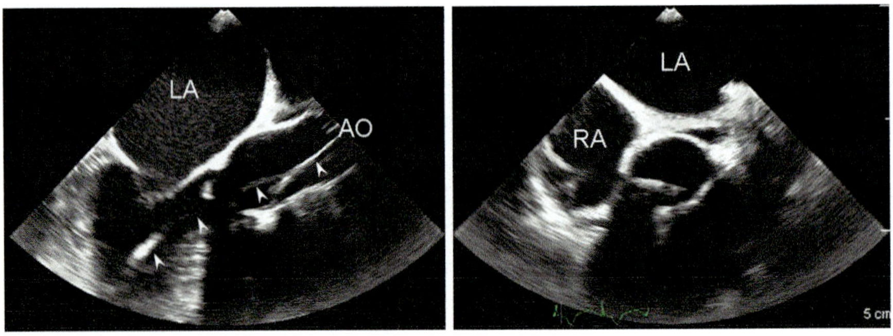

Fig. 1.61 During the transcatheter aortic valve implantation, in an x-plane view, the guiding catheter (arrow heads) advanced across the flailed aortic cusp

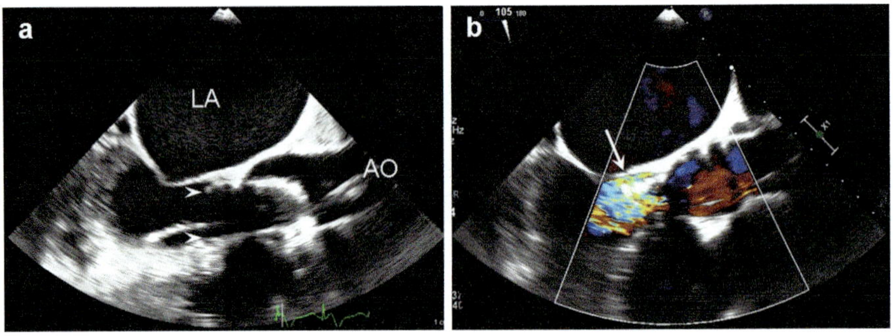

Fig. 1.62 The CoreValve (31 mm, arrow heads, **a**) was then delivered and deployed. However, severe paravalvular leakage (arrow, **b**) was noted due to downward displacement of CoreValve with failed attempt in reposition

Fig. 1.63 Afterward, a valve-in-valve implantation was performed. A SAPIEN valve (29 mm, arrow heads) was advanced and deployed within the previous implanted CoreValve

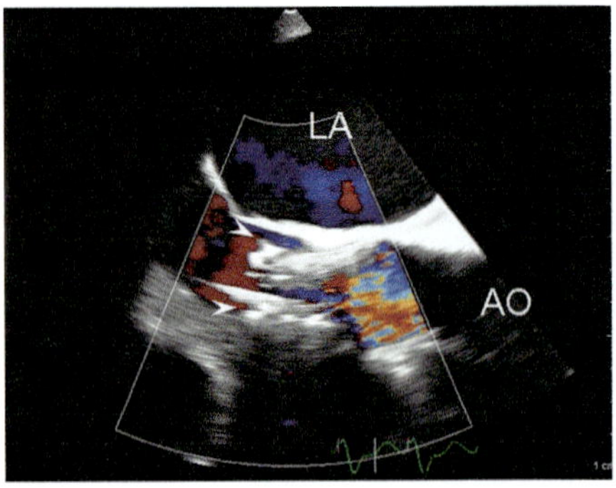

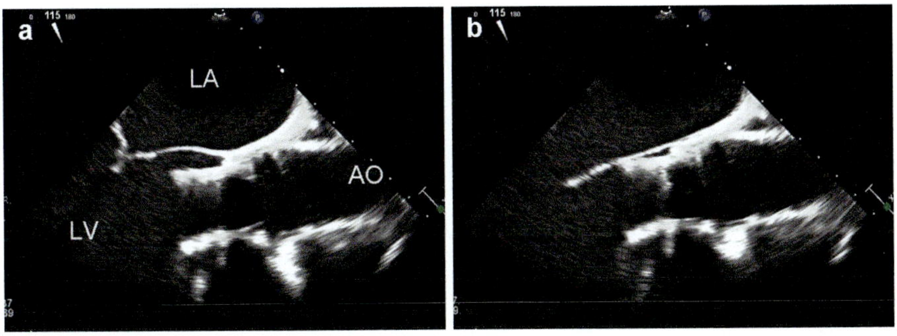

Fig. 1.64 After implantation of both of the transcatheter heart valves, in a midesophageal long-axis view, the inner SAPIEN valve presented normal function in systole (**a**) and diastole (**b**)

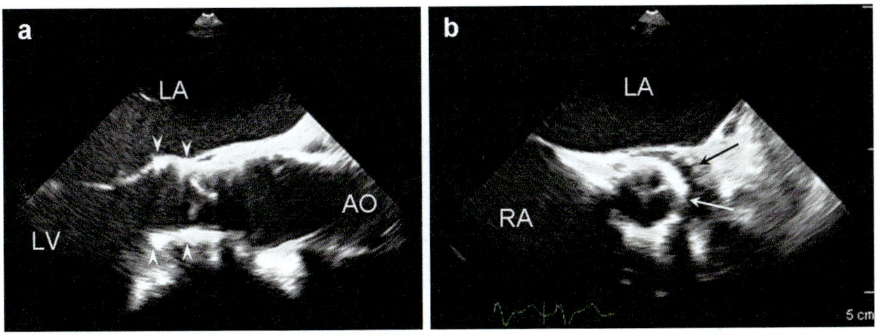

Fig. 1.65 In an x-plane view, left panel showed the position of the CoreValve (between left arrow heads) was deeper in to the ventricle than the SAPIEN valve (between right arrow heads); in right panel, the SAPIEN valve (white arrow) was within the CoreValve (black arrow)

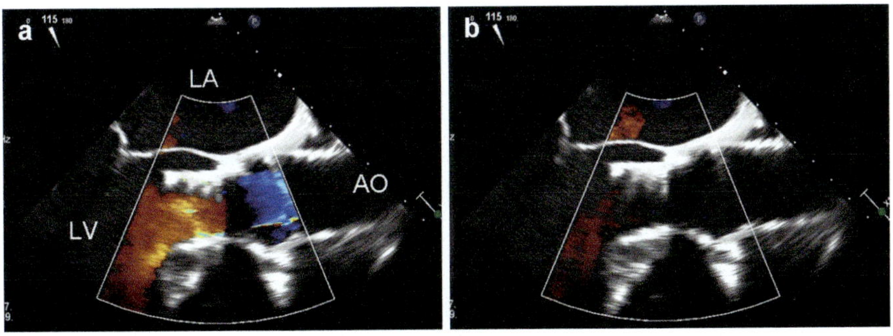

Fig. 1.66 Color Doppler after the procedure. There was no turbulent flow across the prosthetic valve (**a**) in systole, and only trivial leakage was present in diastole (**b**)

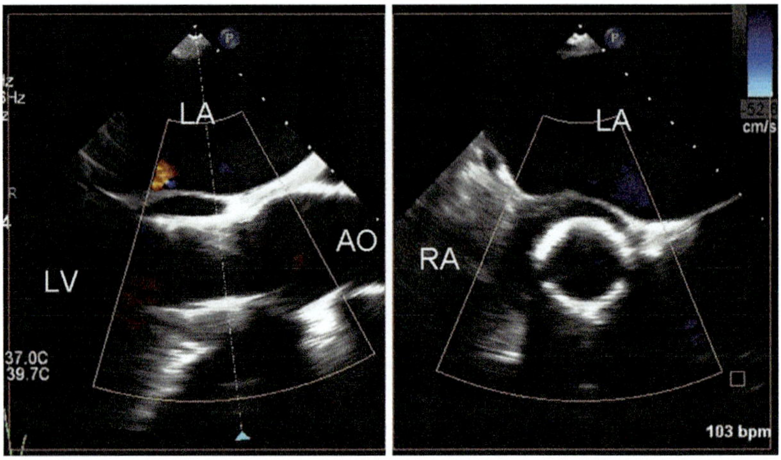

Fig. 1.67 In x-plane color Doppler after the procedure, neither turbulent flow across the prosthetic valve nor significant leakage was demonstrated

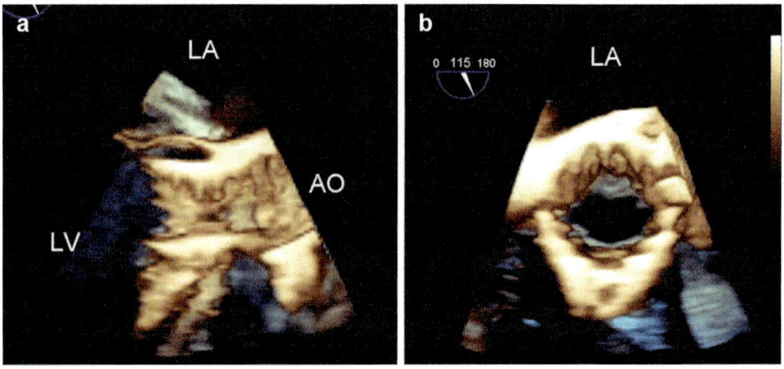

Fig. 1.68 Three dimensional long- (**a**) and short-axis views (**b**) showed normal function of the inner SAPIEN valve

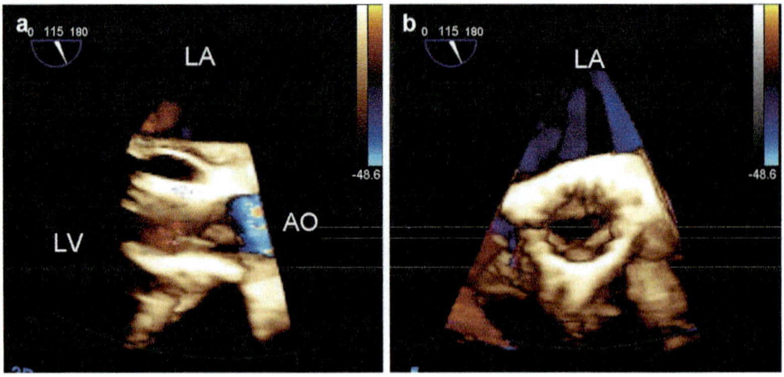

Fig. 1.69 Three dimensional color Doppler of long- (**a**) and short-axis views (**b**) showed neither turbulent flow across the prosthetic valve nor significant leakage

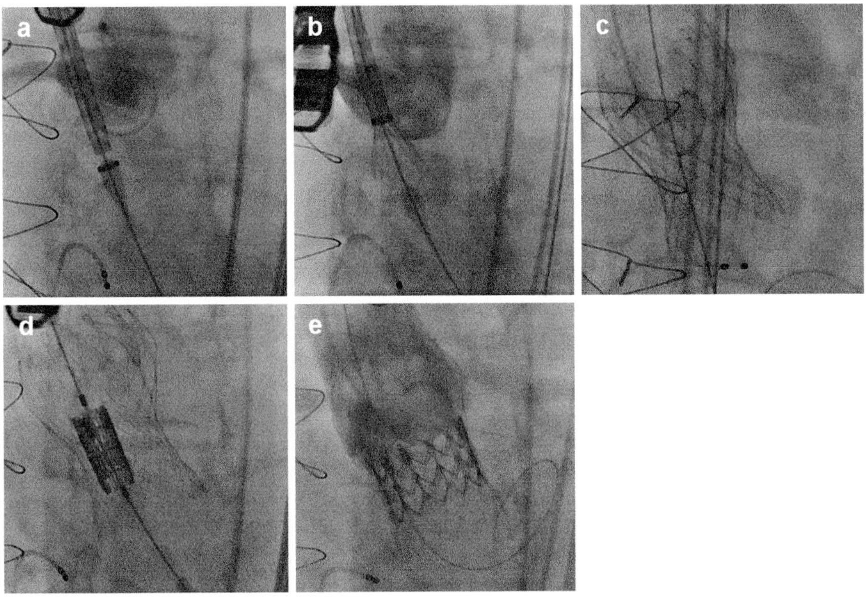

Fig. 1.70 Aortic root angiography during transcatheter aortic valve implantation. (**a**) The crimped CoreValve aligned within the native aortic valve. (**b**) Then the CoreValve started to deploy from the proximal part of the frame to the distal. (**c**) After device deployment, the guiding wire remained within the CoreValve. (**d**) The SAPIEN valve was delivered by the balloon inflation in to the CoreValve. (**e**) The SAPINE valve was then expanded by the balloon at the level of the native aortic valve annulus

Fig. 1.71 In the chest X-ray, the graft in the ascending aorta from previous surgery, the CoreValve, and the SAPIEN valve were visible

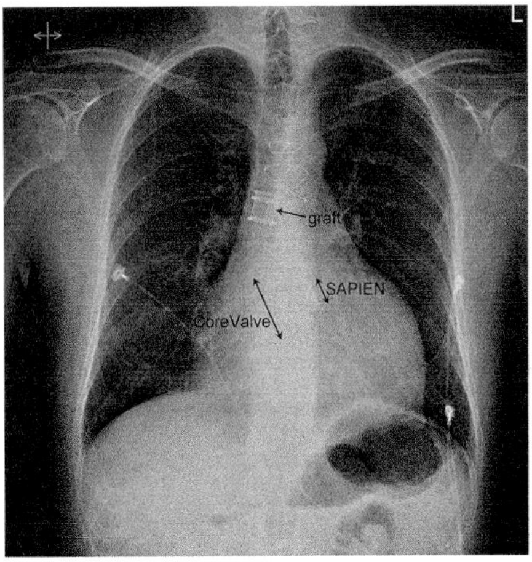

1.9 Demonstration of Left Circumflex During SAPIEN Valve Implantation

A 65-year-old female patient had a history of hypertrophy cardiomyopathy without regular medical treatment. She suffered from orthopnea and lost consciousness while admitted to our emergency room where pulmonary edema and critical aortic stenosis were noted. Therefore, transcatheter aortic valve implantation was indicated by the heart team (Figs. 1.72, 1.73, 1.74, 1.75, 1.76, 1.77, 1.78, 1.79, 1.80, and 1.81; Videos 1.72a, 1.72b, 1.73a, 1.73b, 1.74, 1.75, 1.76, 1.77, 1.78, 1.79, 1.80, and 1.81).

The location of the coronary arteries should be carefully accessed to avoid obstruction in prosthesis implantation or ligation during suture of thoracotomy. However, the coronary arteries cannot be clearly visualized in every single individual by transesophageal echocardiography; therefore, computed tomography should be taken as a tool to measure the locations of the coronary arteries.

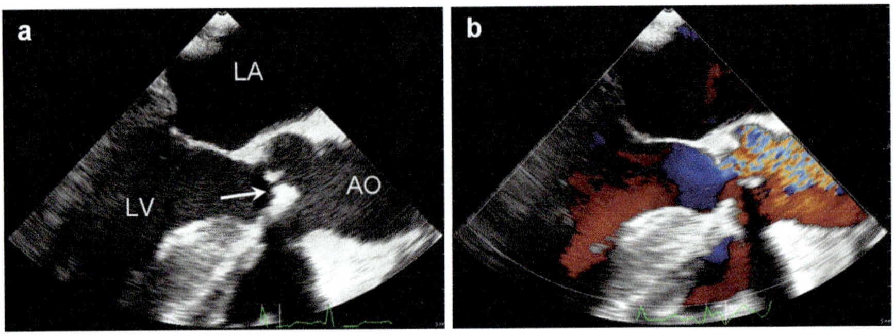

Fig. 1.72 In transesophageal echocardiographic mid-esophageal long-axis view, calcified aortic valve (arrow, **a**) reduced cusp separation and caused turbulent left ventricular outflow in color Doppler (**b**)

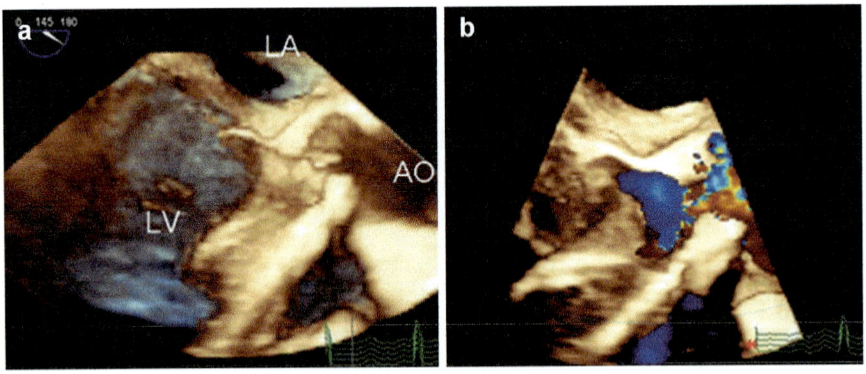

Fig. 1.73 In three dimensional transesophageal echocardiographic mid-esophageal long-axis view, calcified aortic valve reduced cusp separation (**a**) and caused turbulent left ventricular outflow (**b**)

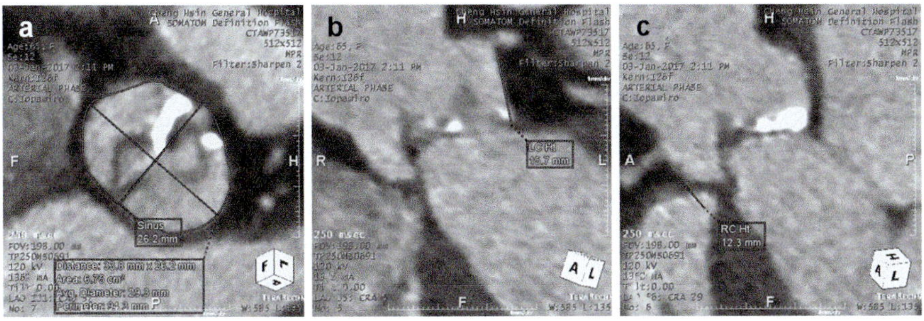

Fig. 1.74 Computed tomographic cross section (**a**) revealed the diameter, perimeter, and area of calcified bicuspid aortic valve. (**b** and **c**) The location and height of the left and right coronary artery were revealed

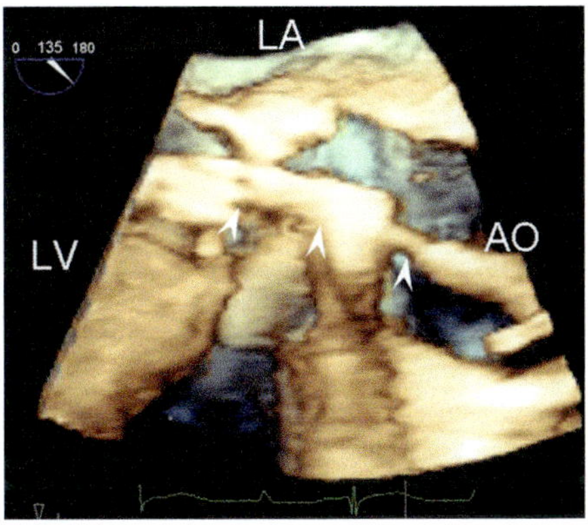

Fig. 1.75 During the transcatheter aortic valve implantation, the guiding sheath (arrow heads) advanced cross the aortic valve

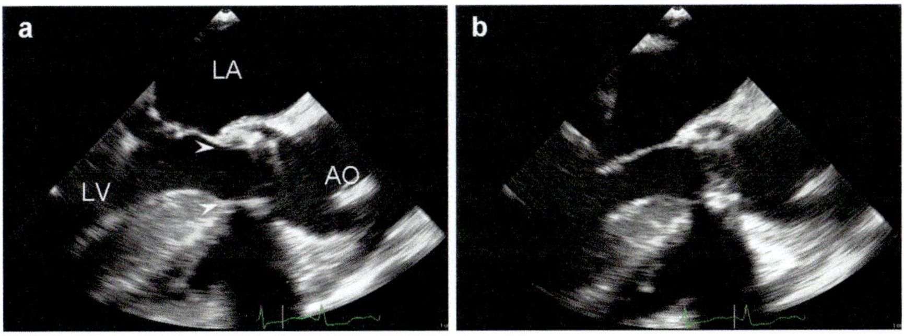

Fig. 1.76 After the transcatheter aortic valve implantation, the SAPIEN valve (arrow heads) presented normal function in systole (**a**) and diastole (**b**)

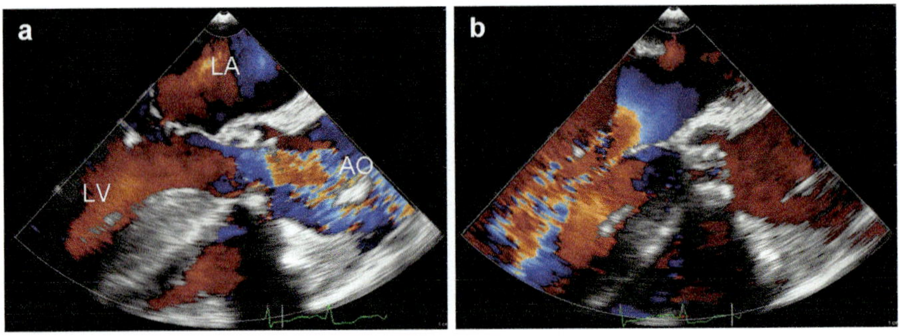

Fig. 1.77 Color Doppler long-axis view after the transcatheter aortic valve implantation. There was no turbulent flow across the SAPIEN valve (**a**), and only trivial paravalvular leakage was present (**b**)

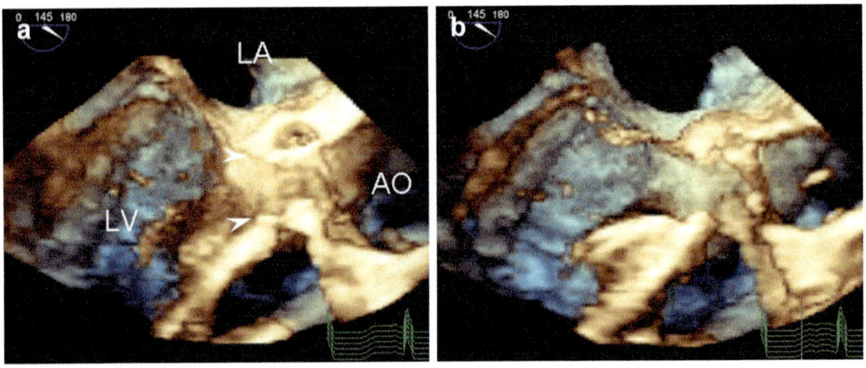

Fig. 1.78 In three dimensional images after the implantation, the SAPIEN valve (arrow heads) was well positioned and presented normal function in systole (**a**) and diastole (**b**)

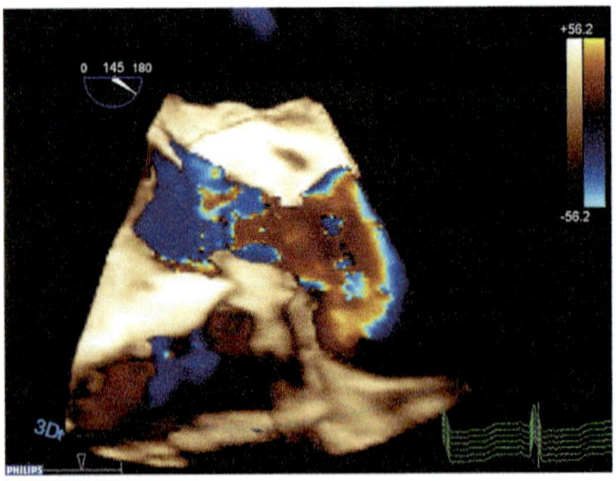

Fig. 1.79 Three dimensional color Doppler long-axis view after the transcatheter aortic valve implantation. There was no turbulent flow across the SAPIEN valve, and only trivial paravalvular leakage was present

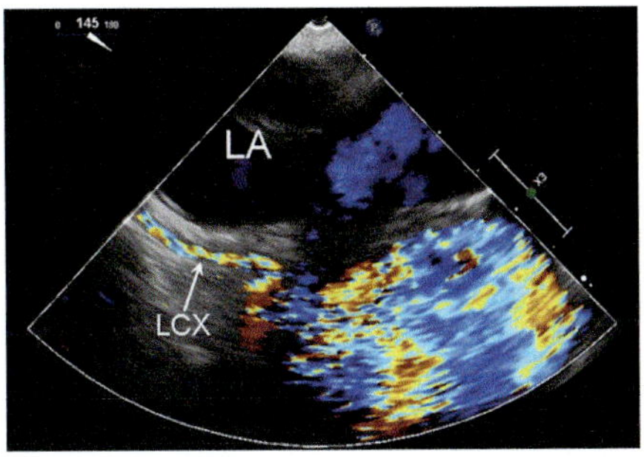

Fig. 1.80 The left circumflex (LCX) was visualized in mid esophageal view with color Doppler at the level of sinus of Valsalva

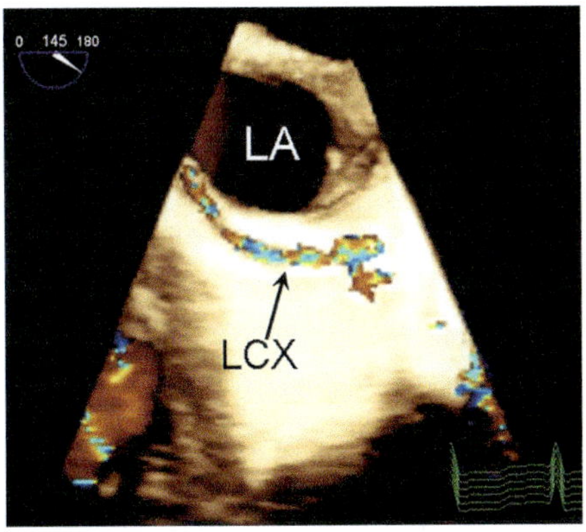

Fig. 1.81 The left circumflex (LCX) was visualized in three dimensional mid esophageal view with color Doppler at the level of sinus of Valsalva

1.10 Improvement of Left Ventricular Function After SAPIEN Valve Implantation

An 81-year-old male patient had a history of critical aortic stenosis, coronary artery disease, hypertension, and hyperlipidemia. He complained of progressive dyspnea on exertion for moths. Auscultation shows a grade 3/6 systolic murmur over apex with radiation to aortic area. Thus, he was admitted for interventional treatment (Figs. 1.82, 1.83, 1.84, 1.85, 1.86, 1.87, 1.88, 1.89, 1.90, 1.91, 1.92, and 1.93; Videos 1.82, 1.83, 1.84, 1.85a, 1.85b, 1.86, 1.87, 1.88a, 1.88b, 1.89, 1.90, 1.91, 1.92, and 1.93).

The hemodynamic benefits of transcatheter aortic valve implantation are reflected by favorable effects on left ventricular function. Furthermore, transcatheter aortic valve implantation had positive effects on left ventricular remodeling and improved neurohormonal activity, myocardial hypertrophy, and diastolic function.

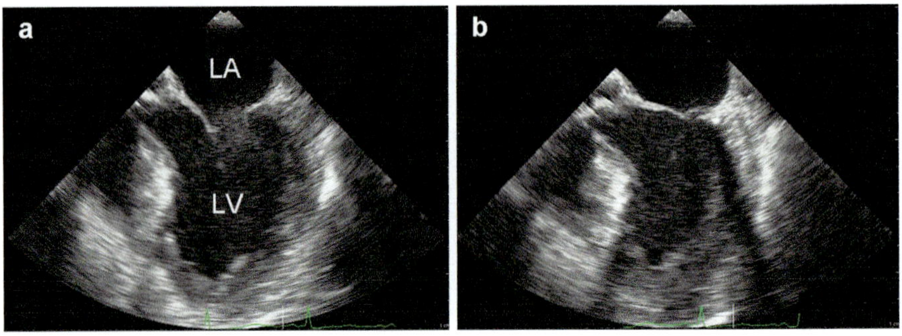

Fig. 1.82 In transesophageal echocardiographic midesophageal four-chamber approach in diastole (**a**) and systole (**b**), left ventricle showed impaired systolic function

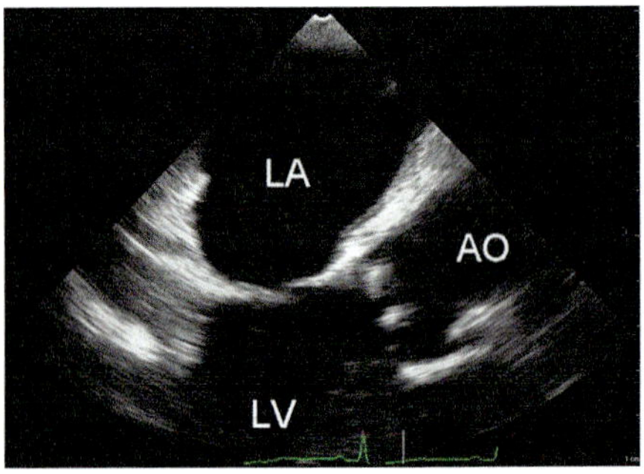

Fig. 1.83 In mid-esophageal long-axis view, the calcified aortic valve reduced cusp separation

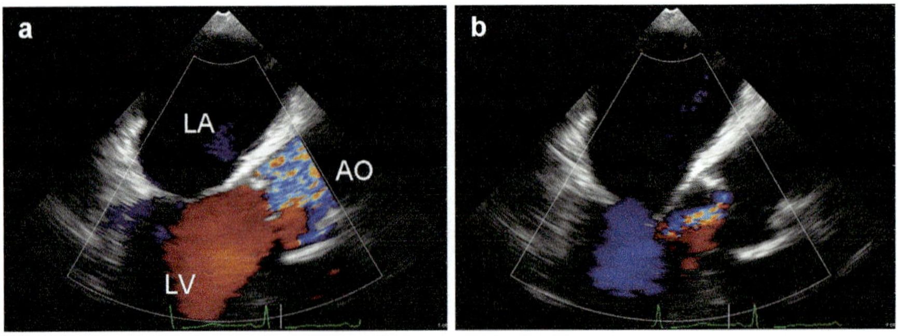

Fig. 1.84 With color Doppler, the thickened aortic valve induced turbulent left ventricular outflow in systole (**a**) and mild regurgitation in diastole (**b**)

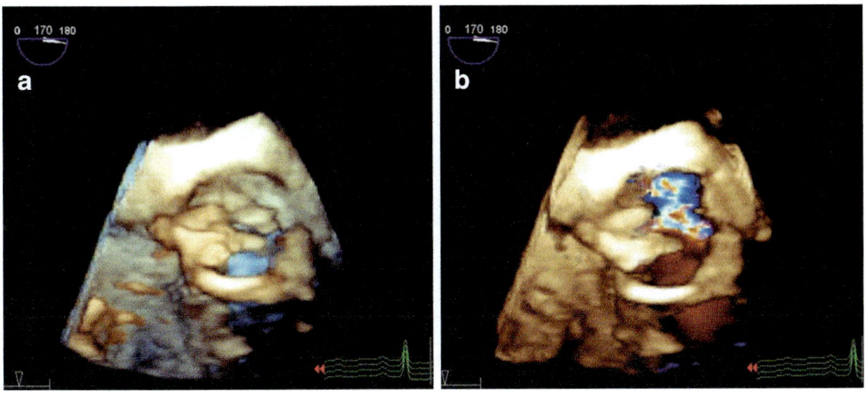

Fig. 1.85 Three dimensional echocardiogram of aortic valve with color Doppler showed severe calcification reduced the aortic orifice (**a**) and caused turbulent left ventricular outflow (**b**)

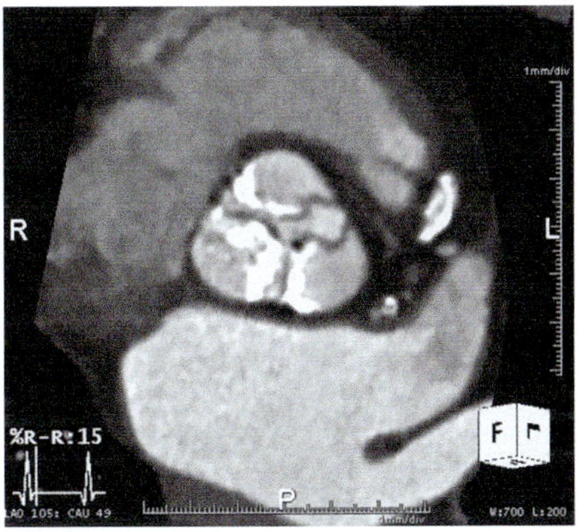

Fig. 1.86 Computed tomographic cross-section of the sinus of Valsalva showed severe calcification of every cusp which reduced the aortic orifice

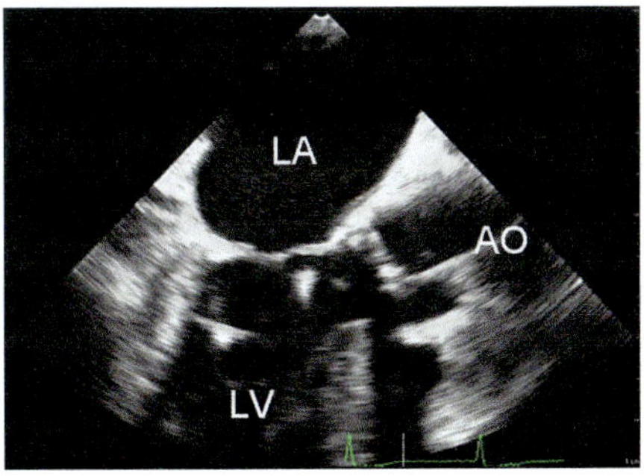

Fig. 1.87 During the transcatheter aortic valve implantation, the guiding sheath advanced cross the aortic valve

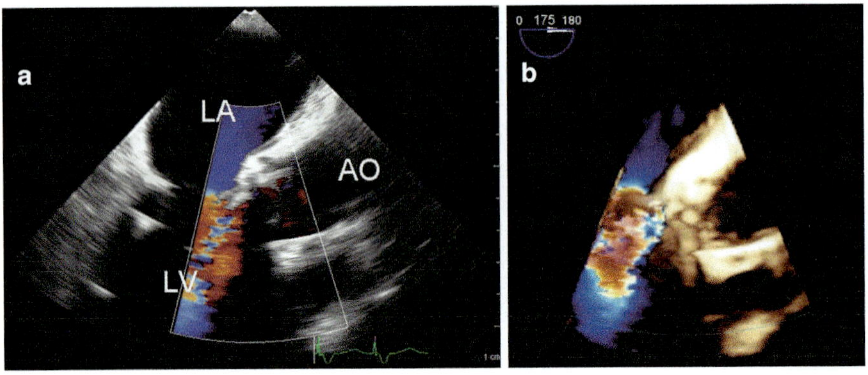

Fig. 1.88 When the SAPIEN valve was delivered and first expanded, two (**a**) and three dimensional (**b**) color Doppler showed mild paravalvular regurgitation

Fig. 1.89 When the SAPIEN valve was fully expanded, it presented normal function

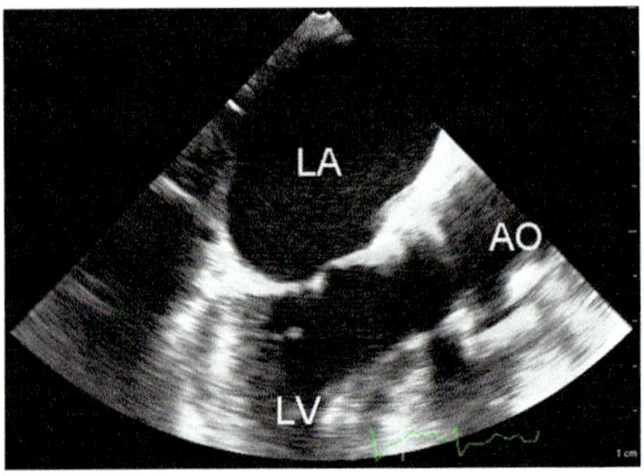

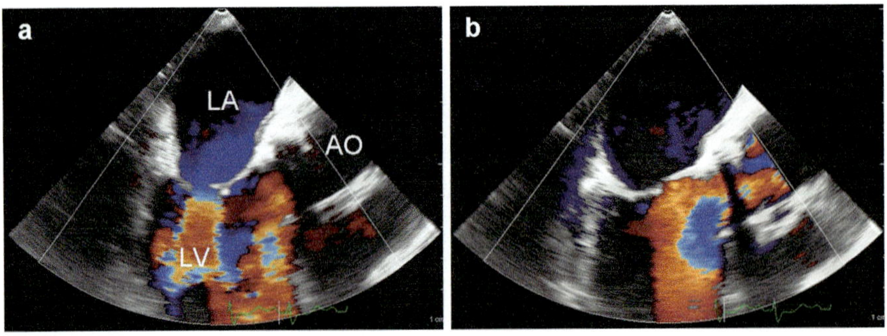

Fig. 1.90 When the SAPIEN valve was fully expanded, there was no turbulent flow across it (**a**) and the paravalvular regurgitation declined to trivial (**b**)

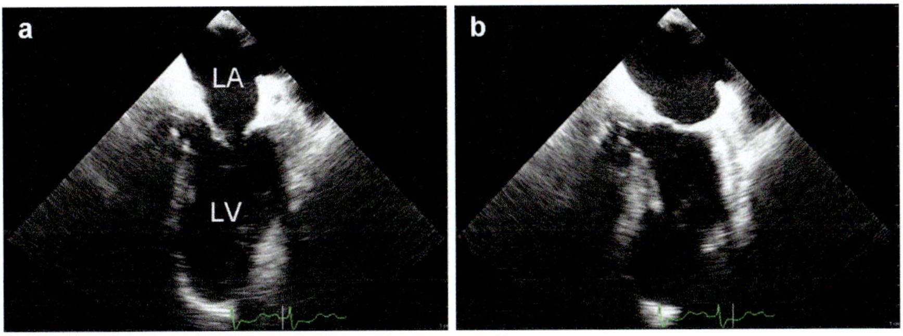

Fig. 1.91 Midesophageal four-chamber approach in diastole (**a**) and systole (**b**). When the whole procedure was done, left ventricular systolic function improved to normal range

Fig. 1.92 In three dimensional mid-esophageal long-axis views r, the ejection fraction improved and the SAPIEN valve was well positioned

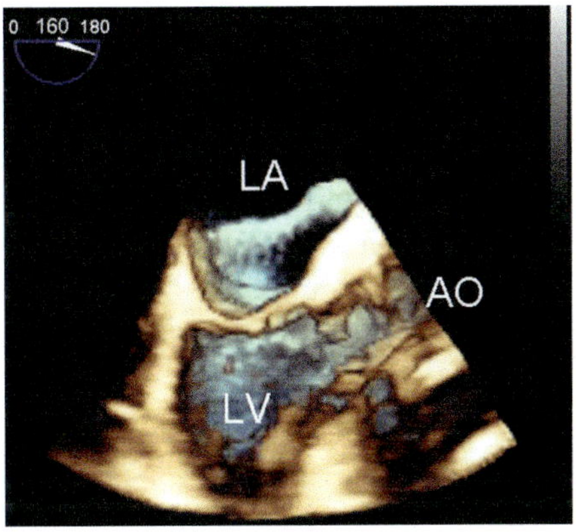

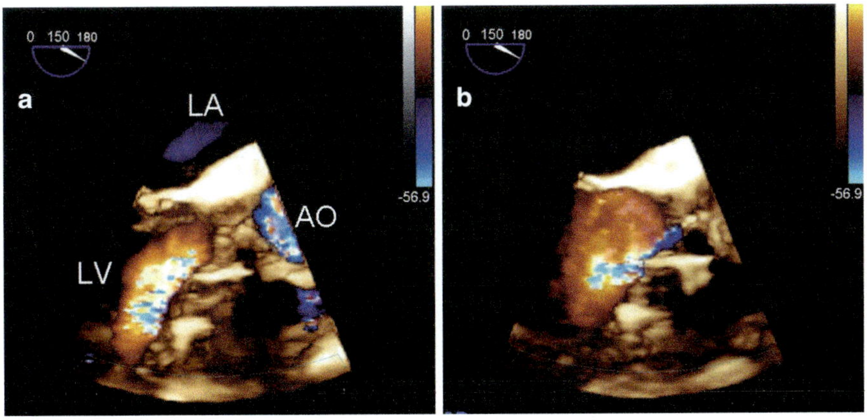

Fig. 1.93 Three dimensional color Doppler long-axis view after the transcatheter aortic valve implantation. There was no turbulent flow across the SAPIEN valve in systole (**a**), and only trivial paravalvular leakage in diastole (**b**)

1.11 Occasional Find of Atheroma During CoreValve Implantation

An 85-year-old male patient had a history of hypertension, hyperlipidemia, chronic renal failure and triple vessel coronary artery disease. He also had valvular heart disease with both aortic stenosis and regurgitation under regular medical treatment. He suffered from orthopnea and chest tightness for days; therefore he admitted for further evaluation and transcatheter aortic valve implantation was indicated (Figs. 1.94, 1.95, 1.96, 1.97, 1.98, 1.99, 1.100, 1.101, 1.102, 1.103, 1.104, 1.105, and 1.106; Videos 1.94, 1.95, 1.96, 1.97, 1.98, 1.99, 1.100a, 1.100b, 1.101a, 1.101b, 1.102, 1.103, 1.104a, 1.104b, 1.105, and 1.106).

Transesophageal echocardiography is helpful to detect and grade the severity of aortic atherosclerosis. Besides, it can also define the location and size of aortic atheroma to decrease the risk of thrombolytic complications and stroke. Atheroma appears as irregular hyperechoic thickening along the intimal surface on ultrasound imaging. The risk of stroke after transfemoral aortic valve implantation due to subsequent embolization of scrap from aortic arch atheroma is low. Despite silent cerebral ischemia could be detected in almost every patient undergoing transcatheter aortic valve implantation, these foci were not associated with apparent neurological events or measurable deterioration of neurocognitive function. In this case, the atheroma produces into the lumen greater than 5 mm, but the patient did not receive further treatment after the occasional discovery during the procedure.

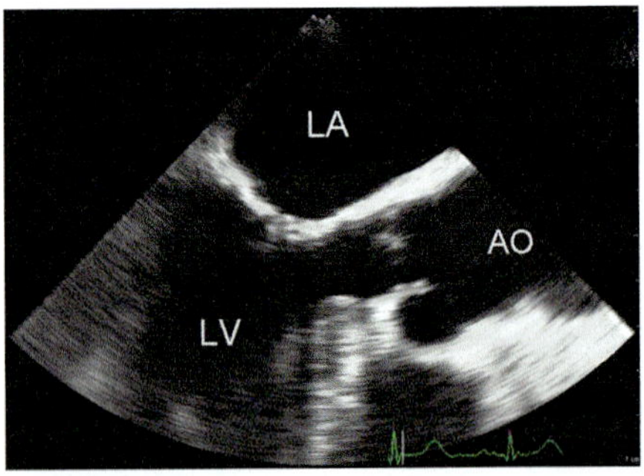

Fig. 1.94 In transesophageal echocardiographic mid-esophageal long-axis view, there were thickened aortic and mitral valve with reduced cusp separation

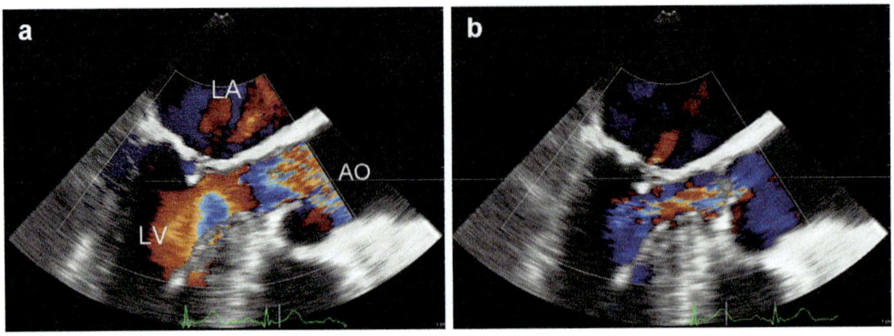

Fig. 1.95 With color Doppler, the thickened aortic valve induced turbulent left ventricular outflow in systole (**a**) and moderate regurgitation in diastole (**b**)

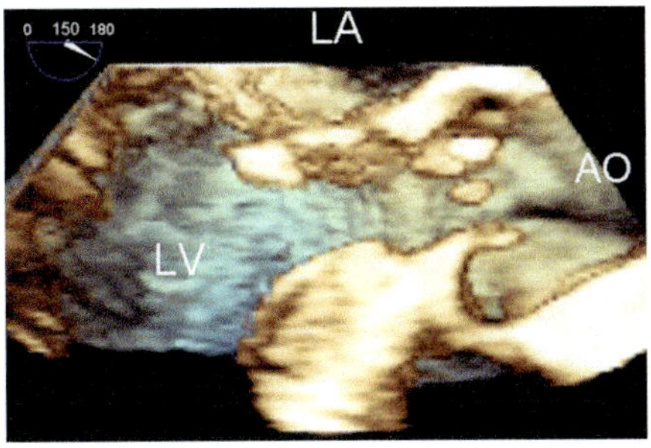

Fig. 1.96 Three dimensional long-axis view showed thickened aortic valve with reduced cusp separation

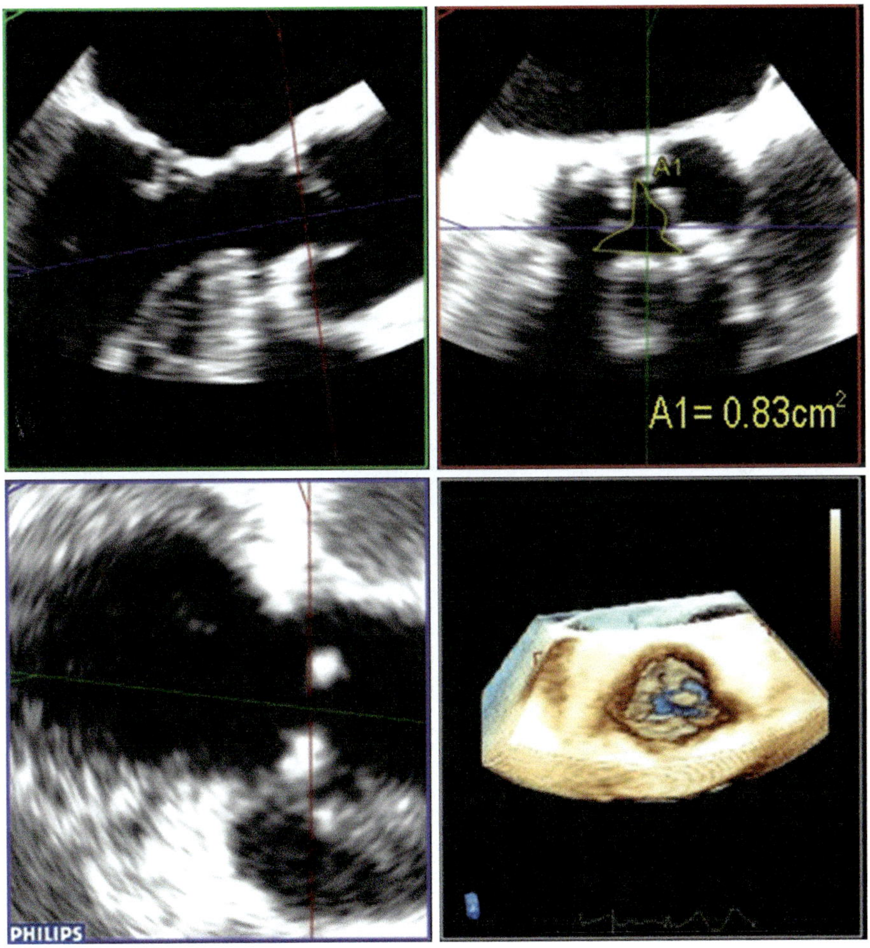

Fig. 1.97 Through multi-planar reconstruction of the three dimensional image, the orifice of the aortic valve was 0.83 cm^2

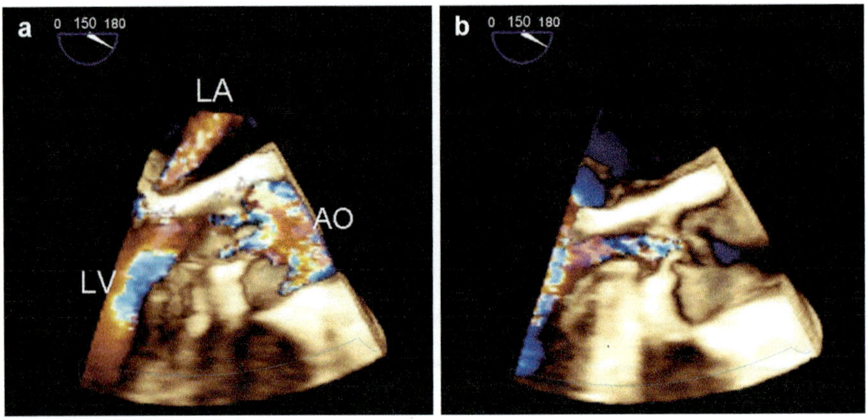

Fig. 1.98 Three dimensional color Doppler showed turbulent left ventricular outflow in systole (**a**) and moderate aortic regurgitation in diastole (**b**)

Fig. 1.99 During the transcatheter aortic valve implantation, the guiding sheath (arrow heads) was advanced cross the aortic valve and into the left ventricular cavity for CoreValve delivery

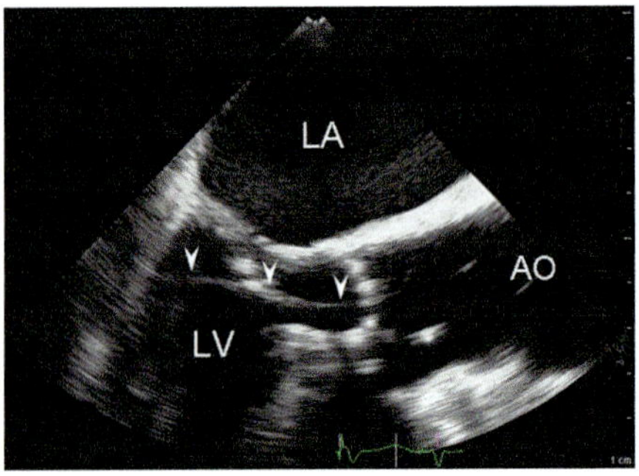

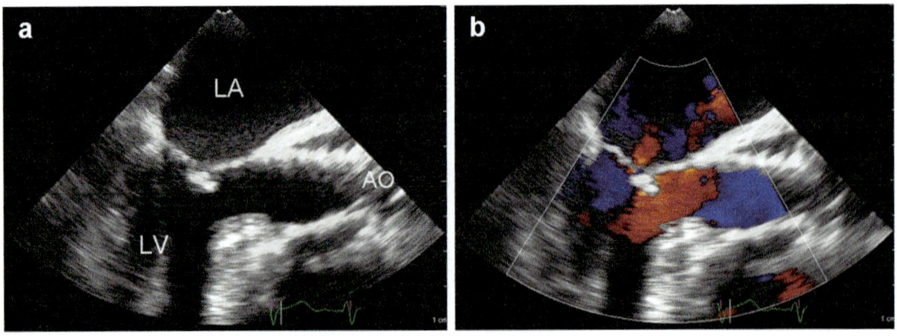

Fig. 1.100 After the CoreValve was deployed and released (**a**), there was merely trivial paravalvular regurgitation (**b**)

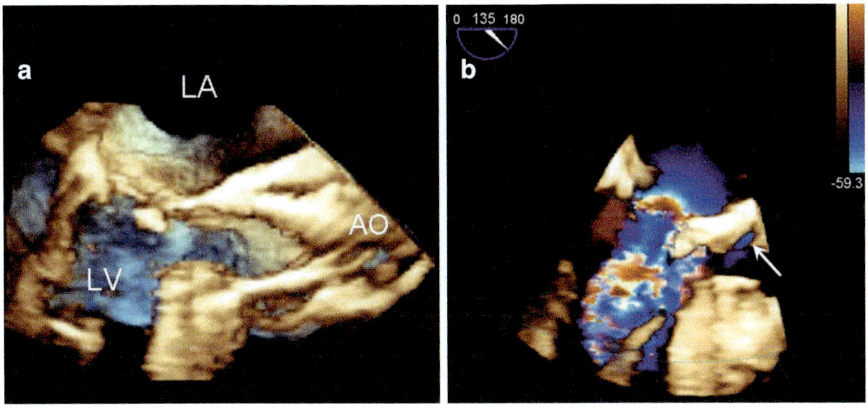

Fig. 1.101 In three dimensional images, the CoreValve was well positioned (**a**) with trivial paravalvular regurgitation occurring (arrow, **b**)

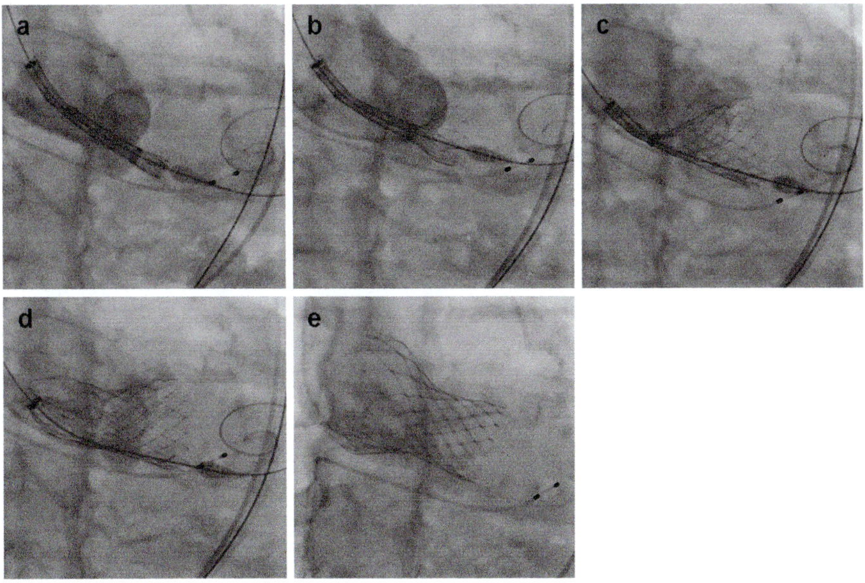

Fig. 1.102 Aortic root angiography during implantation of the CoreValve. (**a**) The crimped CoreValve aligned within the aortic valve. (**b**) Then the CoreValve started to deploy from the proximal part of the frame to the distal (**c** and **d**). (**e**) After deployment had been completed, the CoreValve was detached form the catheter and the pigtail was withdrawn

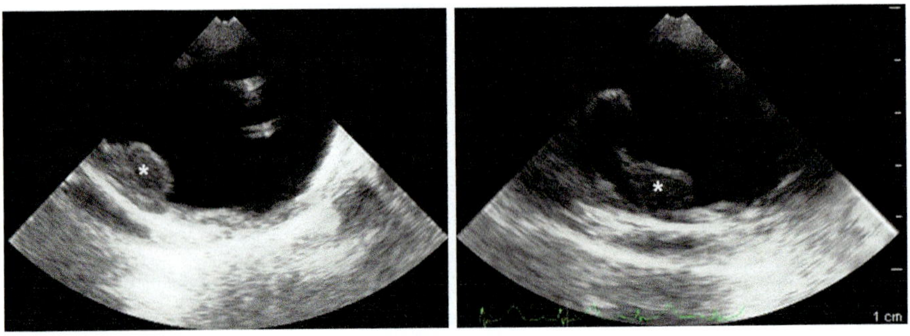

Fig. 1.103 In transesophageal echocardiographic x-plane view of the proximal descending aorta, atherosclerosis with atheroma (asterisk) was revealed occasionally

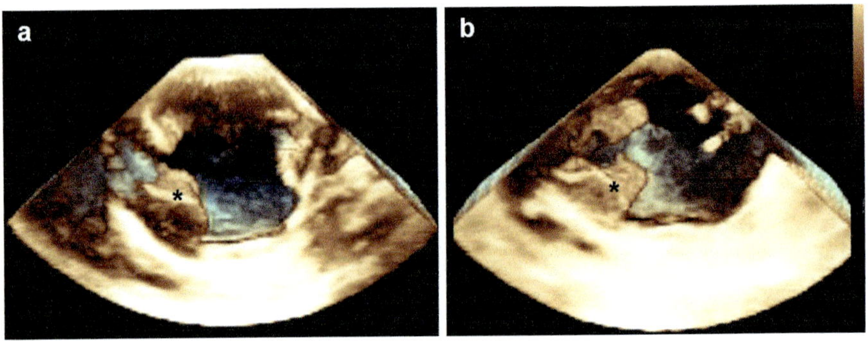

Fig. 1.104 Three dimensional views of the proximal descending aorta during the procedure (**a** and **b**) demonstrated atherosclerosis with atheroma (asterisk)

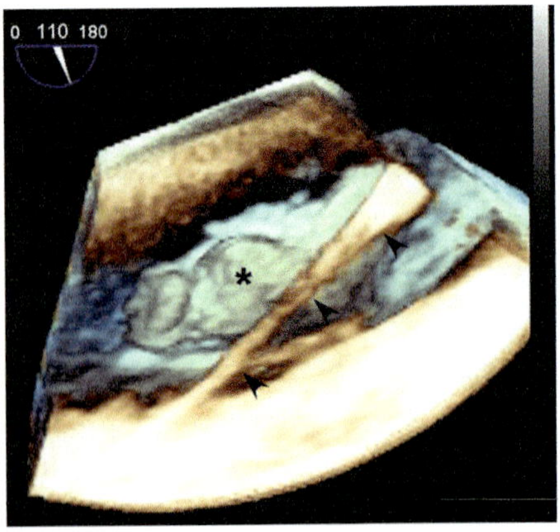

Fig. 1.105 During the procedure, the guidewire (arrow heads) advanced into the descending aorta and crossed the zone of the atheroma (asterisk)

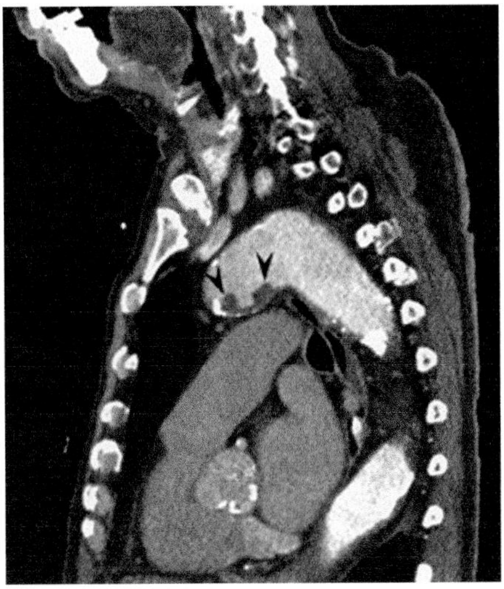

Fig. 1.106 For the purpose of certification, a previous computed tomography was reviewed. In this sagittal view, atherosclerosis with atheroma (arrow heads) had been demonstrated

Suggested Readings

1. Maurizio T, Andrew S, Francesco M, et al. First-in-man case report of the use of an Edwards-Sapien valve to treat a regurgitant CoreValve aortic valve prosthesis. Catheter Cardiovasc Interv. 2010;75:51–5.
2. Philipp K, Stephan CK, Marc S, et al. Silent and apparent cerebral ischemia after percutaneous transfemoral aortic valve implantation: a diffusion-weighted magnetic resonance imaging study. Circulation. 2010;121:870–8.
3. Peter LH, Justus TS, Uta H, et al. Transapical valve implantation after David operation and stenting of the descending aorta. Ann Thorac Surg. 2010;90:2035–7.
4. Namal W, Jian Y, Josep RC, et al. Transcatheter aortic valve implantation in patients with bicuspid aortic valve stenosis. J Am Coll Cardiol Interv. 2010;3:1122–5.
5. Michael G, Michael L, Waldemar B, et al. Hemodynamic results and changes in myocardial function after transcatheter aortic valve implantation. Am Heart J. 2010;159:926–32.
6. Gian U, Marco B, Angelo R, et al. The valve-in-valve technique for treatment of aortic bioprosthesis malposition: an analysis of incidence and 1-year clinical outcomes from the Italian CoreValve registry. J Am Coll Cardiol. 2011;57:1062–8.
7. John DC, John GW. Structural heart disease interventions. Philadelphia: Lippincott Williams & Wilkins; 2012. Chap. 18–20.
8. David H, Jeffrey J, Michael J, et al. Transcatheter aortic-valve replacement with a self-expanding prosthesis. N Engl J Med. 2014;370:1790–8.
9. John ML, Jason HR. Interventional procedures for adult structural heart disease. Philadelphia: Elsevier; 2014. Chap. 6, 7.
10. Vaquerizo B, Spaziano M, Alali J, et al. Three-dimensional echocardiography vs. computed tomography for transcatheter aortic valve replacement sizing. Eur Heart J Cardiovasc Imaging. 2015;17:15–23.
11. Khalique OK, Hamid NB, Kodali SK, et al. Improving the accuracy of effective orifice area assessment after transcatheter aortic valve replacement: validation of left ventricular outflow tractdiameter and pulsed-wave Doppler location and impact of three-dimensional measurements. J Am Soc Echocardiogr. 2015;28(11):1283–93.
12. Torsten PV, Susheel KK, Martin BL. Transcatheter aortic valve replacement 2016: a modern-day "through the looking-glass" adventure. J Am Coll Cardiol. 2016;67:1472–87.
13. George DD, Jeffrey IW, Gennaro G, et al. Prosthetic heart valve thrombosis. J Am Coll Cardiol. 2016;68:2670–89.

2 Valve-In-Valve Therapy

2.1 Introduction

Transcatheter valve-in-valve implantation is feasible in failing bioprostheses and offers an alternative to reoperative surgical valve replacement for many high-risk patients.

Bioprosthetic valves are derived from animal or human tissue, in which the most widely used biologic materials are porcine and bovine tissue. Bioprosthetic failure may occur because of stenosis, regurgitation, both of these, or paravalvular leak, to which a main contributor is calcification. In addition, paravalvular regurgitation should be distinguished from valvular one, because it will not respond effectively to valve-in-valve implantation, further percutaneous closure must also be performed cooperatively.

The majority of our experiences with transcatheter valve-in-valve implantations have been performed with the SAPIEN valve, Medtronic CoreValve, and Lotus valve. The options of access route for the procedure depend on the bioprosthetic position and the delivery system availableness. Transarterial or transapical access to aortic valve is feasible, while it is more easily to use transapical access for mitral valve procedures.

This chapter covers diagnoses, techniques and outcomes of cases received aortic, mitral, or double valve-in-valve implantation with various accesses and prostheses. Furthermore, patients with paravalvular regurgitation underwent both valve-in-valve and occluder implantations are also demonstrated.

Electronic supplementary material The online version of this chapter (https://doi.org/10.1007/978-981-10-6937-6_2) contains supplementary material, which is available to authorized users.

M.-C. Hsiung et al., *Atlas of 3D Transesophageal Echocardiography in Structural Heart Disease Interventions*, https://doi.org/10.1007/978-981-10-6937-6_2

2.2 Mitral Valve-In-Ring Implantation of Lotus Valve

A 72-year-old male patient had a history of severe mitral regurgitation then received mitral annuloplasty 12 years ago. He also had coronary artery disease, hyperlipidemia and gouty arthritis under medical treatment. Recently, he suffered from exertional dyspnea and hoarseness. Recurrent mitral regurgitation was noted. As a result, mitral valve-in-valve replacement was arranged (Figs. 2.1, 2.2, 2.3, 2.4, 2.5, and 2.6; Videos 2.1, 2.2a, 2.2b, 2.3a, 2.3b, 2.3c, 2.3d, 2.4a, 2.4b, 2.4c, 2.4d, 2.5, and 2.6).

Mitral valve repair, which includes ring annuloplasty in most cases, is the preferable treatment for mitral regurgitation if feasible. However, failure of the repair with recurrence of significant may occur. Reoperation is the standard cure for these patients, but can possibly carry prohibitive risk in elderly patients. Experiences have shown that transcatheter mitral valve replacement after failure of mitral valve surgery with ring annuloplasty is feasible, which decreases the rate of threatened complications.

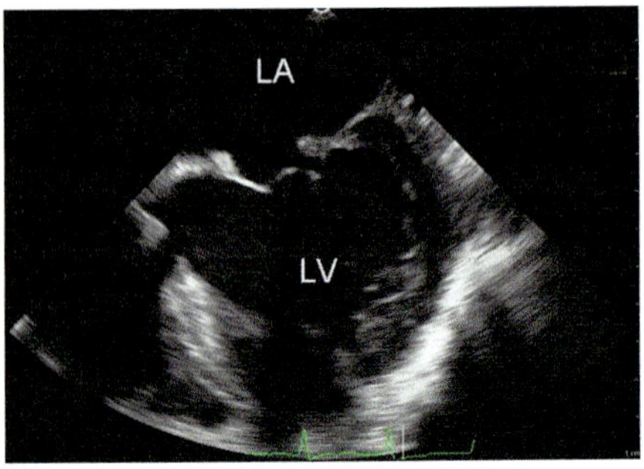

Fig. 2.1 Transesophageal echocardiography, mid-esophageal four-chamber view. The patient had received mitral annuloplasty before. Ventricular dysfunction along with tethering and rupture of mitral leaflet was demonstrated

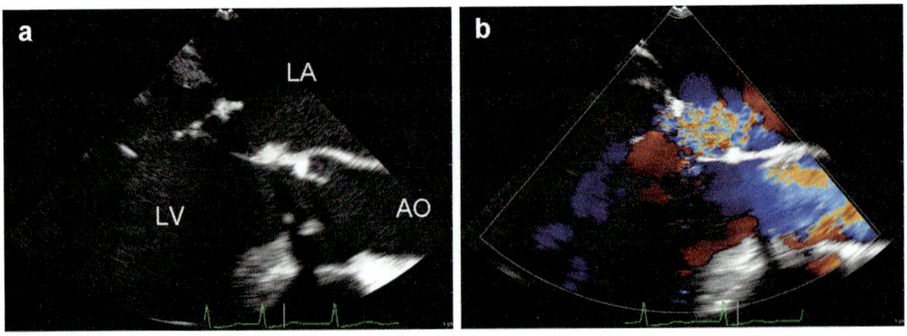

Fig. 2.2 In mid-esophageal long-axis view in systole (**a**), tethering and rupture of the leaflets made the valve incapable to close properly, which induced severe mitral regurgitation in color Doppler (**b**)

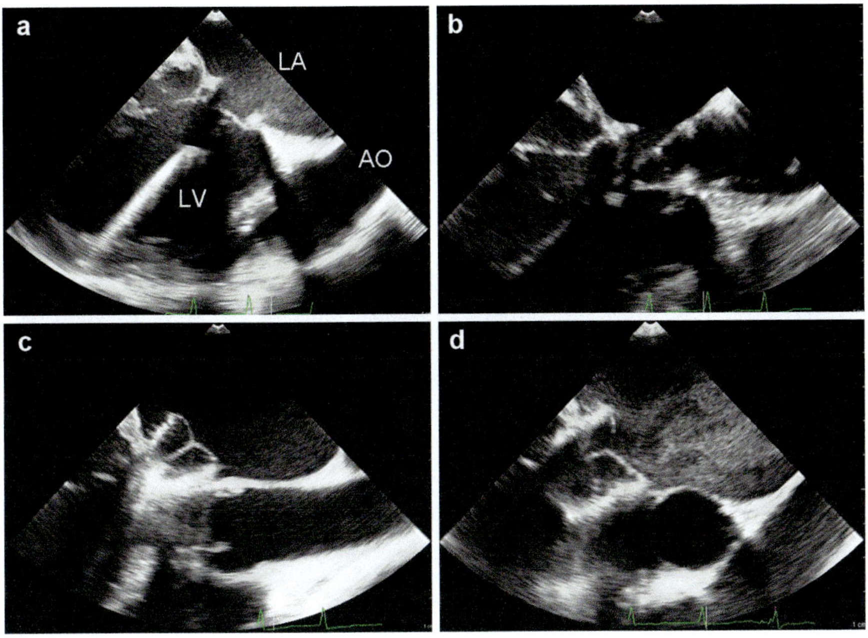

Fig. 2.3 During the valve-in-valve replacement, retrograde transapical approach was used and the puncturing needle accessed straightforward for the mitral annulus (**a**). (**b**) The guiding catheter advanced into the mitral annuloplasty ring. (**c**) A Lotus valve was positioned but not yet fully deployed. (**d**) The Lotus valve was deployed with normal function

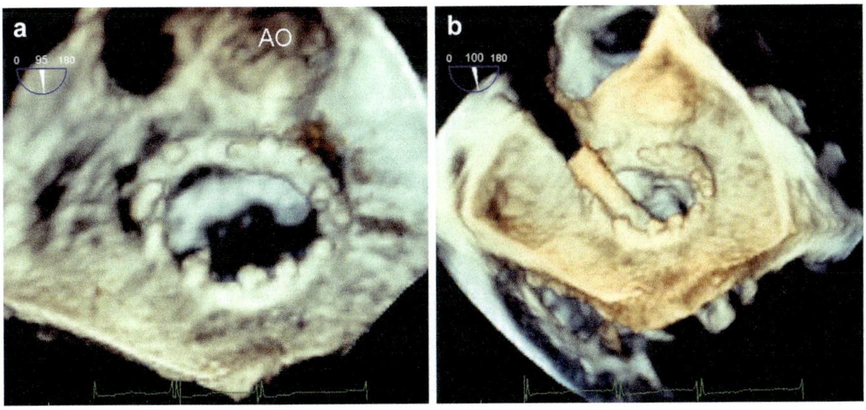

Fig. 2.4 Three-dimensional mitral en face view. (**a**) The patient had received mitral annuloplasty and leaflets dysfunction was demonstrated. (**b**) During the mitral valve-in-ring implantation, a guiding catheter advanced into the mitral annulus. (**c**) A Lotus valve was delivered and deployed within the mitral annuloplasty ring. (**d**) After the whole procedure was done, the Lotus valve presented normal function from ventricular perspective

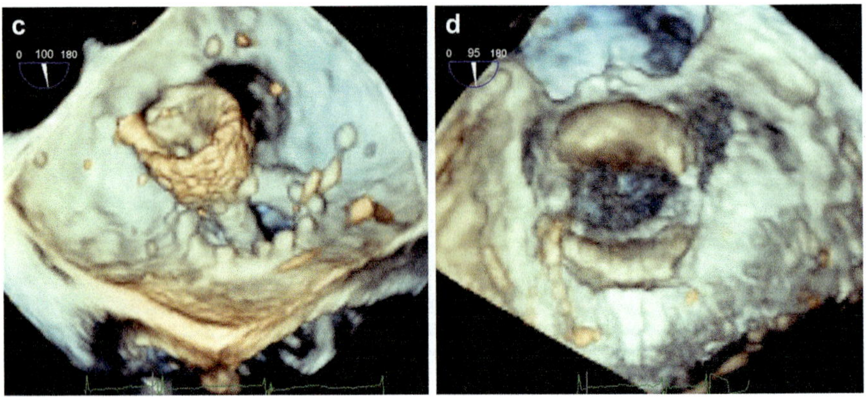

Fig. 2.4 (continued)

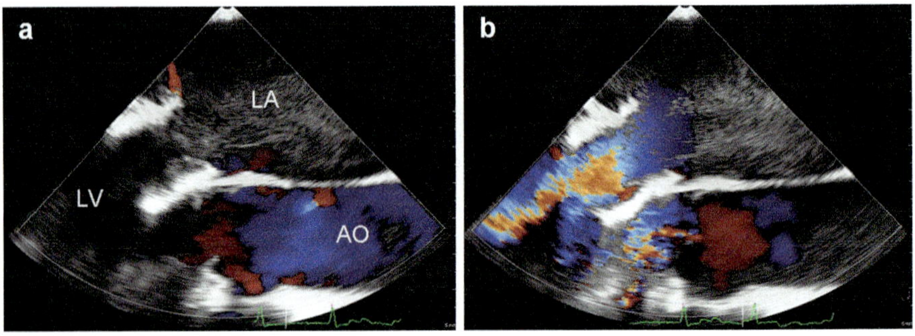

Fig. 2.5 Mid-esophageal long-axis color Doppler after the procedure. There was trivial leakage presented in systole (**a**) and no mosaic flow across the transcatheter mitral prosthesis in diastole (**b**)

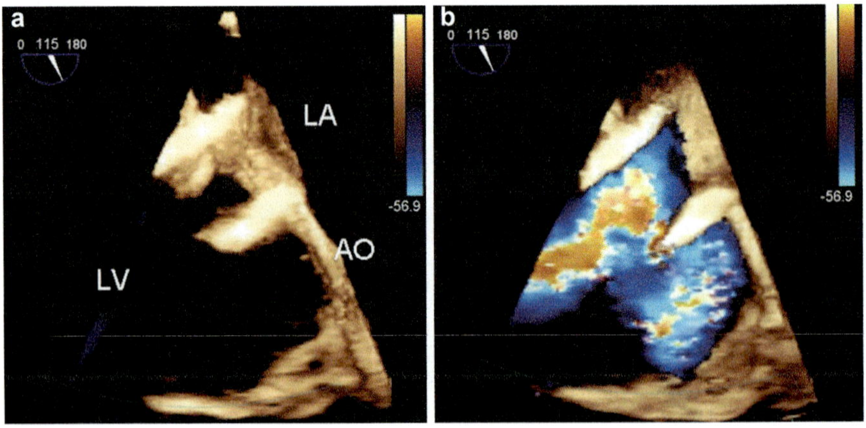

Fig. 2.6 Three dimensional color Doppler after the procedure. There was trivial leakage presented in systole (**a**) and no mosaic flow across the transcatheter mitral prosthesis in diastole (**b**)

2.3 Mitral Valve-In-Valve Implantation of Lotus Valve

A 67-year-old female patient had received mitral replacement and coronary artery bypass graft five years ago. Two years after the operation, she developed severe valvular mitral regurgitation due to the mitral prosthesis structural dysfunction, but refused a redo surgery. Recently, symptoms of dyspnea on exertion and chest tightness worsened. Therefore a mitral valve-in-valve replacement was indicated (Figs. 2.7, 2.8, 2.9, 2.10, 2.11, 2.12, 2.13, 2.14, 2.15, 2.16, and 2.17; Videos 2.7, 2.8, 2.9, 2.10, 2.11, 2.12, 2.13, 2.14, 2.15, 2.16, and 2.17).

Failure of bioprosthetic valves may arise due leaflet failure or nonleaflet failure or both. Leaflet failures are the result of leaflet degeneration which includes wear and calcification, or destruction, caused by endocarditis. In general, the outcome of failure due to calcification is valvular stenosis, and failure due to leaflet destruction results in regurgitation. In failure due to wear, which is frequently associated with calcification and abnormal leaflet coaptation, mix of stenosis and regurgitation is common.

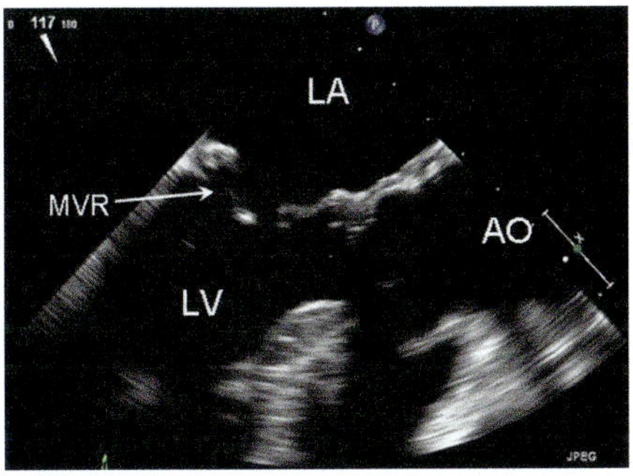

Fig. 2.7 Transesophageal echocardiography, mid-esophageal long-axis view. The patient had received mitral valve replacement (MVR) with bovine valve before. The bioprosthetic valve failed to open and close properly

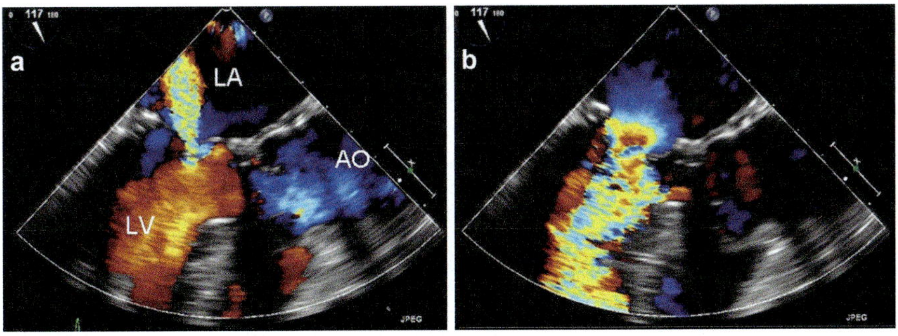

Fig. 2.8 In color Doppler, severe mitral regurgitation was demonstrated in systole (**a**); besides, flow across the mitral prosthesis was mosaic in diastole (**b**)

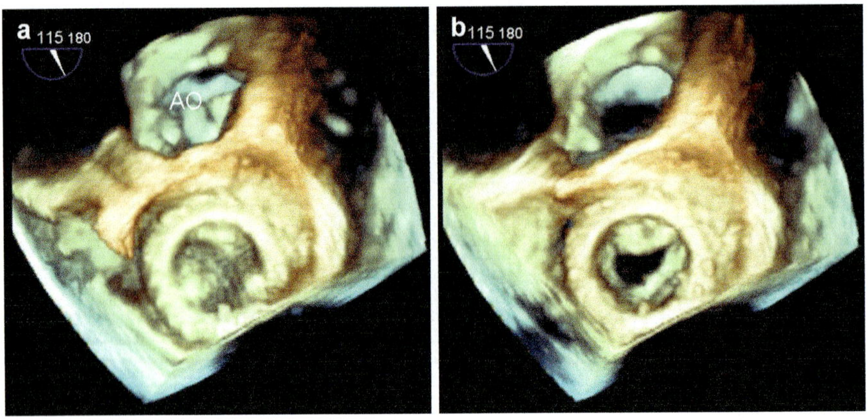

Fig. 2.9 In three-dimensional en face view in systole (**a**) and diastole (**b**), the leaflets were thickened and failed to open and close properly

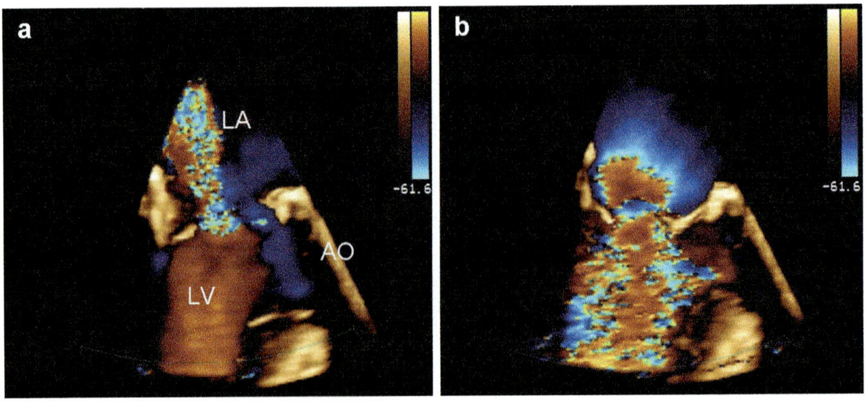

Fig. 2.10 In three-dimensional color Doppler, (**a**) Severe mitral regurgitation was demonstrated in systole. (**b**) flow across the mitral prosthesis was mosaic in diastole

Fig. 2.11 During the transcatheter valve-in-valve implantation, the delivery catheter advanced into the bioprosthetic mitral valve

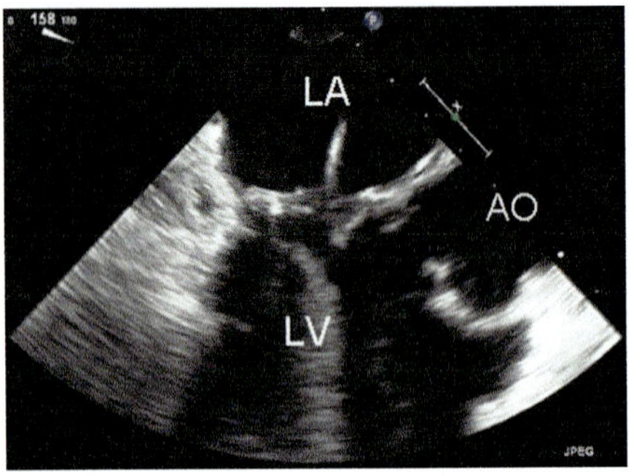

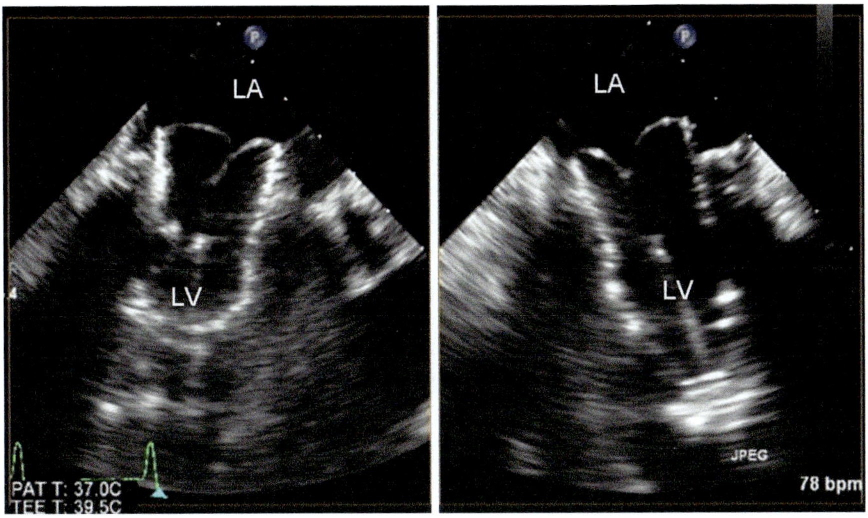

Fig. 2.12 In x-plane view after implantation, the Lotus valve (27 mm) was well positioned and deployed

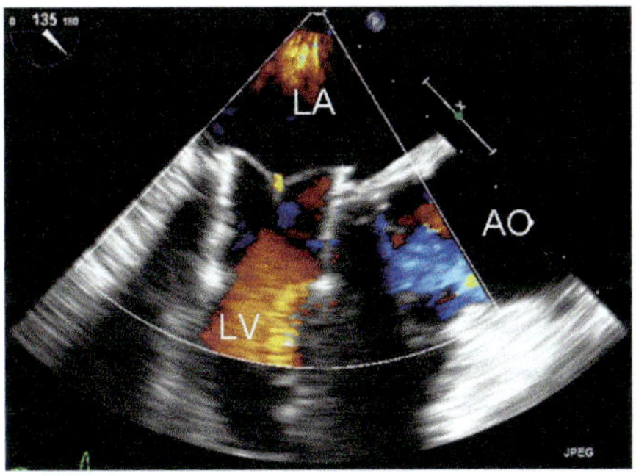

Fig. 2.13 Color Doppler after the procedure. There was trivial leakage in systole

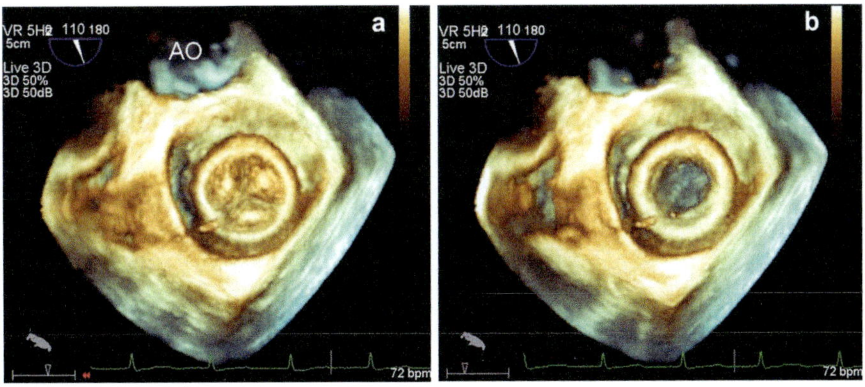

Fig. 2.14 In three-dimensional en face view during the procedure, the Lotus valve was advanced into the mitral prosthesis (**a**), but not fully extended yet (**b**)

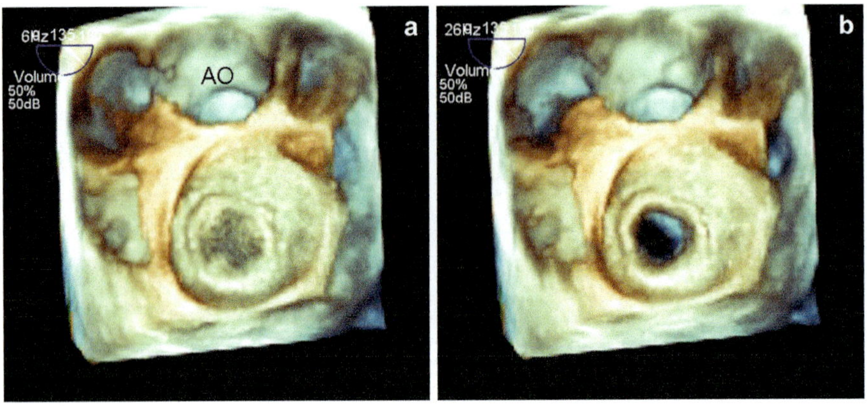

Fig. 2.15 After the procedure, the frame of a Lotus valve was seen within the sewing ring of the failed prosthesis (**a**). The leaflets were wide-open in diastole (**b**)

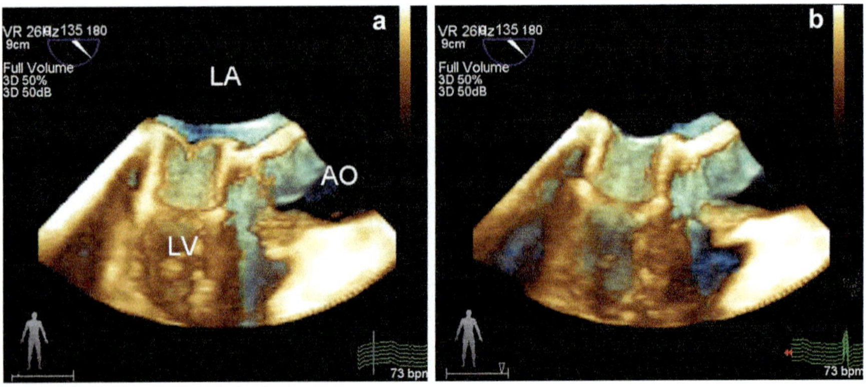

Fig. 2.16 Three-dimensional long-axis view in systole (**a**) and diastole (**b**) after implantation, the Lotus valve was well positioned and deployed

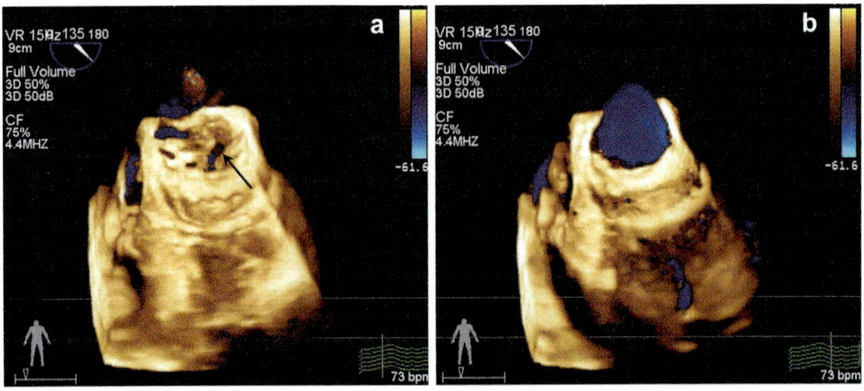

Fig. 2.17 Three dimensional color Doppler after the procedure. There was trivial leakage (arrow, **a**) in systole and no mosaic flow across the valve-in-valve mitral prosthesis in diastole (**b**)

2.4 Aortic Valve-In-Valve Implantation of CoreValve

A 64-year-old female patient with valvular heart disease had received aortic and mitral valve replacement six years ago. Three years later, she underwent redo mitral valve replacement due to mitral prosthesis dysfunction. This time, she was sent to our emergency room for epigastric pain. Auscultation showed a grade 3/6 systolic murmur. Echocardiography showed severe aortic regurgitation. Infective endocarditis was diagnosed afterward. Therefore, antibiotic therapy and further surgical intervention were suggested (Figs. 2.18, 2.19, 2.20, 2.21, 2.22, 2.23, 2.24, 2.25, and 2.26; Videos 2.18, 2.19, 2.20, 2.21, 2.22, 2.23, 2.24a, 2.24b, 2.25a, 2.25b, and 2.26).

Of all heart valves, the aortic valve has the highest rate of surgical valve replacement. As a result, failing bioprostheses in the aortic position are increasingly encountered as a target for valve-in-valve procedures.

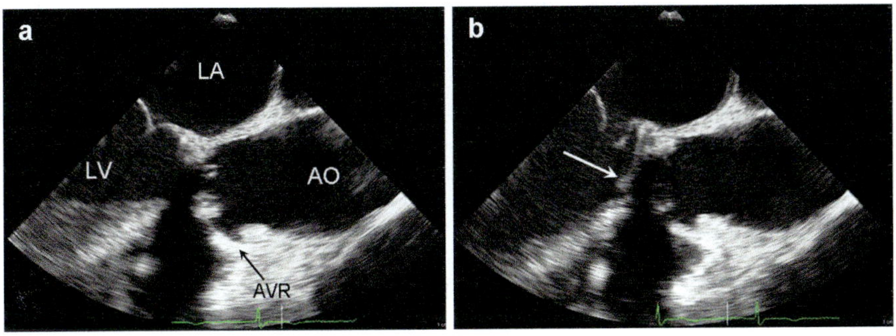

Fig. 2.18 Transesophageal echocardiographic mid-esophageal long-axis view. (**a**) The patient had received mitral and aortic valve replacement (AVR, 21 mm porcine valve) before. (**b**) A highly mobile echo-density (arrow) was seen attaching to the bioprosthetic aortic leaflet and prolapsed into the left ventricle in diastole

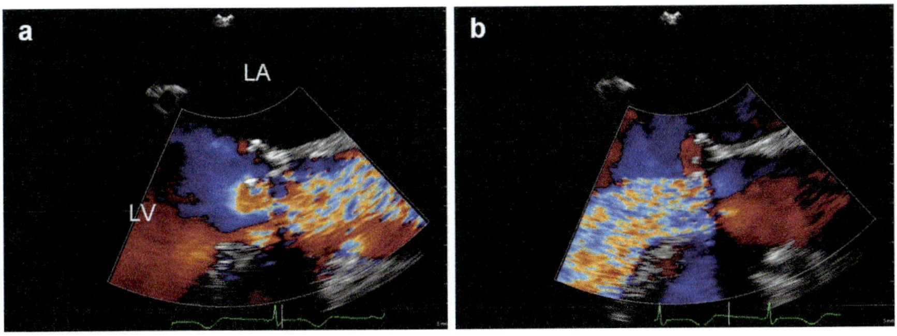

Fig. 2.19 In color Doppler, flow across the aortic prosthesis was mosaic in systole (**a**). Severe aortic regurgitation was demonstrated in diastole (**b**)

Fig. 2.20 In three dimensional long-axis view, previous surgical aortic and mitral prostheses were demonstrated

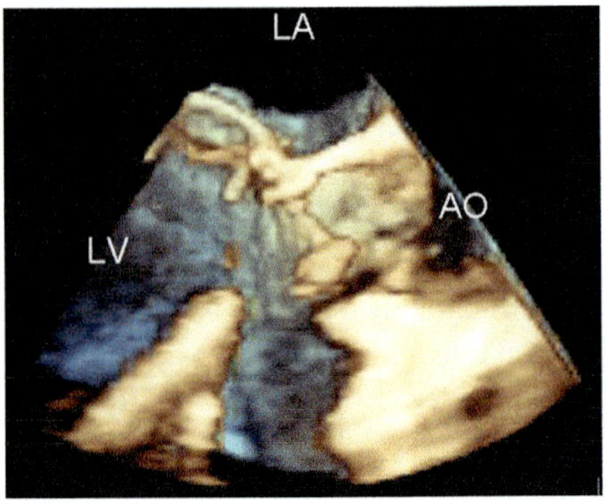

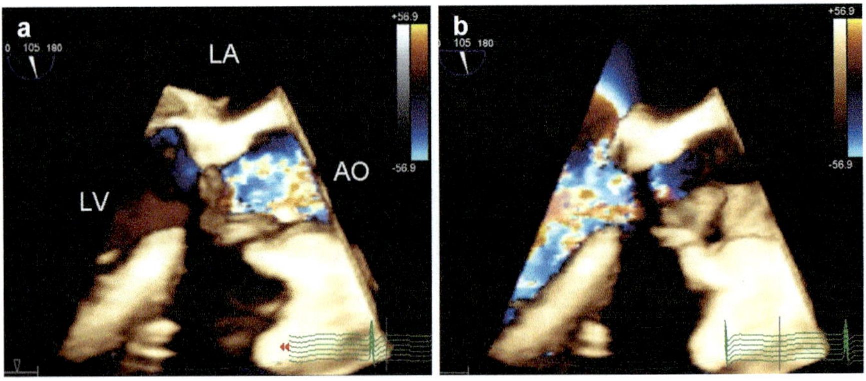

Fig. 2.21 In three dimensional color Doppler, flow across the aortic prosthesis was mosaic in systole (**a**). Severe aortic regurgitation was demonstrated in diastole (**b**)

Fig. 2.22 During transcatheter aortic valve-in-valve implantation, crimped CoreValve (asterisk) was advanced into the bioprosthesis

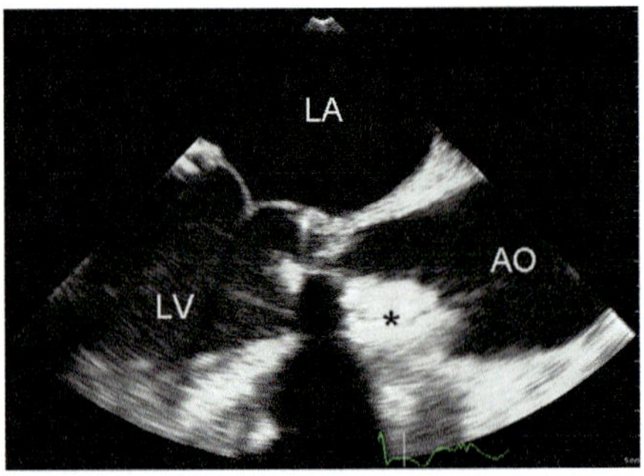

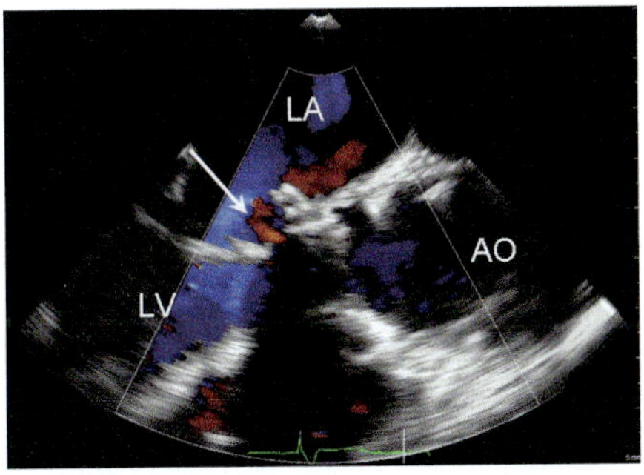

Fig. 2.23 When the CoreValve first expanded, color Doppler showed mild paravalvular regurgitation (arrow)

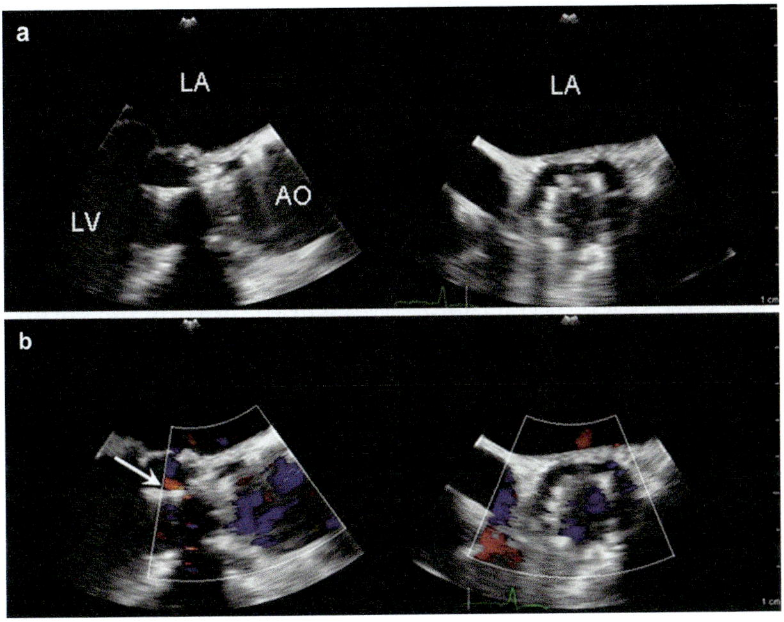

Fig. 2.24 X-plane views after release of the CoreValve. The device was well positioned and worked normally (**a**). Only trivial paravalvular leakage (arrow) was present in color Doppler (**b**)

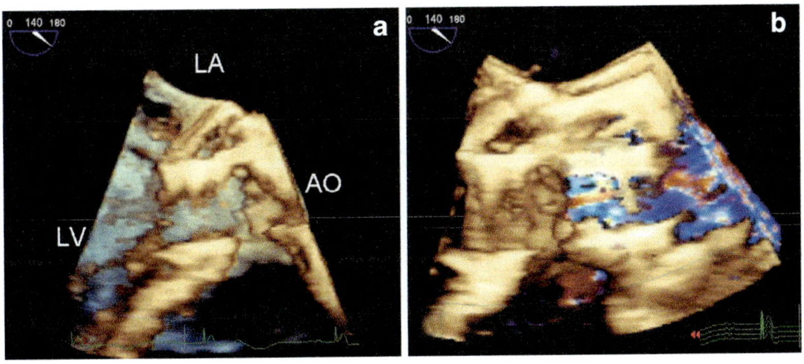

Fig. 2.25 Three dimensional long-axis views after the valve-in-valve implantation. The CoreValve was well positioned and deployed (**a**), and only trivial paravalvular leakage was present in color Doppler (**b**)

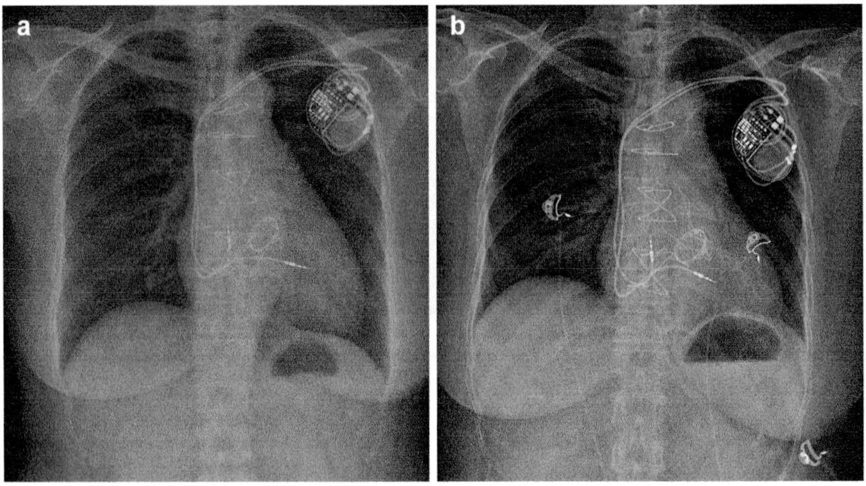

Fig. 2.26 Chest X-rays after the aortic and mitral valve replacement (**a**) and the subsequent transcatheter aortic valve-in-valve implantation (**b**). Retained surgical wires of median sternotomy, and CoreValve within bioprosthetic aortic annulus were demonstrated

2.5 Aortic and Mitral Valve-In-Valve Implantation of SAPIEN Valves in One Session

A 67-year-old male patient was admitted for exertional dyspnea and general weakness. He had a history of coronary artery bypass graft and surgical replacement of the aortic and the mitral valve with bioprostheses (21 and 29 mm) 7 years ago. He also had hypertension, atrial fibrillation and depressed ventricular function. Echocardiography showed severe aortic and mitral stenosis and moderate mitral regurgitation due to degeneration of the prostheses. Therefore the patient was scheduled for transcatheter double valve-in-valve implantation (Figs. 2.27, 2.28, 2.29, 2.30, 2.31, 2.32, 2.33, and 2.34; Videos 2.27, 2.28, 2.29a, 2.29b, 2.29c, 2.29d, 2.30, 2.31a, 2.31b, 2.31c, 2.32, 2.33, and 2.34).

Imaging will play a major role in the developing era of transcatheter interventions. These therapies will enable treatments of patients with valvular disease which are not operable. The heart valves are complex structures that can be evaluated excellently with echocardiography but not with fluoroscopy. Whereas, the visualization of the catheter and the stent of the prosthesis are not optimal with echocardiography due to artifacts created by the catheter material.

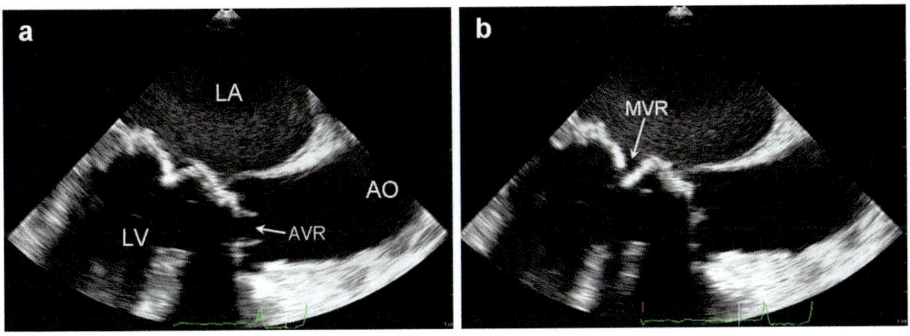

Fig. 2.27 In transesophageal echocardiographic mid-esophageal long-axis view, the patient had received aortic and mitral valve replacement (AVR, MVR) with bioprosthesis before, which had degenerated and failed to open properly. Aortic and mitral stenosis were demonstrated in systole (**a**) and diastole (**b**) respectively

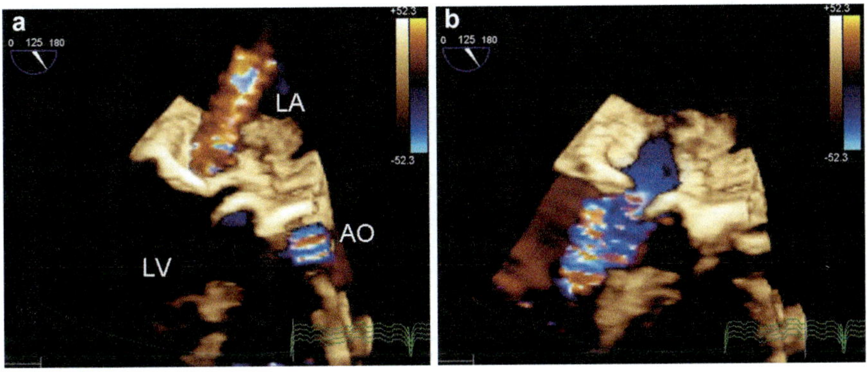

Fig. 2.28 In three-dimensional color Doppler, (**a**) moderate mitral regurgitation and aortic stenosis were demonstrated in systole. (**b**) Flow across the mitral prosthesis was mosaic in diastole

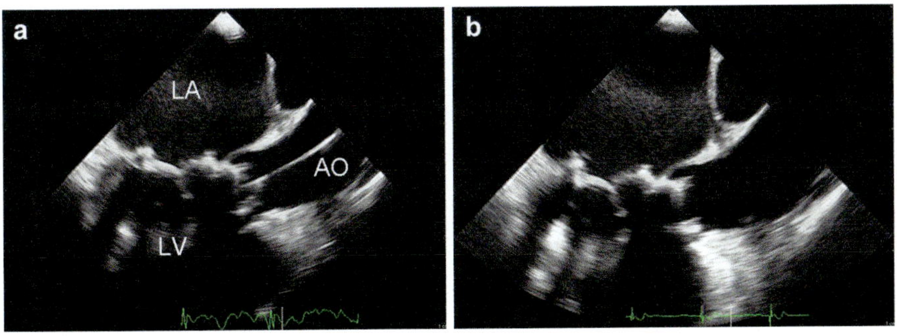

Fig. 2.29 Both of the valves were treated in one session through a transapical access. Aortic valve implantation was performed first. The guiding catheter advanced into the degenerated aortic prosthesis (**a**), and a SAPIEN valve (23 mm) was implanted within it (**b**). Afterward, guiding catheter of mitral implantation advanced into the mitral annulus for another SAPIEN valve (29 mm) to deploy (**c**). After the implantations of both aortic and mitral valve were done, they presented normal function (**d**)

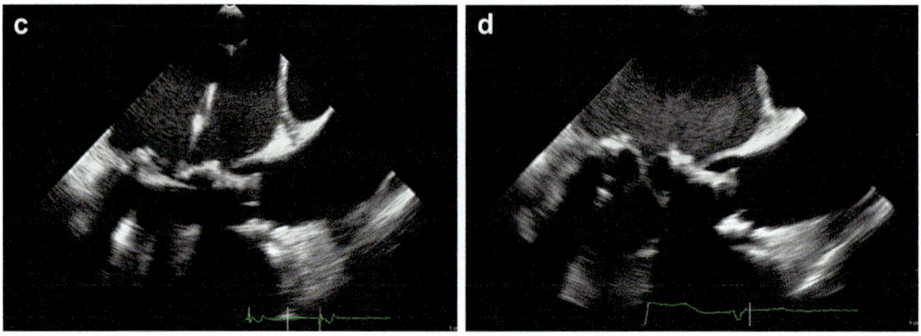

Fig. 2.29 (continued)

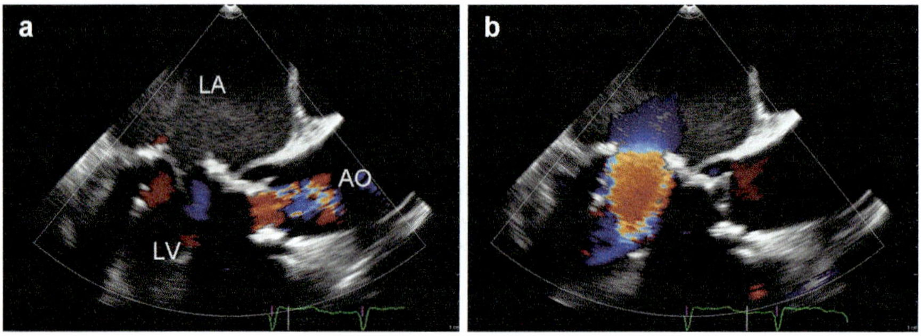

Fig. 2.30 In color Doppler after the procedure, there was trivial leakage and no mosaic flow across the valve-in-valve aortic and mitral prostheses in systole (**a**) and diastole (**b**)

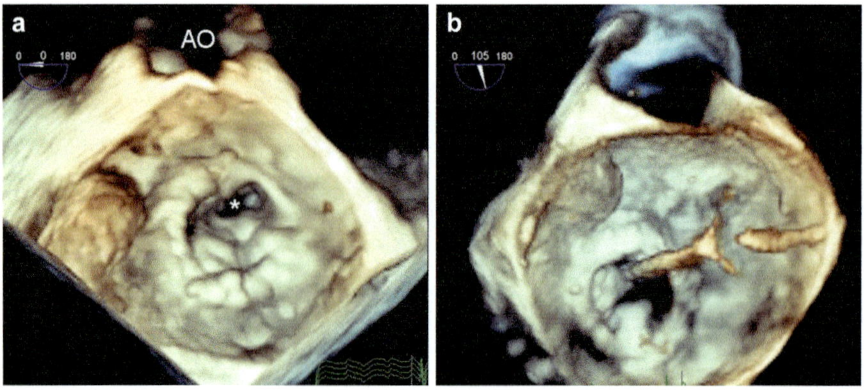

Fig. 2.31 Three-dimensional en face views of mitral valve. (**a**) The degenerated mitral bioprosthesis developed small valve area (asterisk). (**b**) During the valve-in-valve procedure, the guiding catheter advanced into the mitral annulus. (**c**) After expansion, the SAPIEN prosthesis was well positioned

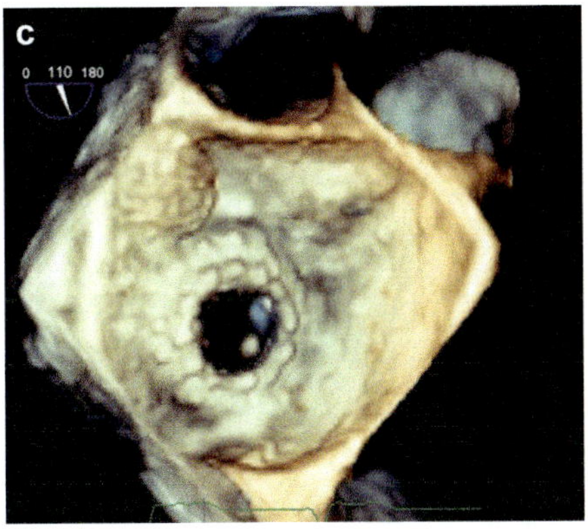

Fig. 2.31 (continued)

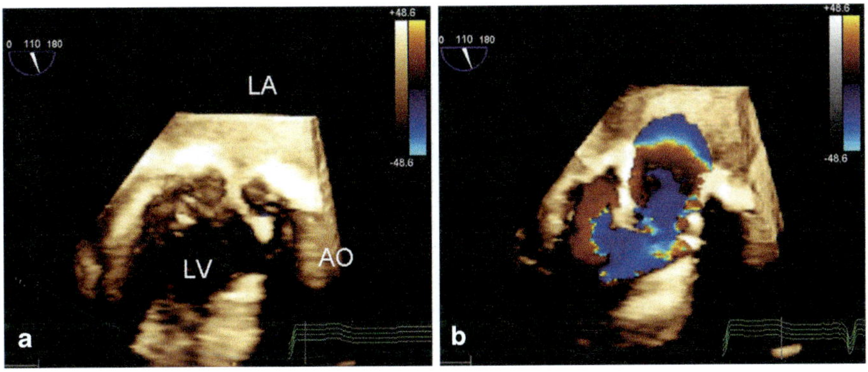

Fig. 2.32 Three dimensional color Doppler after the procedure. There was scarcely no leakage presented in systole (**a**) and no mosaic flow across the valve-in-valve prosthesis (**b**)

Fig. 2.33 During the procedure, there was thrombus seen in the left atrial appendage

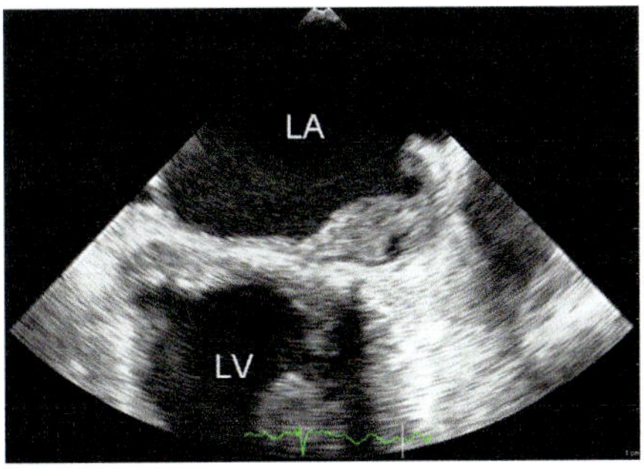

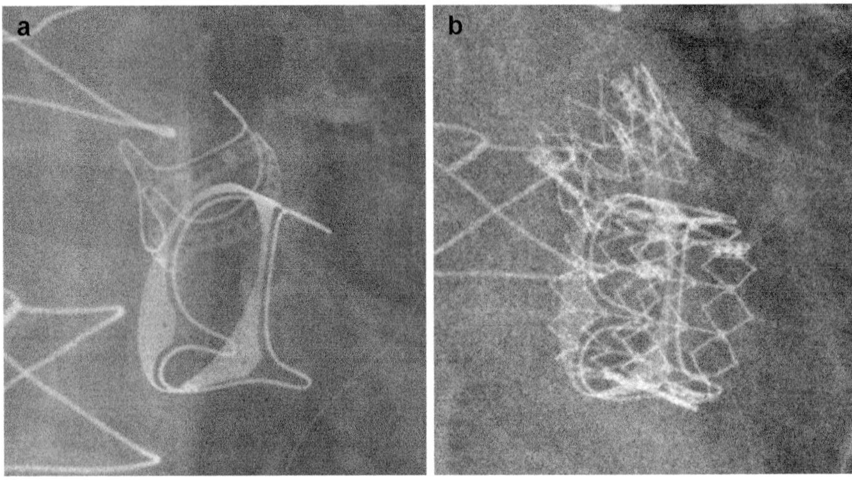

Fig. 2.34 Chest X-rays after the aortic and mitral valve replacement (**a**) and the subsequent transcatheter aortic and mitral valve-in-valve implantation (**b**). The SAPIEN valves within bioprosthetic aortic and mitral annulus were demonstrated

2.6 Occluder and Mitral Valve-In-Valve Implantation for Paravalvular Leakage

A 64-year-old female patient with valvular heart disease had received mitral and tricuspid valve replacement four times (the last time was seven years ago). She suffered from pancytopenia and severe anemia recently. Echocardiography revealed mitral prosthesis failure with severe paravalvular leakage. Therefore a percutaneous paravalvular leakage closure and mitral valve in valve implantation were indicated (Figs. 2.35, 2.36, 2.37, 2.38, 2.39, 2.40, 2.41, 2.42, 2.43, 2.44, 2.45, and 2.46; Videos 2.35a, 2.35b, 2.36, 2.37, 2.38a, 2.38b, 2.39a, 2.39b, 2.39c, 2.40, 2.41a, 2.41b, 2.42a, 2.42b, 2.43, 2.44, 2.45, and 2.46).

In patients with bioprosthetic valve regurgitation, whether it is transvalvular or paravalvular regurgitation must be clarified. Even though the former may be successfully treated using valve-in-valve therapy, the latter is not suitable for such techniques only. Patients with bioprosthetic paravalvular regurgitation who are deemed unsuitable for reoperation may, however, benefit from other percutaneous techniques like occluder to block the paravalvular leak.

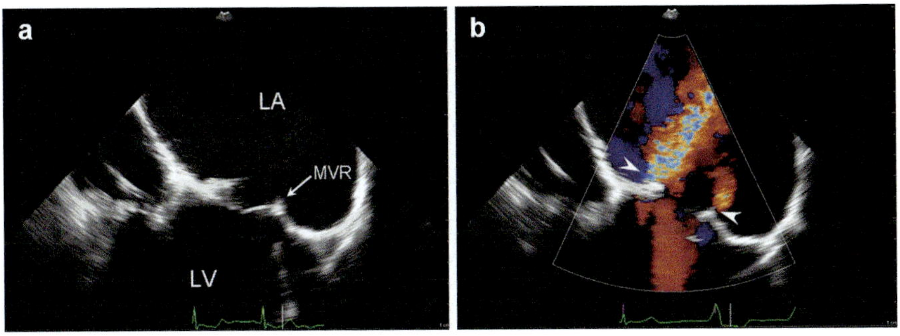

Fig. 2.35 In transesophageal echocardiographic four-chamber view, the patient had received mitral valve replacement (MVR) with bioprosthesis (**a**). In color Doppler, severe paravalvular leakages (arrow heads) were demonstrated around the mitral annulus (**b**)

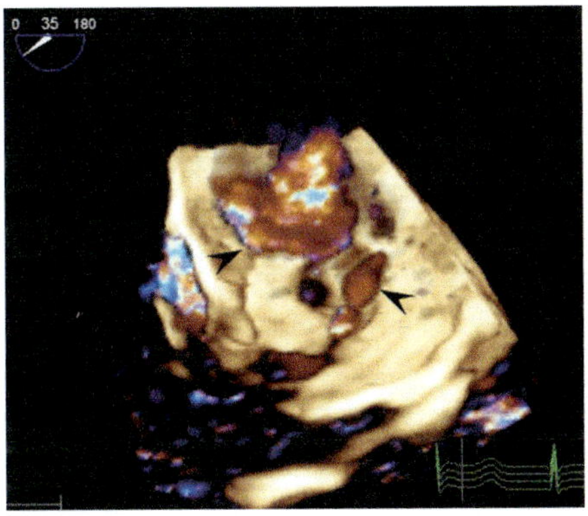

Fig. 2.36 Three dimensional color Doppler viewed from left atrium depicted two separate paravalvular leakages (arrow heads)

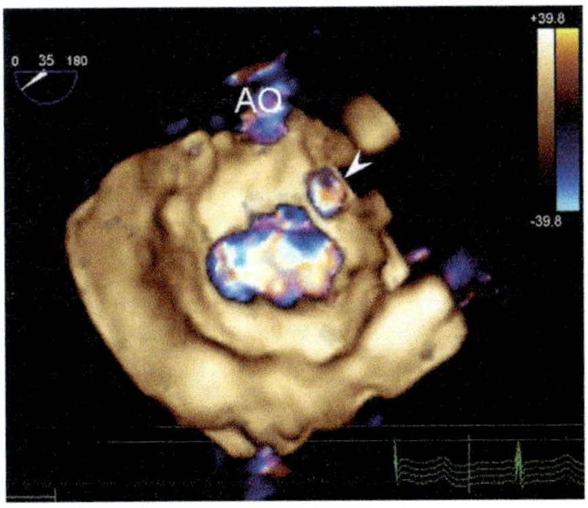

Fig. 2.37 Three dimensional color en face view showed the origin of the residual paravalvular leakage at 2 o'clock position (arrow head)

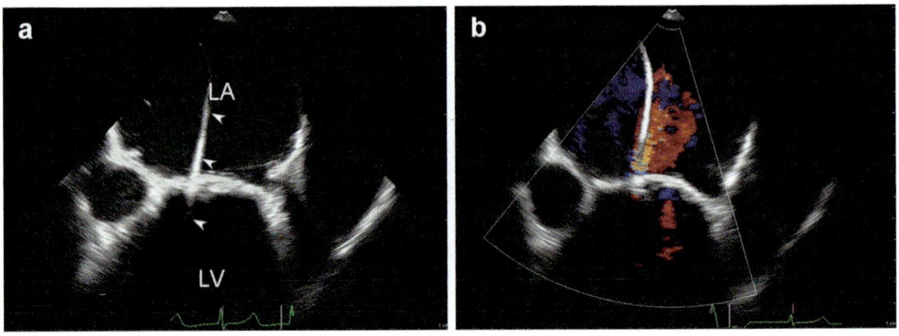

Fig. 2.38 In a mid-esophageal long-axis view during the occluder implantation, the guiding catheter (arrow heads, **a**) crossed the mitral annular plane through the opening of the paravalvular leakage. Color Doppler (**b**) is helpful in demonstrating correct positioning of the occluder delivery system

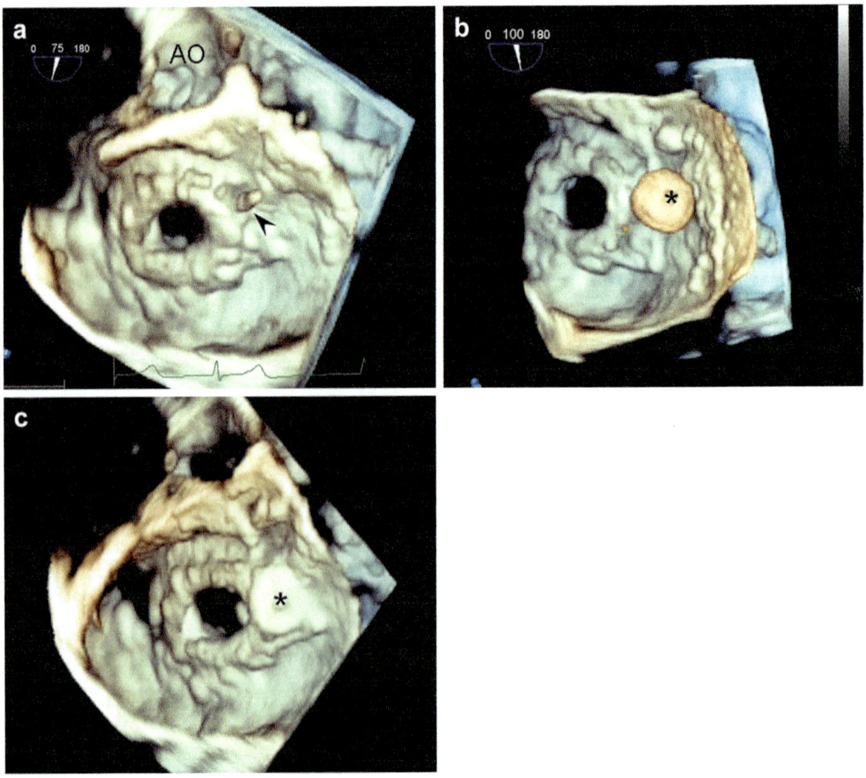

Fig. 2.39 Three dimensional en face views during occluder implantation showed the wire crossing the mitral annulus through the opening of the paravalvular leakage at 2 o'clock position (arrow head, **a**). An occluder (asterisk) was delivered and deployed in the atrial side (**b**) and released after capturing the surrounding tissue (**c**)

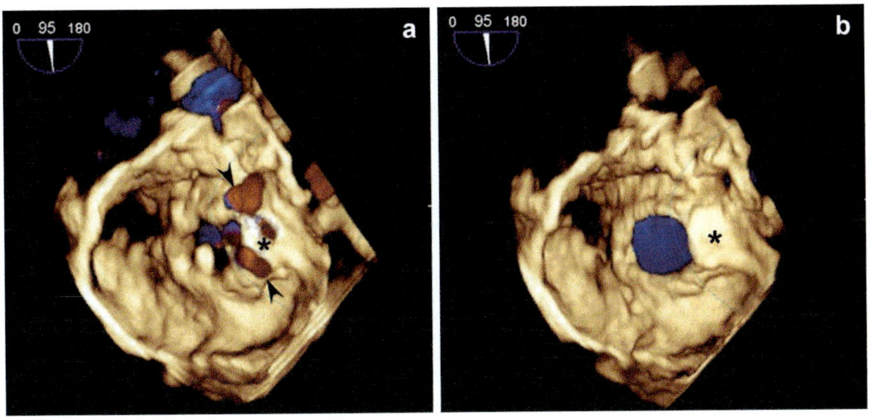

Fig. 2.40 In color Doppler after the percutaneous closure, the final position of the occluder (asterisk, **b**) was confirmed and mild to moderate paravalvular leakages (arrow heads, **a**) were present in systole

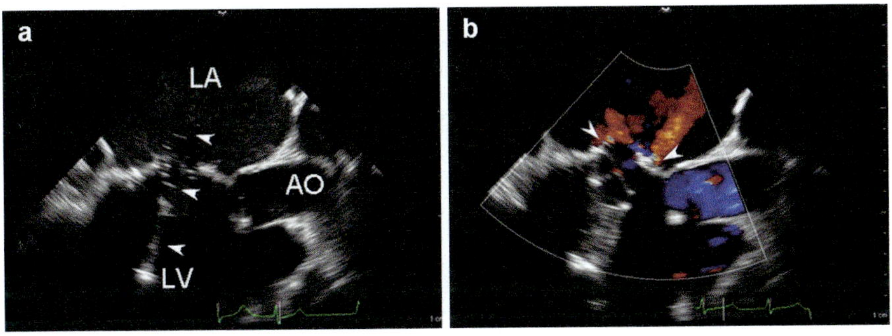

Fig. 2.41 To reduce the persisted paravalvular leakage, transcatheter mitral valve-in-valve implantation was performed. In a mid-esophageal long-axis view, the guiding catheter (arrow heads, **a**) advanced into the bioprosthetic mitral annulus and the Edwards SAPIEN valve (29 mm) was delivered. Before the device was fully expended, paravalvular leakages (arrow heads, **b**) were demonstrated in color Doppler

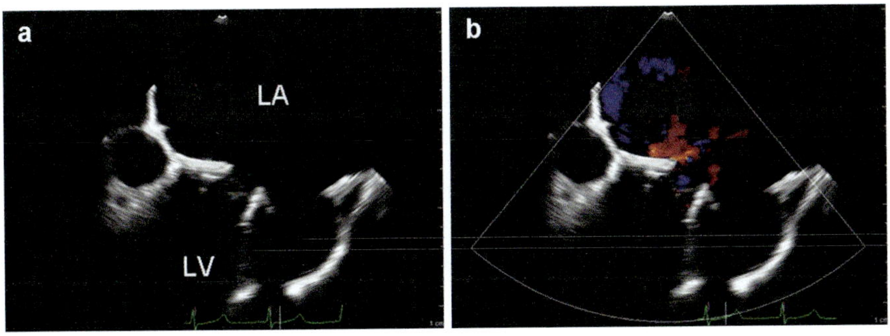

Fig. 2.42 After both the occluder and mitral valve- in-valve implantation were completed, the mitral prosthesis worked well (**a**) and there was trivial paravalvular leakages remaining (**b**)

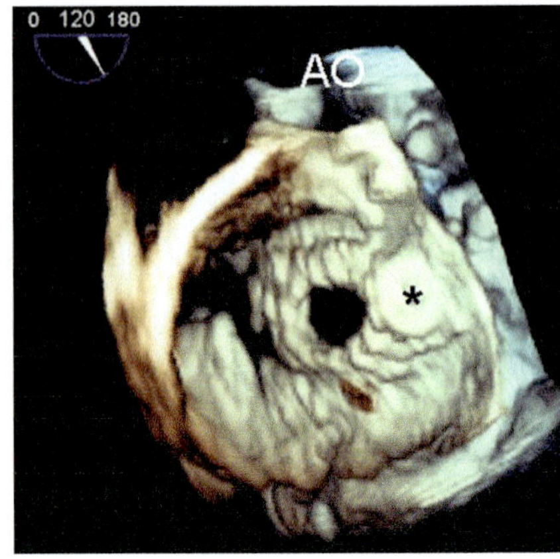

Fig. 2.43 Three dimensional en face view after the whole procedure showed the occluder (asterisk) was in the adequate position and the Edwards SAPIEN valve was within the bioprosthetic mitral annulus

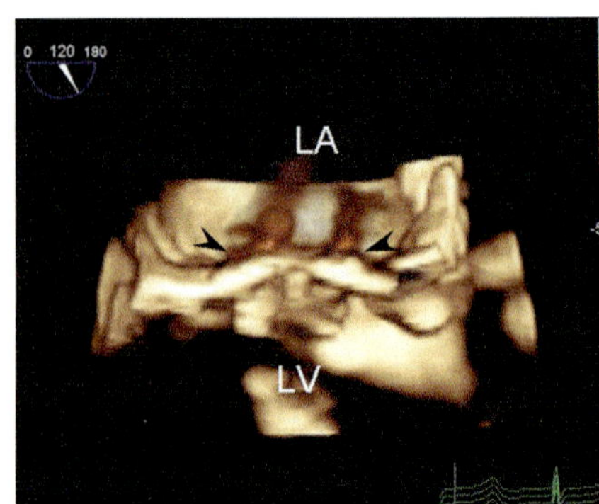

Fig. 2.44 Three dimensional color Doppler after the whole procedure showed trivial paravalvular leakages remaining (arrow heads)

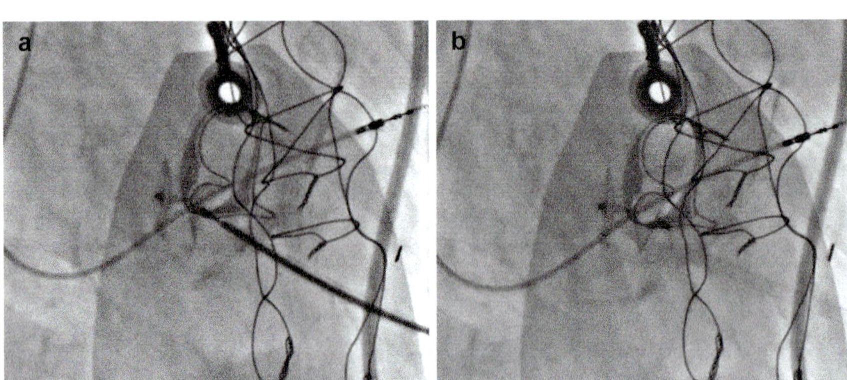

Fig. 2.45 Fluoroscopy during the occluder implantation. (**a**) Both disks of the occluder were deployed and still attached to the delivery cable. (**b**) The device was released. Its position was at the edge of the bioprosthetic mitral annulus

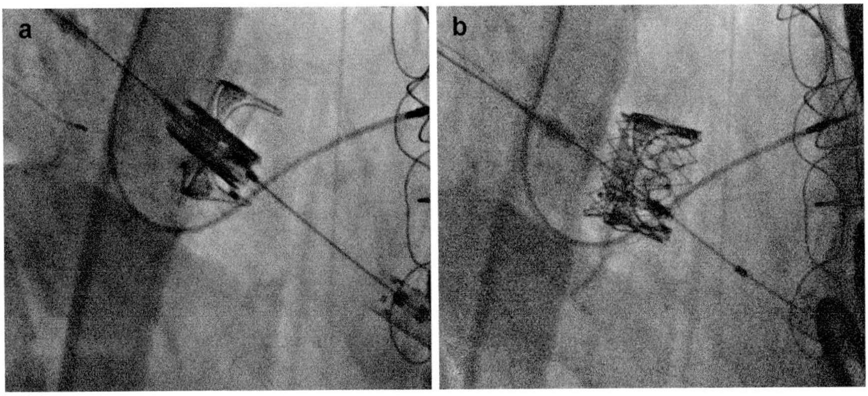

Fig. 2.46 Fluoroscopic images during transcatheter SAPIEN valve implantation. (**a**) The guiding catheter delivered the crimped SAPIEN valve through the surgical mitral bioprosthesis. (**b**) The SAPIEN valve was expanded with the correct implant height

2.7 Double Occluders and Mitral Valve-In-Valve Implantation for Paravalvular Leakage

A 72-year-old male patient with rheumatic heart disease with severe mitral regurgitation had undergone surgical mitral valve replacement for three times due to recurrent events of valvular and paravalvular leakage. The first replacement was done in 1997; the redo surgery was performed in 2005; the last time was in 2012. However, four years after the third operation, he suffered from dyspnea, swelling bilateral lower limbs, and hemolytic anemia. Recurrent moderate paravalvular leakage was revealed. Therefore transcatheter mitral valve in valve replacement was arranged (Figs. 2.47, 2.48, 2.49, 2.50, 2.51, 2.52, 2.53, 2.54, and 2.55; Videos 2.47a, 2.47b, 2.48, 2.49, 2.50a, 2.50b, 2.51, 2.52a, 2.52b, 2.53, 2.54a, 2.54b, and 2.55).

Transcatheter interventions are emerging as attractive alternatives to reoperative surgery for high-risk patients with severe bioprosthetic mitral valve degeneration. The success of these procedures relies on real-time image guidance. Transesophageal echocardiography is crucial in identifying the exact location, size, and origin of the paravalvular leakage jet and in guiding and monitoring the stepwise occlusion. Three dimensional assessments can provide extra certainty of the catheter position and permit guidance of complex cardiac structures.

The locations of the paravalvular leaks are essential for access site determination. For mitral paravalvular leaks between 6 and 9 o'clock, the transseptal approach is efficient. Nevertheless, when leaks are between 10 and 1 o'clock, as in this patient, the transapical approach is a preferred route. Furthermore, when a large crescent–shape leak is present, it is better to use two smaller devices in order to cover most of the defect rather than use a single large device.

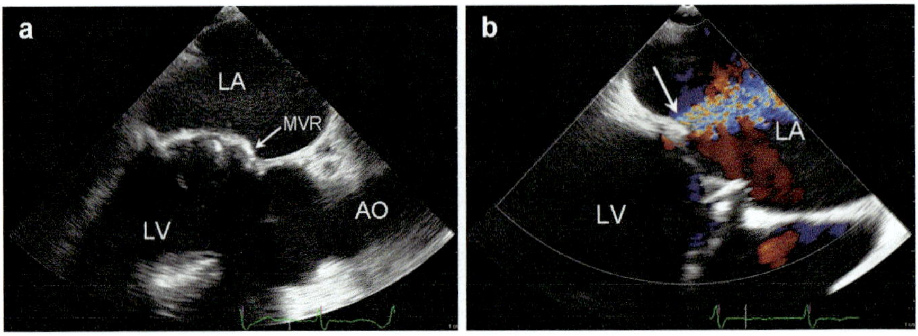

Fig. 2.47 In transesophageal echocardiographic mid-esophageal long-axis view (**a**), the patient had received mitral valve replacement (MVR) with bovine valve before. In color Doppler (**b**), moderate paravalvular leakage (arrow) was demonstrated

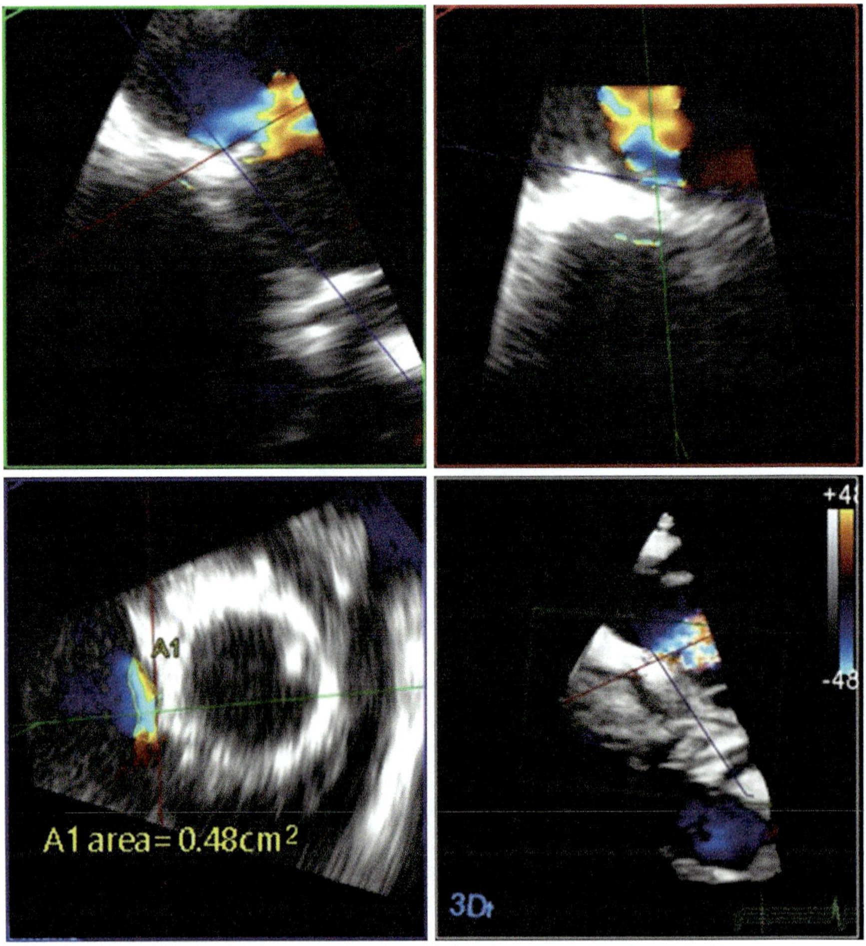

Fig. 2.48 Through multi-plane reconstruction, the origin of the paravalvular leakage between 8 and 10 o'clock position was measured 0.48 cm^2, which approximately accounted for 20% of the mitral annulus circumference

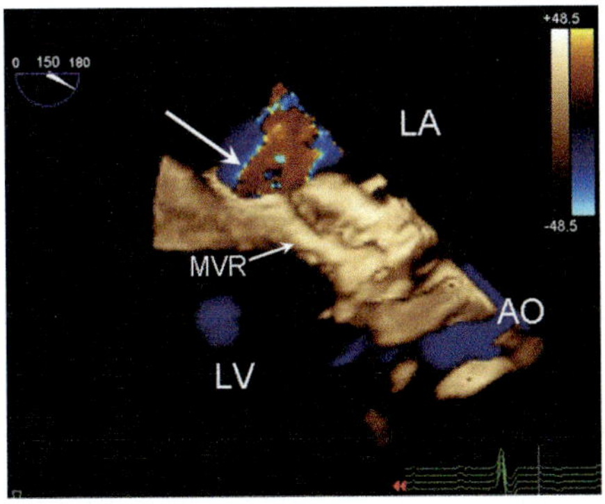

Fig. 2.49 In three dimensional long-axis view with color Doppler, moderate paravalvular leakage (arrow) was demonstrated around the posterior aspect of the mitral prosthesis

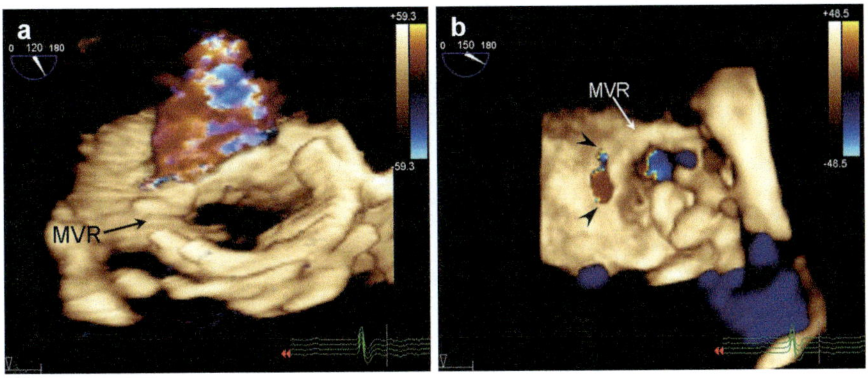

Fig. 2.50 In three dimensional color Doppler images viewed from the left atrium toward left ventricle (**a**) and the opposite aspect (**b**), a large turbulent paravalvular jet and the orifice of it (arrow heads) were demonstrated

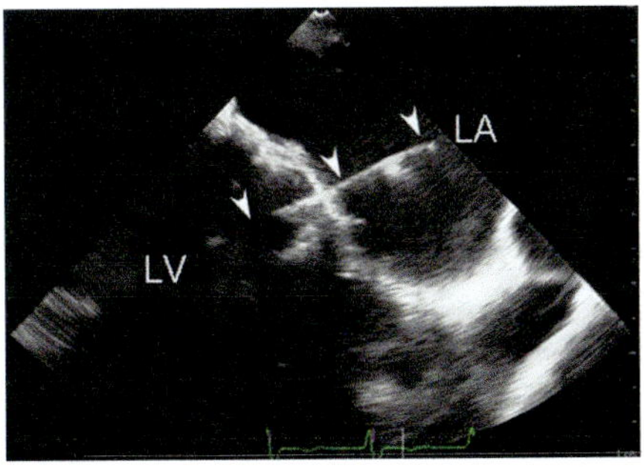

Fig. 2.51 During the transcatheter mitral valve-in-valve implantation, the guiding catheter (arrow heads) advanced into the bioprosthetic mitral valve

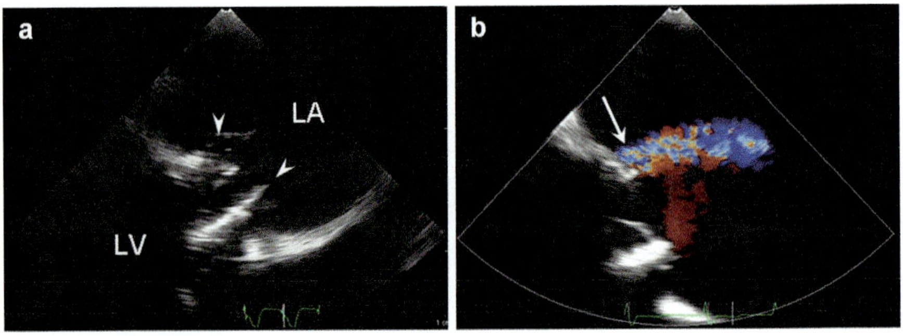

Fig. 2.52 The Edwards SAPIEN valve was delivered and expended (**a**, arrow heads). However, paravalvular leakage (arrow, **b**) persisted after the mitral valve-in-valve implantation

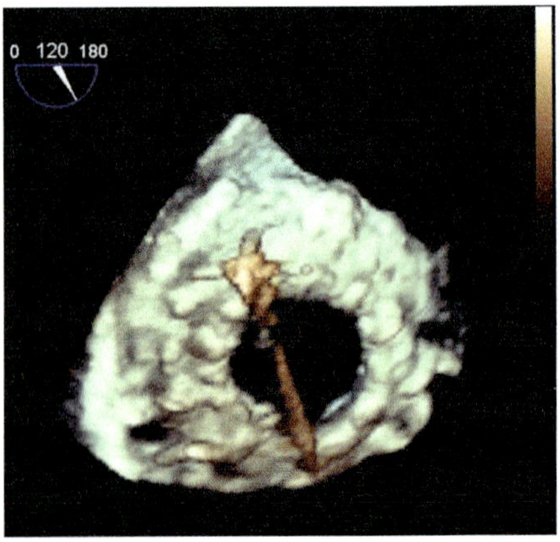

Fig. 2.53 To close the leak, occluder implantation was indicated. In three-dimensional transesophageal echocardiography en face view, the wire crossed the mitral annulus through the opening of the paravalvular leakage

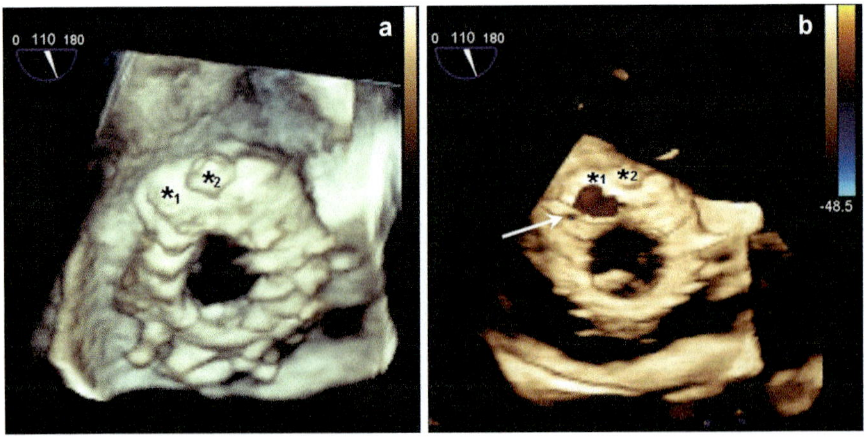

Fig. 2.54 Two occluders were deployed (**a**, asterisk[1], asterisk[2]). In color Doppler, mild paravalvular leakage (arrow, **b**) was present near the occluders (*[1], *[2])

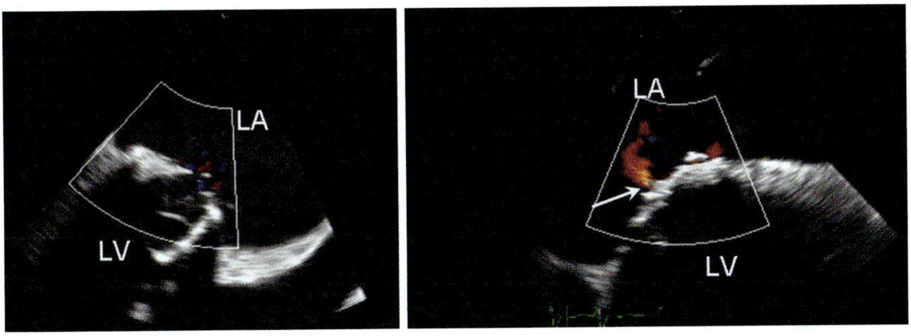

Fig. 2.55 Confirmation in two-dimensional X-plane color Doppler showed mild paravalvular leakage (arrow)

2.8 Recapture of Lotus Valve During Mitral Valve-In-Valve Implantation

A 22-year-old male patient with hypertrophic obstructive cardiomyopathy had received myectomy and mitral valve replacement nine years ago. He developed exertional dyspnea and cough recently. After medical treatments, symptoms worsen. Auscultation showed regular rhythm with grade 2/6 systolic murmur over apex region. Echocardiography showed dysfunction of the prosthetic mitral valve with regurgitation and stenosis. According to the condition, mitral valve-in-valve replacement was arranged (Figs. 2.56, 2.57, 2.58, 2.59, 2.60, 2.61, 2.62, 2.63, 2.64, and 2.65; Videos 2.56, 2.57, 2.58, 2.59, 2.60a, 2.60b, 2.60c, 2.60d, 2.61, 2.62a, 2.62b, 2.62c, 2.62d, 2.63a, 2.63b, 2.64a, 2.64b, and 2.65).

The Lotus valve system is a fully repositionable device designed to facilitate optimal position of the valve. The valve's position can be adjusted at any point during valve expansion. Upon full expansion, flow dynamics can be assessed prior to release of the valve. If the implant needs to be repositioned or retrieved, it can be partially or completely withdrawn back into the sheath. When the final position is established, the device is deployed and detached from the delivery system.

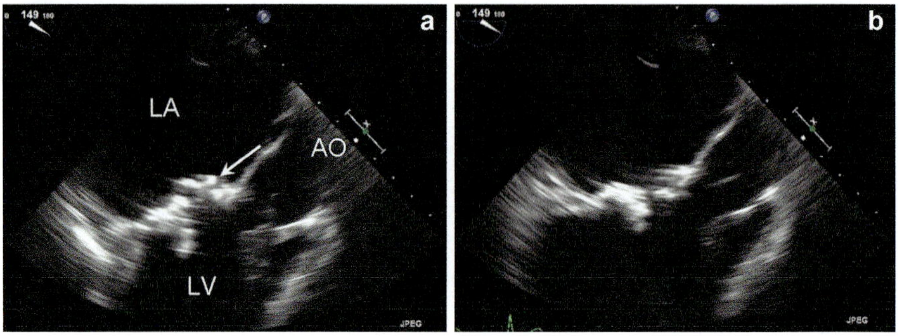

Fig. 2.56 Transesophageal echocardiography, mid-esophageal long-axis view. The patient had received mitral valve replacement with porcine valve before. The leaflet of the bioprosthetic valve flailed into the left atrium (arrow, **a**) in systole and opened restrictively in diastole (**b**)

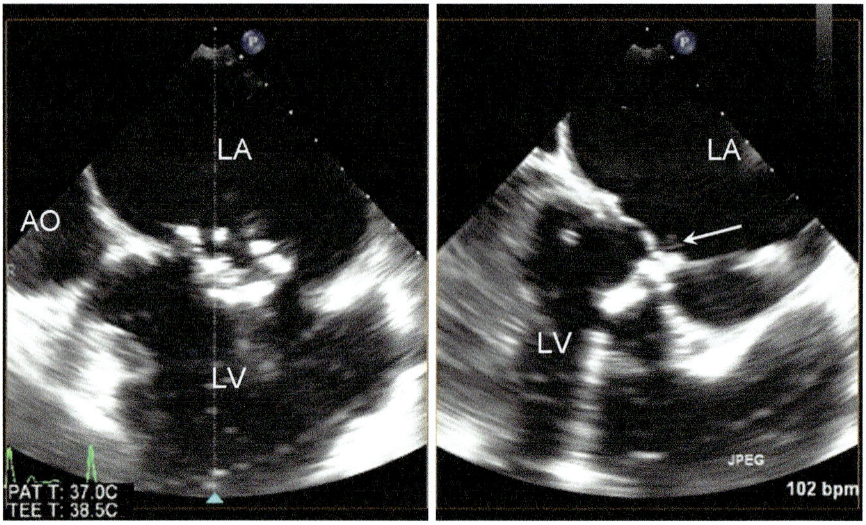

Fig. 2.57 Transesophageal x-plane view. The patient had received mitral valve replacement with porcine valve before. *Flailed leaflets* (arrow) were demonstrated on the atrial side of the mitral bioprosthesis

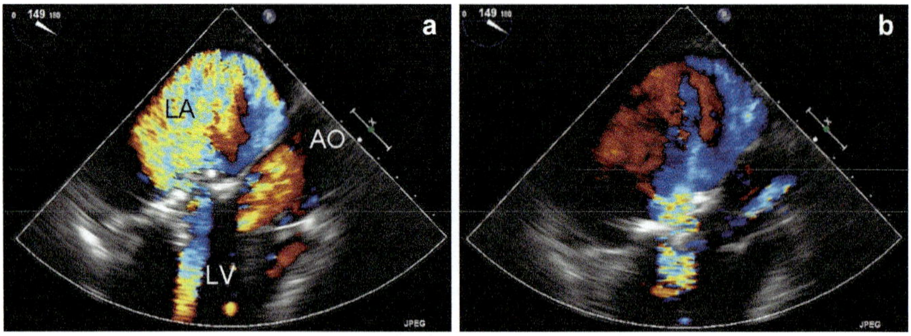

Fig. 2.58 With color Doppler, severe mitral regurgitation was revealed in systole (**a**) and mosaic flow across the mitral prosthesis was demonstrated in diastole (**b**)

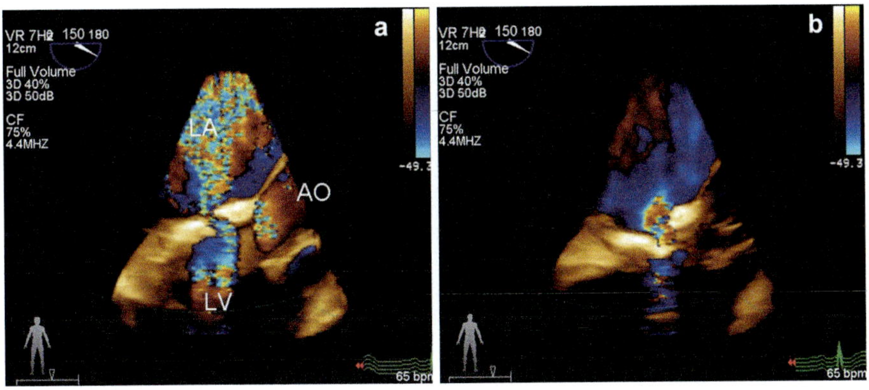

Fig. 2.59 Three dimensional color Doppler, severe mitral regurgitation was revealed in systole (**a**) and mosaic flow across the mitral prosthesis was demonstrated in diastole (**b**)

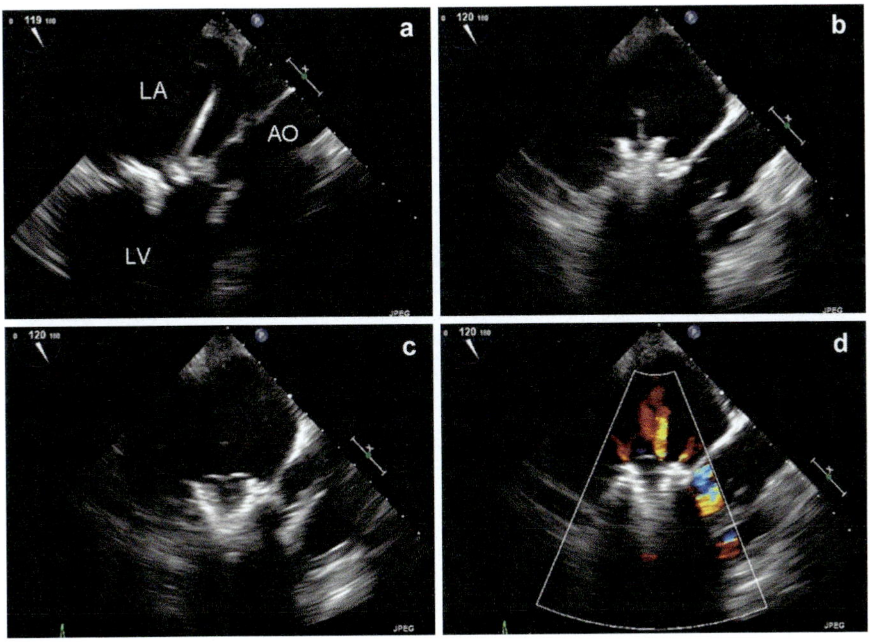

Fig. 2.60 During the transcatheter valve-in-valve implantation, the guiding catheter advanced into the bioprosthetic mitral valve (**a**) and delivered the crimped Lotus valve (**b**). After the deployment of the Lotus valve (**c**), mild valvular and paravalvular leakage were demonstrated by color Doppler (**d**). It might be caused by the improper positioning of the transcatheter heart valve; therefore a repositioning of the device was indicated

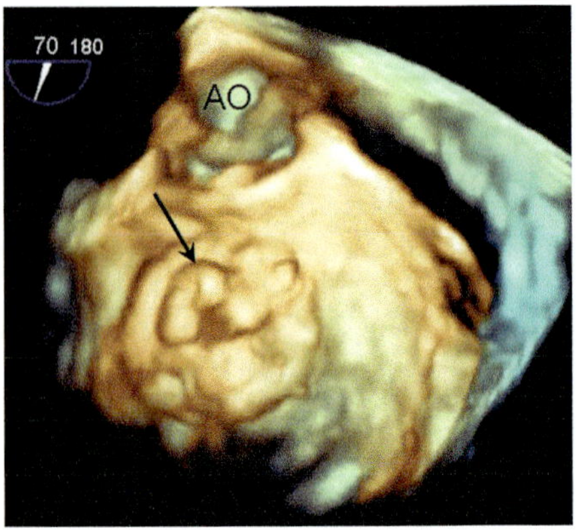

Fig. 2.61 In three dimensional en face view, flailed leaflets (arrow) were present in systole

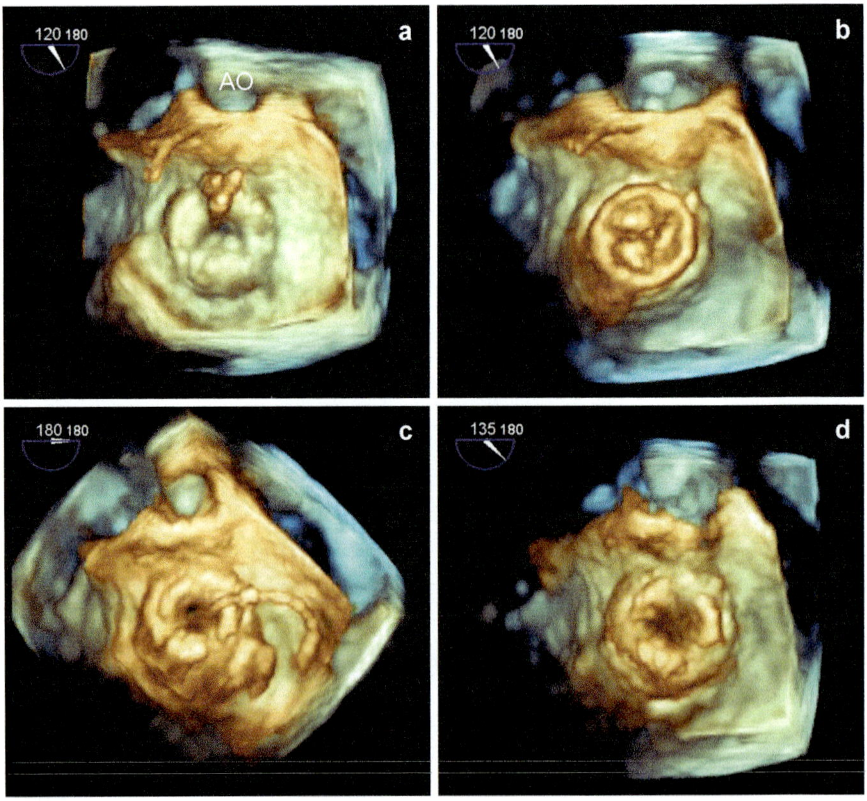

Fig. 2.62 Three dimensional en face views during the procedure. (**a**) During the first time of the Lotus valve positioning, the guiding catheter advanced into the bioprosthetic mitral valve and device was deployed while its position was too high for the annular plane (**b**). During the repositioning, the Lotus valve was recaptured (**c**) and deployed again in a relatively lower position (**d**)

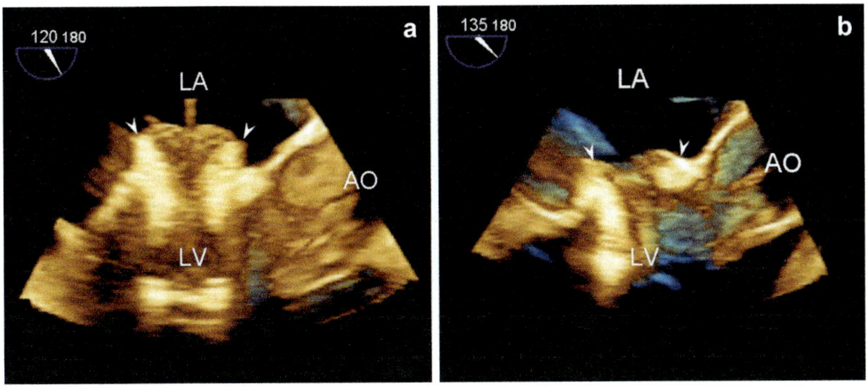

Fig. 2.63 In three dimensional long-axis views, the position of the Lotus valve (arrow heads) in the first deployment (**a**) is deeper into the left atrium than the later one (**b**)

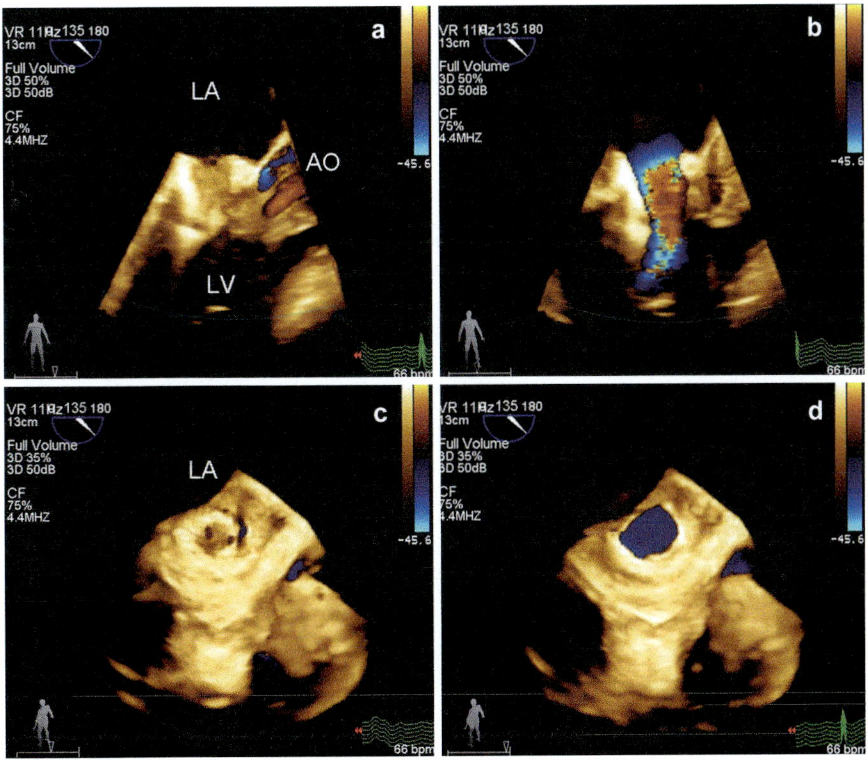

Fig. 2.64 Long- (upper panel) and short-axis (lower panel) views of three dimensional color Doppler after the procedure. There was trivial leakage presented in systole (**a** and **c**) and no mosaic flow across the valve-in-valve mitral prosthesis (**b** and **d**)

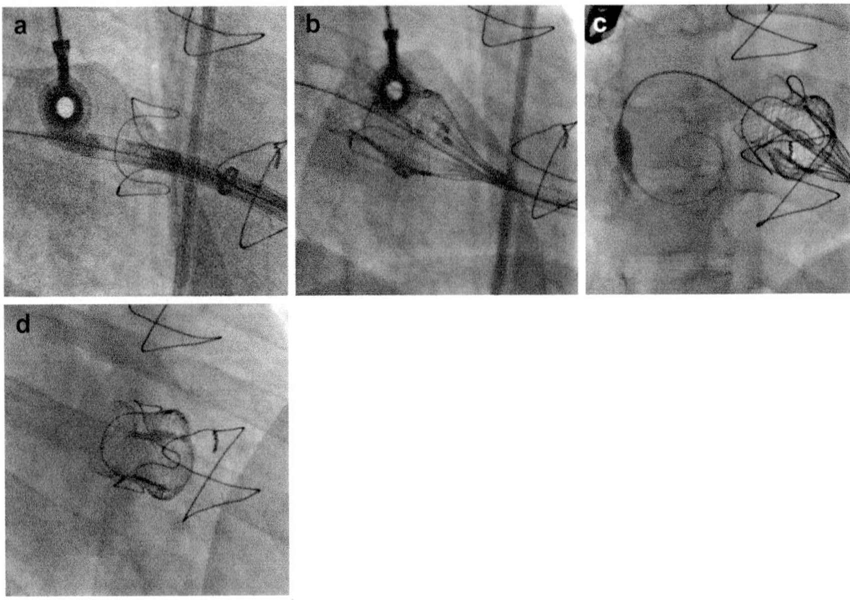

Fig. 2.65 Fluoroscopic images during positioning of a transcatheter Lotus valve. (**a**) The guiding catheter delivered the crimped Lotus valve through the wire frame of a degenerated surgical mitral bioprosthesis. (**b**) The Lotus valve was expanded. (**c**) Due to improper position, the Lotus valve was recaptured before released. (**d**) After the whole procedure had been done, the device was detached from the delivery system

Suggested Readings

1. John W, David W, Jian Y, et al. Transcatheter valve-in-valve implantation for failed bioprosthetic heart valves. Circulation. 2010;121:1848–57.
2. Anson C, Ronen G, Jian Y, et al. Transcatheter transapical mitral valve-in-valve implantations for a failed bioprosthesis: a case series. J Thorac Cardiovasc Surg. 2011;141:711–5.
3. Ronen G, Anson C, Jian Y, et al. Transcatheter valve-in-valve implantation for failed surgical bioprosthetic valves. J Am Coll Cardiol. 2011;58:2196–209.
4. John C, John W. Structural heart disease interventions. Philadelphia: Lippincott Williams & Wilkins; 2012. Chap. 18–20.
5. Fleur D, Dominique H, Francesco M, et al. Transcatheter valve-in-ring implantation after failure of surgical mitral repair. Eur J of Cardio-Thorac Surg. 2013;44:e8–e15.
6. John ML, Jason HR. Interventional procedures for adult structural heart disease. Philadelphia: Elsevier; 2014. Chap. 13.
7. Danny D, John W, Sabine B, et al. Transcatheter aortic valve implantation in failed bioprosthetic surgical valves. JAMA. 2014;312(2):162–70.
8. Manuel W, Konstantin A, Sems MT, et al. Pushing limits- further evolutions of transcatheter valve procedures in the mitral position, including valve-in-valve, valve-in-ring, and valve-in-native-ring. J Thorac Cardiovasc Surg. 2014;147:210–9.
9. Jean-Michel P, Maria DT, Rishi P, et al. Transcatheter valve-in-valve and valve-in-ring for treating aortic and mitral surgical prosthetic dysfunction. JACC: Cardiovasc Interv. 2015;66:2019–37.

10. Liam M, Robert G, Siobhan L, et al. First reported use of the repositionable Lotus valve system for a failing surgical aortic bioprosthesis. JACC: Cardiovasc Interv. 2015;8(2):e19–20.
11. Nicolas A, Aurelie V, Jean-François P, et al. Combined structural heart disease interventions to treat a failed bioprosthesis: the Janus procedure. JACC: Cardiovasc Interv. 2016;9:1968–9.
12. Andreas S, Thomas KJ, Elizabeth P, et al. Two-in-one using 3D: mitral paravalvular leakage closure with concomitant transcatheter valve-in-valve implantation. J Cardiothorac Vasc Anesth. 2016. pii: S1053-0770(16)30379-2. (In Press).
13. Joanna C, Nana T, Anelechi CA, et al. Relation of mitral valve surgery volume to repair rate, durability, and survival. JACC: Cardiovasc Interv. 2017;69:2397–406.

MitraClip

3

3.1 Introduction

Interventional therapies for mitral regurgitation have found a role for patients at high operative risk. The MitraClip is a novel percutaneous therapy which uses a catheter-based system to deliver a clip-like implant to provide apposition between mitral anterior and posterior leaflets. The MitraClip is introduced from a percutaneous, transvenous, and a transseptal approach to reach the mitral valve. Being placed in the central portions of the anterior and posterior leaflets, it acts to anchor prolapse or flail segments to reduce mitral regurgitation.

The traditional imaging tool in catheterization room of fluoroscopy is limited in this procedure, owing to the fact that fluoroscopy cannot visualize the mitral leaflets. As a result, the procedure should be guided by simultaneous transesophageal echocardiographic imaging. The imaging skills, both two and three dimensional, are decisive to technical success.

This chapter provides techniques and the outcomes of MitraClip procedure. One of the cases received both transcatheter aortic valve implantation and MitraClip at the same session. Another one developed mitral stenosis after the procedure, and the last got valvular tear after double MitraClip devices deployment.

3.2 Transcatheter Aortic Valve Implantation and MitraClip in One Session

A 91-year-old male patient has a history of valvular heart disease with moderate aortic regurgitation and severe mitral regurgitation. He suffered from exertional

Electronic supplementary material The online version of this chapter (https://doi.org/10.1007/978-981-10-6937-6_3) contains supplementary material, which is available to authorized users.

M.-C. Hsiung et al., *Atlas of 3D Transesophageal Echocardiography in Structural Heart Disease Interventions*, https://doi.org/10.1007/978-981-10-6937-6_3

dyspnea and swelling lower limbs. Auscultation showed regular rhythm with a grade 3/6 systolic murmur over apex and aortic region. Interventional treatments including transcatheter aortic valve implantation and percutaneous mitral valve repair were managed (Figs. 3.1, 3.2, 3.3, 3.4, 3.5, 3.6, 3.7, 3.8, 3.9, 3.10, 3.11, 3.12, 3.13, 3.14, and 3.15; Videos 3.1, 3.2, 3.3a, 3.3b, 3.4a, 3.4b, 3.5, 3.6a, 3.6b, 3.7a, 3.7b, 3.8, 3.9, 3.10a, 3.10b, 3.10c, 3.11, 3.12a, 3.12b, 3.12c, 3.13a, 3.13b, 3.14, and 3.15).

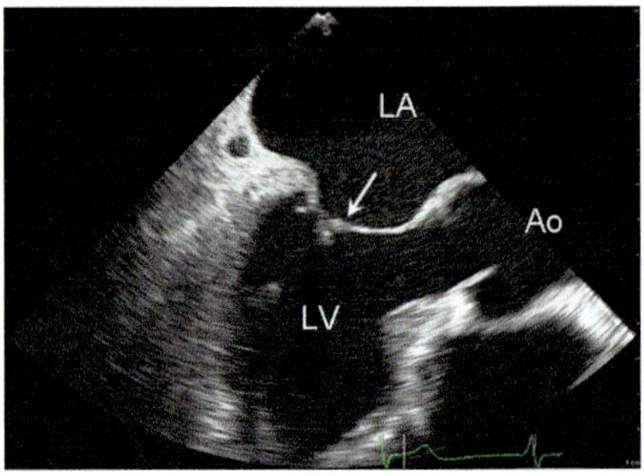

Fig. 3.1 In a mid-esophageal long-axis view, engorged left atrium with mitral annular dilation, degenerative change of mitral (arrow) and aortic leaflets, was demonstrated

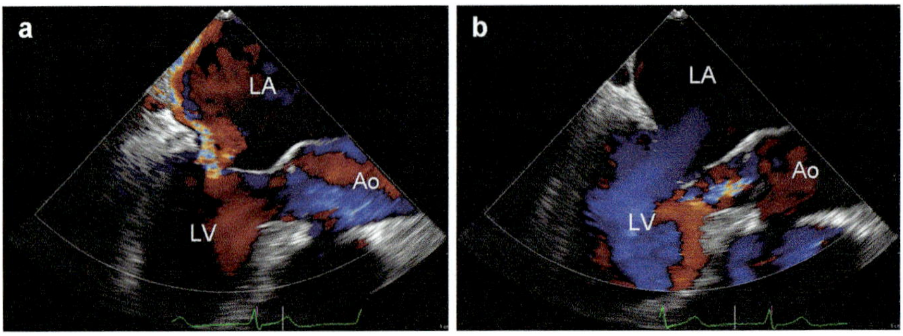

Fig. 3.2 Color Doppler images showed severe mitral regurgitation in systole (**a**) and mild to moderate aortic regurgitation in diastole (**b**). The severity of regurgitation might be underestimated because the patient was under general anesthesia

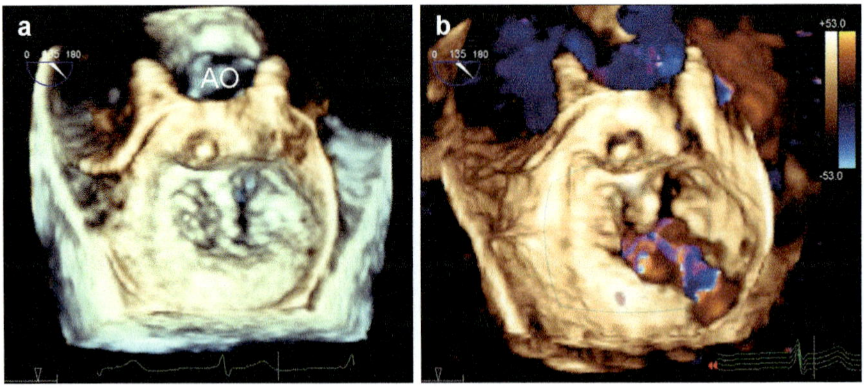

Fig. 3.3 Three dimensional surgical en-face view of the mitral valve showed thickened leaflets (**a**) with severe mitral regurgitation (**b**)

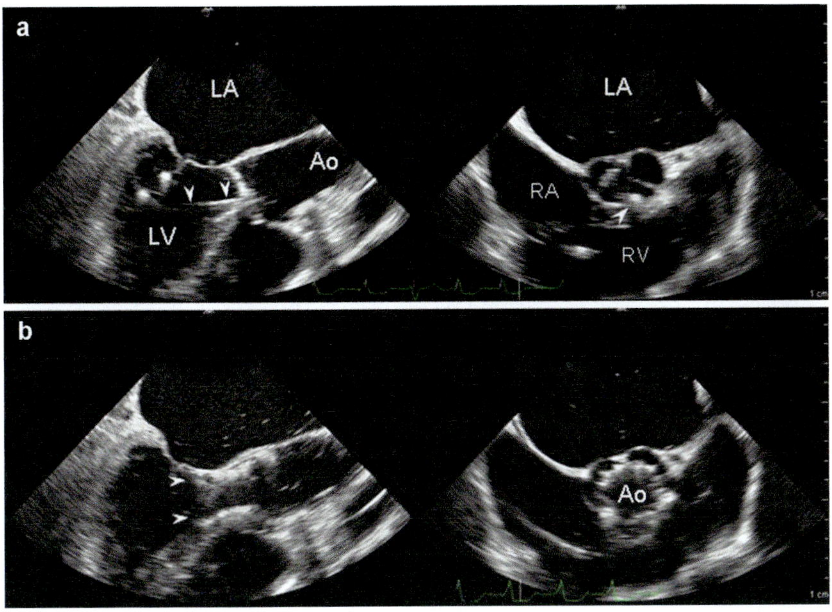

Fig. 3.4 X-plane views during transcatheter aortic valve implantation. (**a**) The guiding catheter (arrow heads) crossed the native aortic valve. (**b**) The CoreValve (31 mm, arrow heads) deployed below the basal sinus border, which lead to paravalvular leakage

Fig. 3.5 The guiding catheter (arrow heads) remained within the first implanted CoreValve, and the second CoreValve was delivered

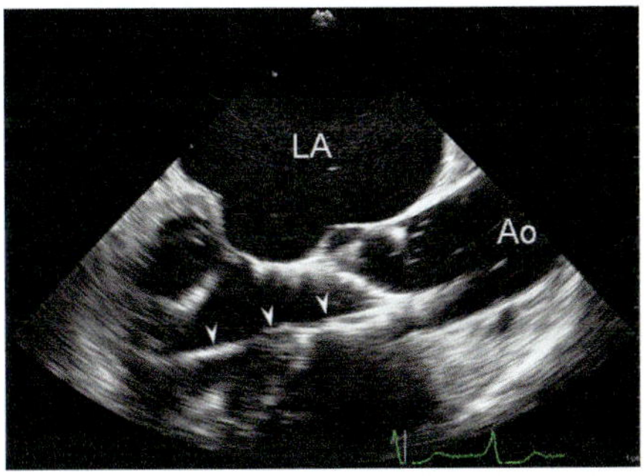

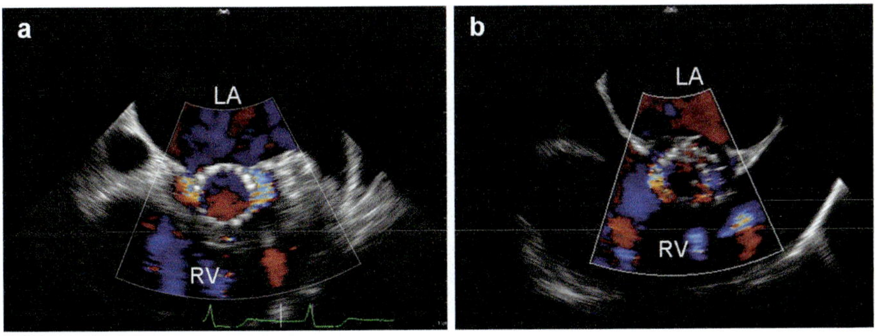

Fig. 3.6 After the first transcatheter aortic valve implantation, severe paravalvular leakage was obtained (**a**). Thus the second CoreValve was implanted inside the first one. Then the leakage reduced to mild consequently (**b**)

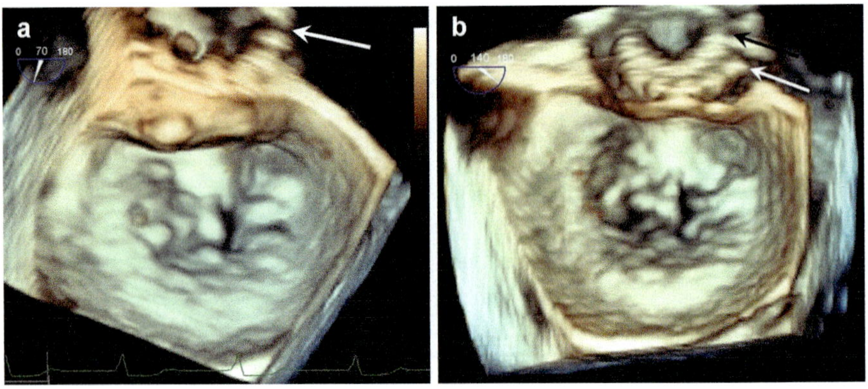

Fig. 3.7 Three dimensional surgical en face view of the mitral valve after the aortic valve implantation (**a**) and the following valve in valve procedure (**b**). The second CoreValve (black arrow) was inside the first one (white arrow)

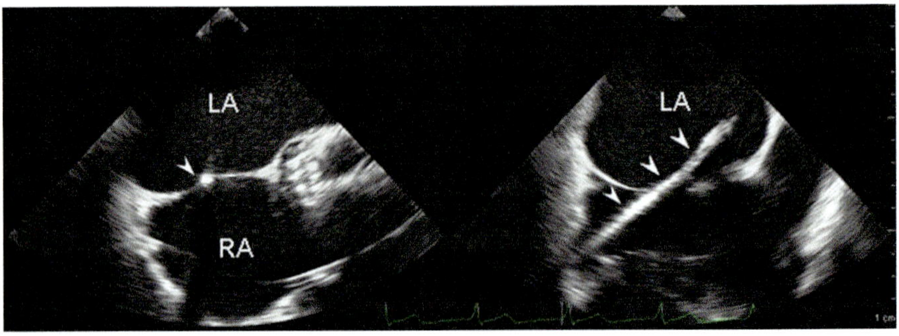

Fig. 3.8 During the MitraClip procedure, transseptal puncture was demonstrated in transesophageal echocardiographic x-plane view (short-axis and bi-caval views). The guiding sheath (arrow heads) advanced into left atrium through the atrial septum

Fig. 3.9 In a three dimensional perspective from the left atrium toward the atrial septum. The catheter tip (arrow) was visualized in the left atrium

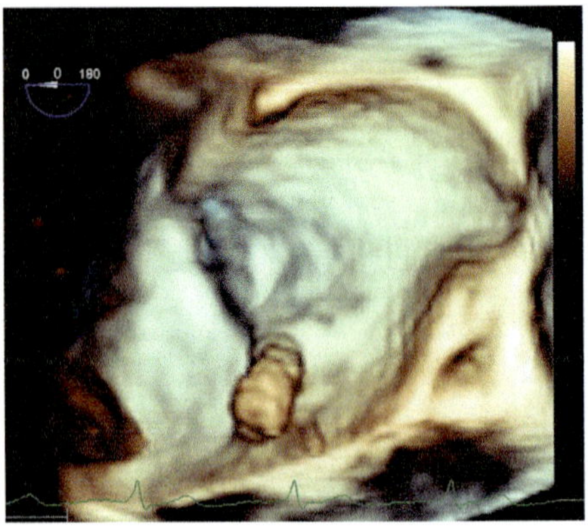

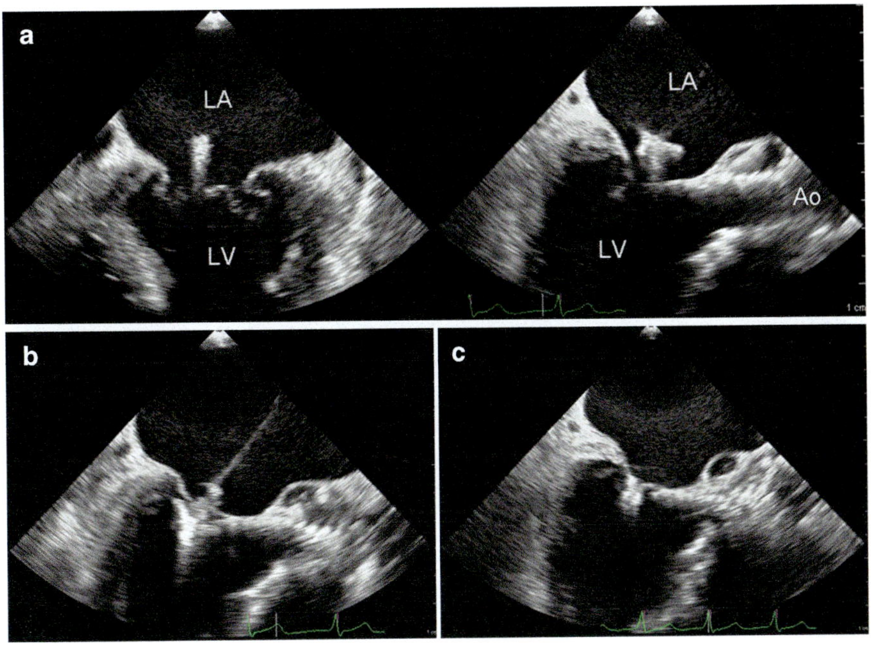

Fig. 3.10 (**a**) The clip was steered toward the mitral valve with its trajectory perpendicular to the mitral annular plane. (**b**) The device advanced into the left ventricle through the origin of mitral regurgitation and the arms of the clip grasped the mitral leaflets. (**c**) The clip was closed and released

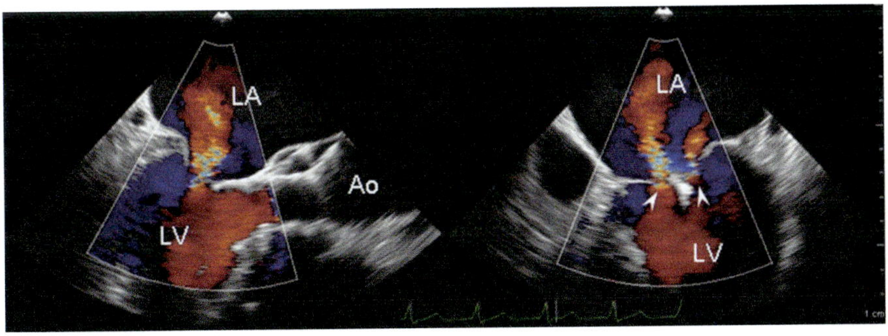

Fig. 3.11 After clip deployment, mitral regurgitation jet was split into two (arrow heads), and the degree decreased to mild to moderate

Percutaneous interventions for valvular heart disease have grown rapidly. Transcatheter aortic valve implantations for aortic stenosis and percutaneous mitral valve repair with the MitraClip have been shown to be comparable with surgery. However, population received combination of these interventions for mixed valvular disease is little. This case demonstrates that patients with double-valve disease can be treated fully percutaneously.

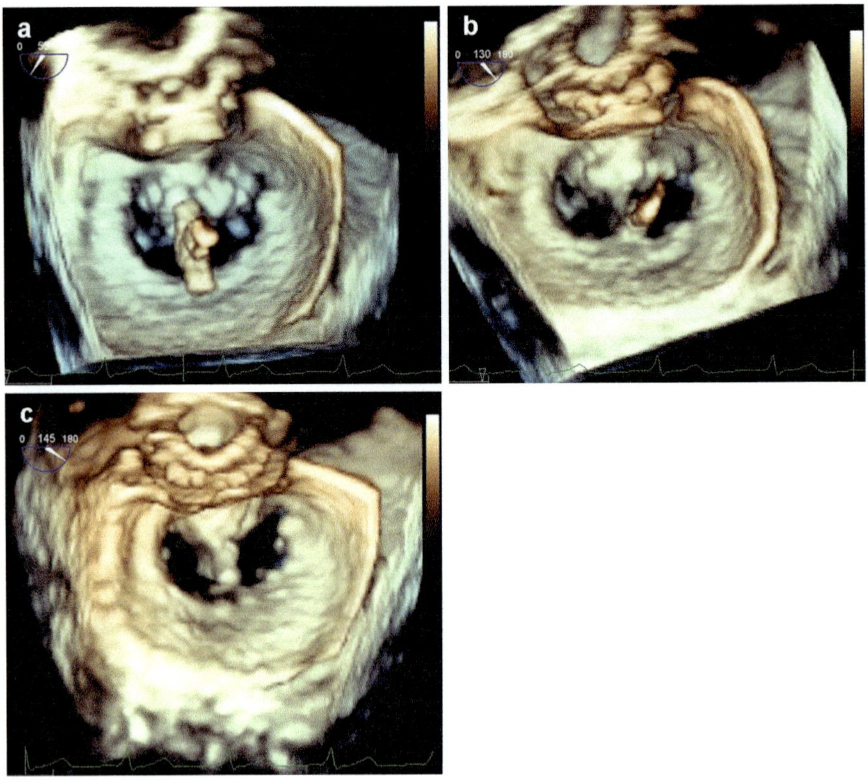

Fig. 3.12 Three dimensional surgical en face view of the mitral valve during the MitraClip procedure. (**a**) The clip advanced into the left ventricle with its arms opened. After closure (**b**) and deployment (**c**) of the clip, the mitral valve became double-orifice

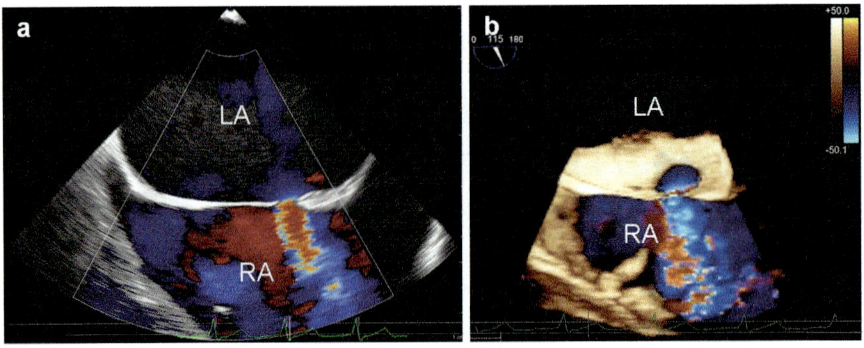

Fig. 3.13 Two (**a**) and three dimensional (**b**) color Doppler after the procedure, an iatrogenic atrial septal defect with left to right shunt was demonstrated

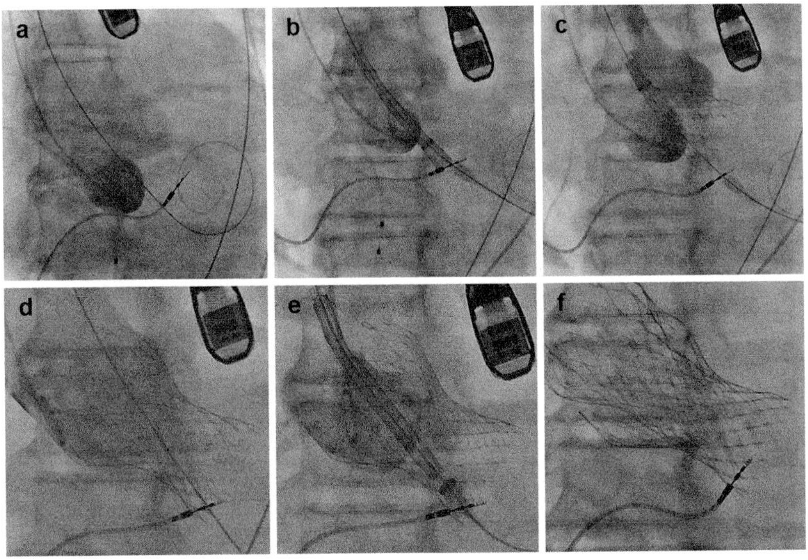

Fig. 3.14 Aortic root angiography during transcatheter aortic valve implantation. (**a**) The guiding wire advanced across the aortic annulus. (**b**) The crimped CoreValve aligned within the native aortic valve. (**c**) Then the CoreValve started to deploy from the proximal part of the frame to the distal. (**d**) After device deployment, the guiding wire remained within the CoreValve. (**e**) The second CoreValve was delivered into the prior implanted CoreValve. (**f**) The second CoreValve then expanded at the level deeper into the ascending aorta than the previous one

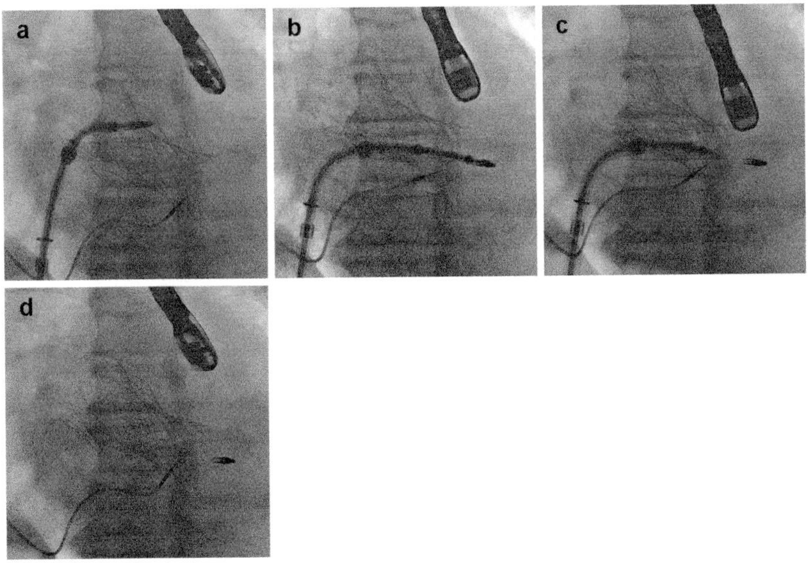

Fig. 3.15 MitraClip procedure under fluoroscopy guidance. (**a**) The clip delivery system advanced across the atrial septum, entering the left atrium. (**b**) The delivery system kept steering toward the mitral valve. (**c**) The MitraClip device was then deployed. (**d**) Once the MitraClip device had been released, the delivery system was retracted and removed

3.3 Mitral Stenosis After the MitraClip Procedure

An 82-year-old male patient had a history of hypertension under medical treatment for years. He developed shortness of breath recently. Auscultation showed regular rhythm with a grade 3 murmur over apex. Valvular heart disease with severe mitral regurgitation was revealed by echocardiography and operations including traditional and transcatheter repair were explained. The patient chose transcatheter one eventually (Figs. 3.16, 3.17, 3.18, 3.19, 3.20, 3.21, 3.22, 3.23, 3.24, 3.25, 3.26, 3.27, 3.28, 3.29, 3.30, and 3.31; Videos 3.16, 3.17a, 3.17b, 3.18a, 3.18b, 3.19a, 3.19b, 3.20, 3.21a, 3.21b, 3.22a, 3.22b, 3.23, 3.24, 3.25, 3.26, 3.27a, 3.27b, 3.28a, 3.28b, 3.29, 3.30, and 3.31).

In general, the more MitraClip device is implanted, the greater mitral regurgitation reduction is. However, it sacrificed to reduce mitral valve area and accordingly cause mitral stenosis. Therefore, mitral valve area should be evaluated to decide the suitability of the MitraClip procedure preoperatively.

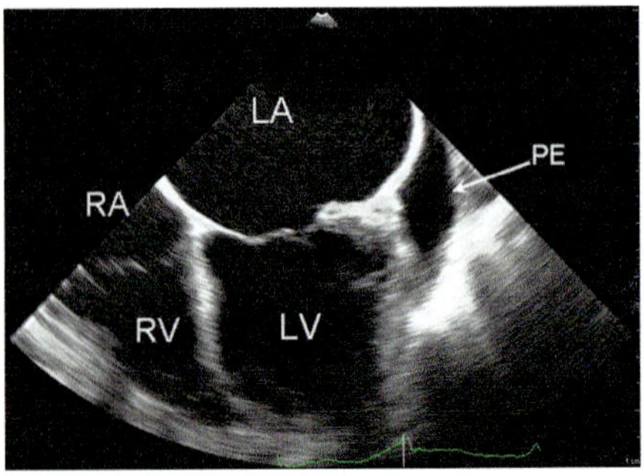

Fig. 3.16 In mid-esophageal four-chamber view, engorged left atrium with mitral annular dilation, degenerative change of mitral leaflets, and pericardial effusion (PE) was demonstrated

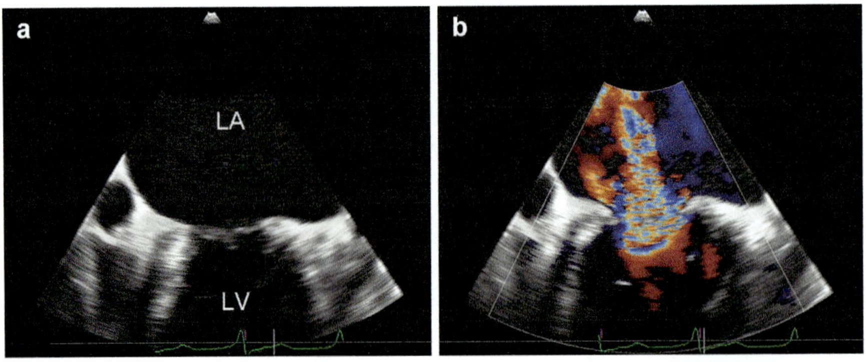

Fig. 3.17 In mid-esophageal four-chamber view (**a**) with color Doppler (**b**), severe mitral regurgitation in systole was revealed

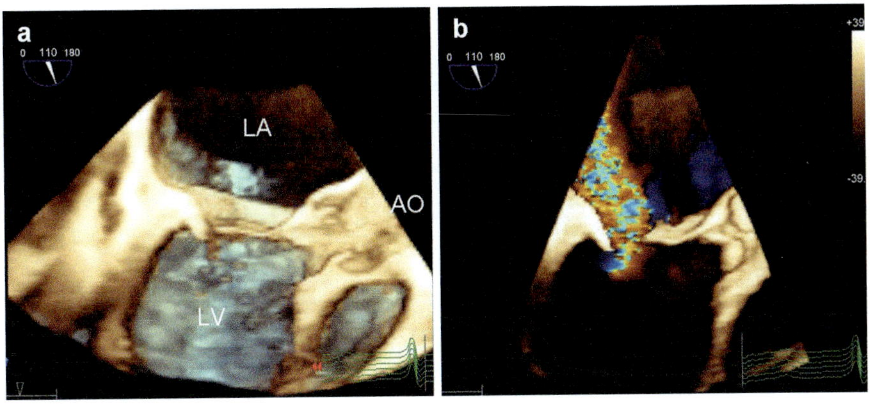

Fig. 3.18 Three dimensional mid-esophageal long-axis view showed thickened and relative larger anterior mitral leaflet (**a**). Severe mitral regurgitation was revealed in color Doppler (**b**)

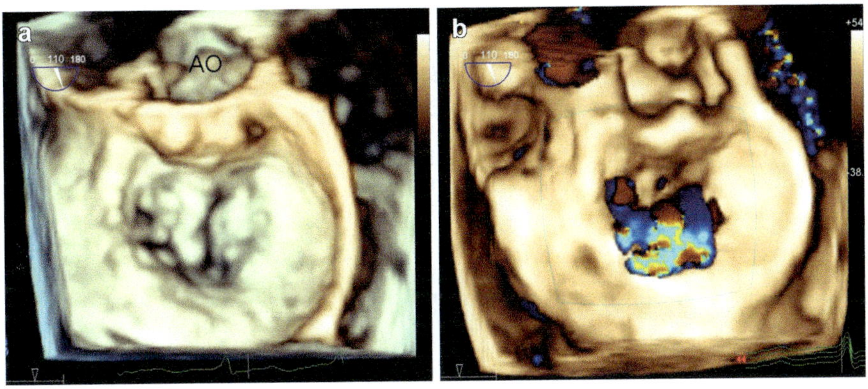

Fig. 3.19 In three dimensional surgical en-face view of the mitral leaflet (**a**) with color Doppler (**b**), thickened and relative larger anterior mitral leaflet with severe mitral regurgitation was revealed

Fig. 3.20 In a three dimensional perspective from the left atrium toward the mitral valve during the MitraClip procedure, transseptal puncture was performed. The catheter tip (arrow) was visualized in the left atrium

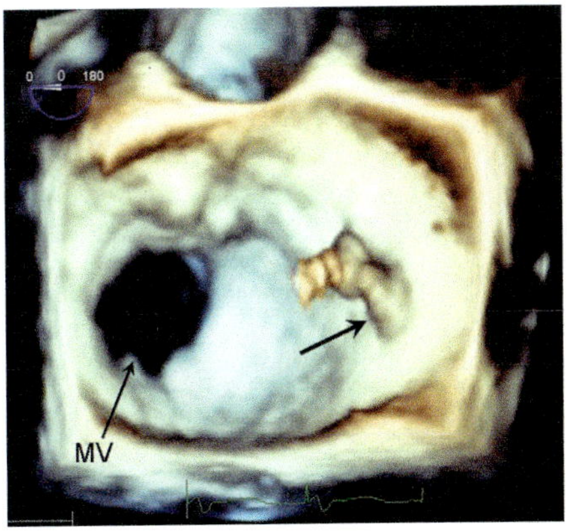

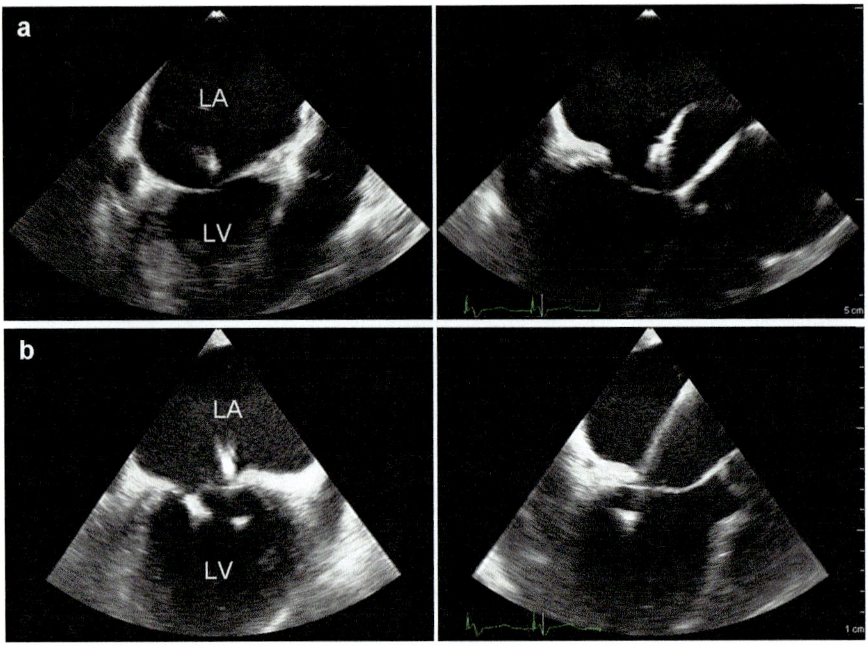

Fig. 3.21 In x-plane view during MitraClip delivering, the guiding catheter crossed the atrial septum and advanced toward the mitral valve (**a**). The mitral valve was used to orient the device in an anteroposterior direction (**b**)

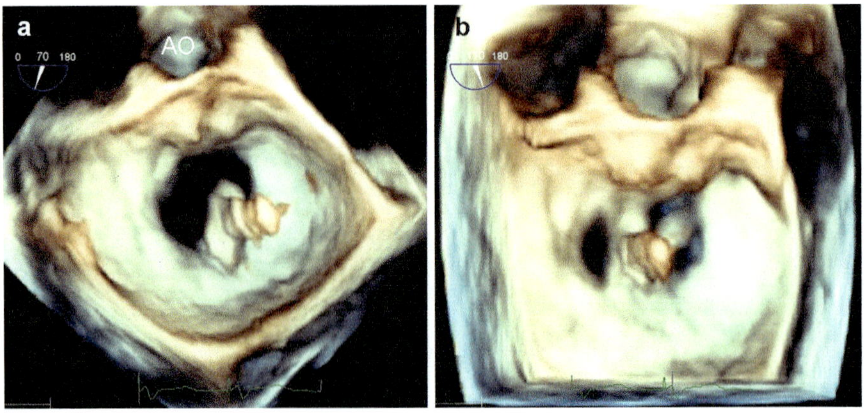

Fig. 3.22 Three dimensional surgical en face view of the mitral valve during the MitraClip procedure. The clip advanced into the left ventricle with the arms opened (**a**). After closure of the clip, the mitral valve became double- orifice (**b**)

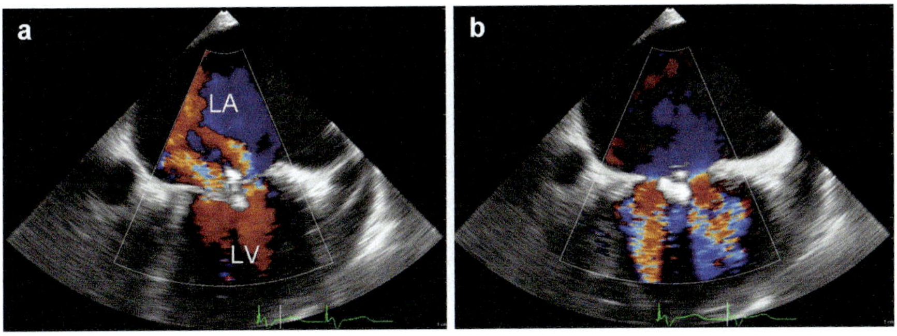

Fig. 3.23 After clip deployment, two-chamber color Doppler showed the mitral regurgitation (**a**) and mitral inflow (**b**) were split into two jets, and the regurgitation degree decreased to moderate

Fig. 3.24 In three dimensional long-axis color Doppler after clip deployment, mitral regurgitation decreased to moderate

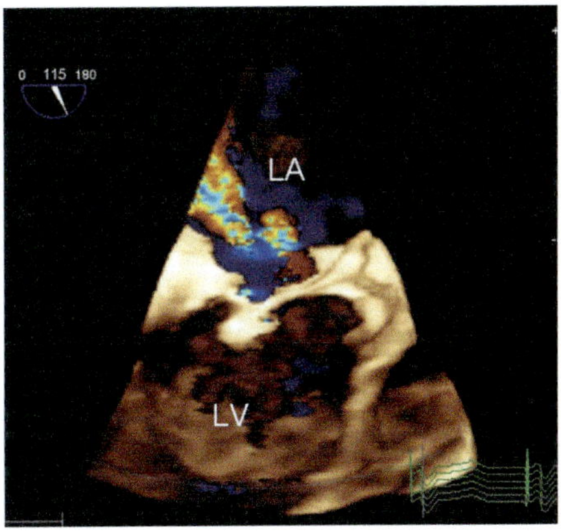

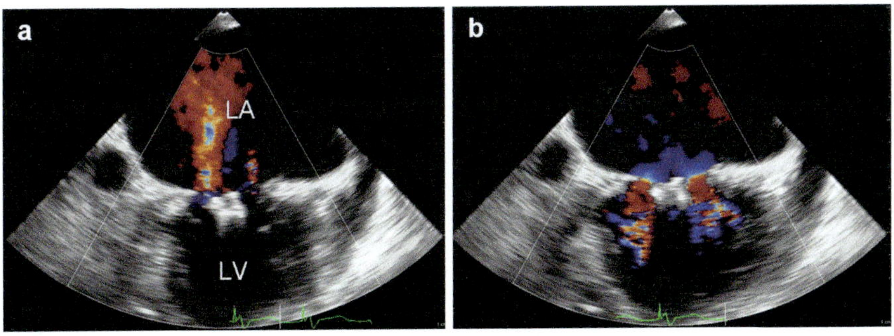

Fig. 3.25 To reduce the remained mitral regurgitation, a second MitraClip was deployed. In two-chamber color Doppler after the procedure, the regurgitation degree lessened to mild to moderate in systole (**a**). The mitral inflow decreased as well due to reduced mitral orifice (**b**)

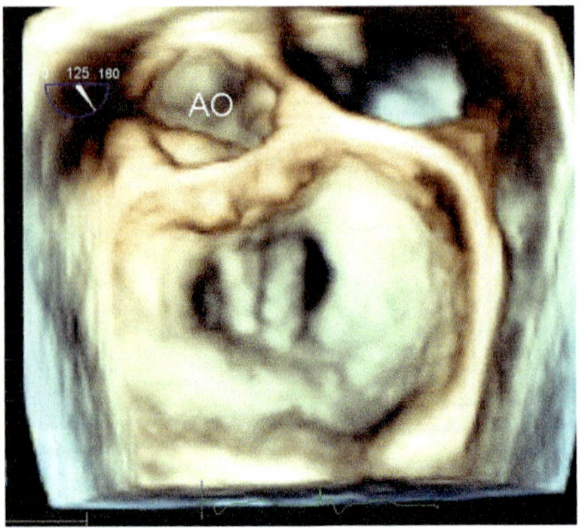

Fig. 3.26 Three dimensional surgical en face view of the mitral valve after double MitraClip deployment. The MitraClip devices settled adjacently in the central portion between the anterior and posterior leaflets, and the mitral valve became narrowed double-orifice

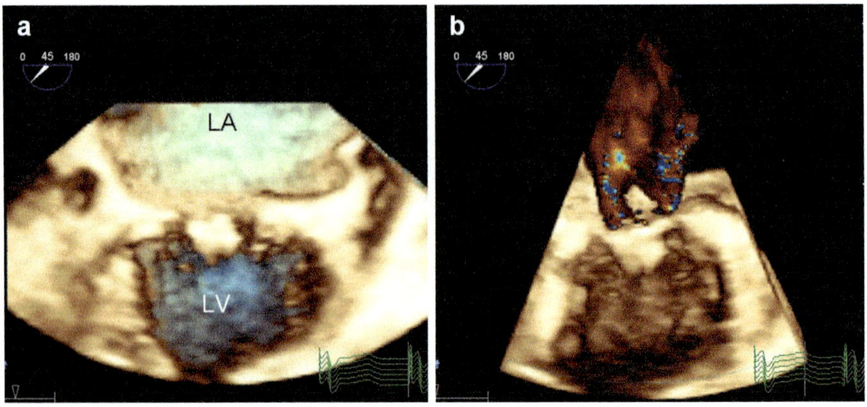

Fig. 3.27 In three dimensional long-axis view (**a**) with color Doppler (**b**) after double clip deployment, mobility of the mitral valve was restricted, and mitral regurgitation decreased to mild to moderate

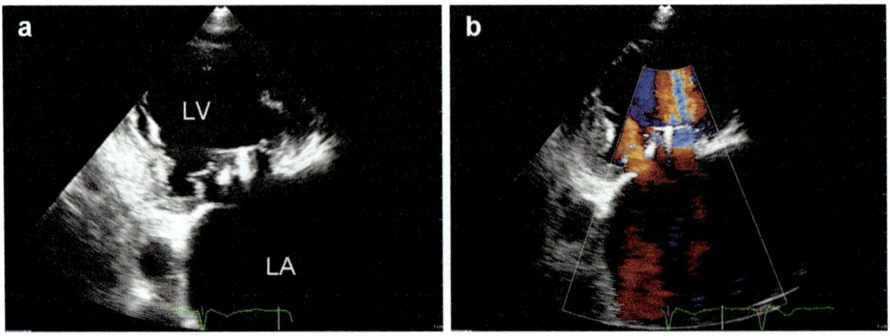

Fig. 3.28 Transthoracic echocardiography was done twenty days following the MitraClip procedure. In apical two-chamber view, two MitraClip devices were revealed on the tip of mitral valve (**a**), which reduced the mitral orifice, lessened the regurgitation and induced mosaic transmitral flow (**b**)

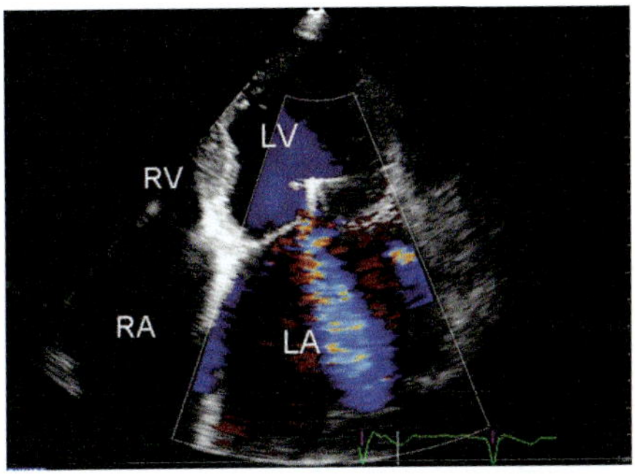

Fig. 3.29 In transthoracic apical four-chamber color Doppler, recurrent mild to moderate mitral regurgitation was demonstrated

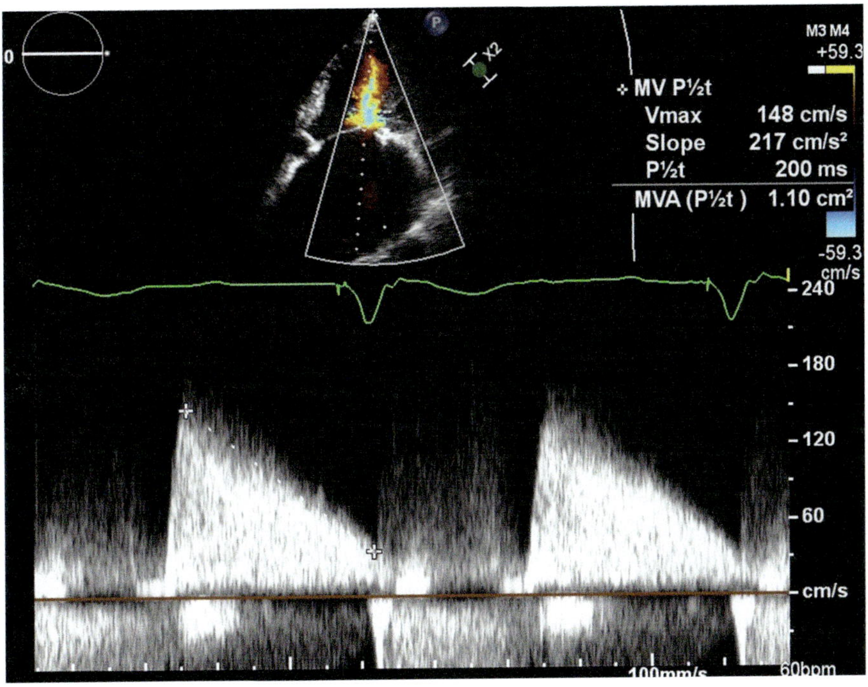

Fig. 3.30 Doppler velocity curves across the mitral valve showed mild mitral stenosis developed after MitraClip implantation. The maximum velocity is 148 cm/s. The pressure half time was 200 ms, corresponding to the mitral valve area of 1.10 cm^2

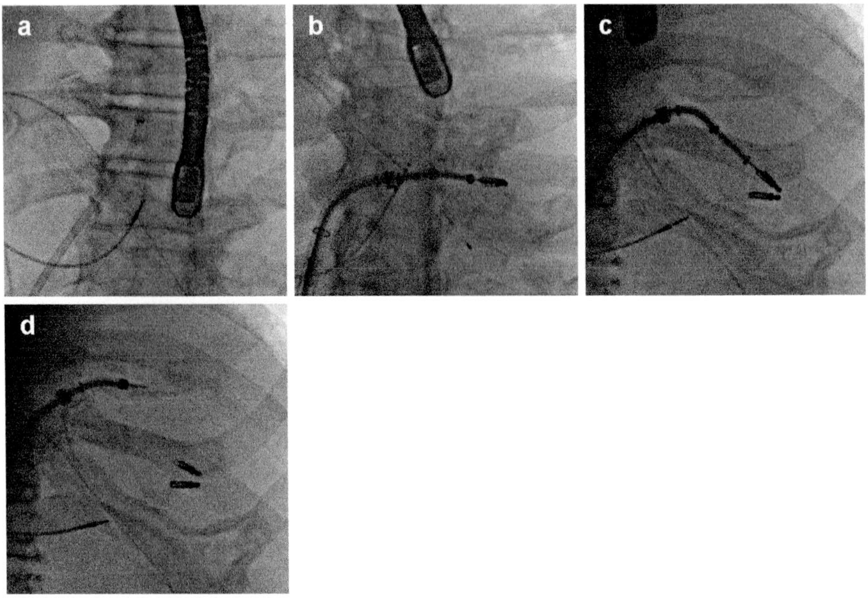

Fig. 3.31 MitraClip procedure under fluoroscopy guidance. (**a**) The guiding sheath advanced across the atrial septum. (**b**) The clip delivery system entered the left atrium and was steered toward the mitral valve. (**c**) The second MitraClip device was delivered after the first one had been deployed. (**d**) Once the double MitraClip devices were both released, the delivery system was retracted and removed

3.4 Mitral Valve Tear After Double MitraClip Procedure

A 72-year-old man had a history of coronary artery disease and had received percutaneous coronary interventions eight times before. He suffered from intermittent orthopnea for four months. Another stent for left circumflex artery was implanted but the symptom remained. Echocardiography revealed valvular heart disease with severe ischemic mitral regurgitation. Therefore, further intervention was indicated (Figs. 3.32, 3.33, 3.34, 3.35, 3.36, 3.37, 3.38, 3.39, 3.40, 3.41, 3.42, 3.43, 3.44, 3.45, 3.46, 3.47, and 3.48; Videos 3.32, 3.33, 3.34, 3.35a, 3.35b, 3.36a, 3.36b, 3.37, 3.38, 3.39, 3.40, 3.41, 3.42a, 3.42b, 3.43a, 3.43b, 3.44a, 3.44b, 3.45a, 3.45b, 3.46, 3.47a, 3.47b, 3.48a, and 3.48b).

This case illustrates that leaflet grasping and clipping attempts during a MitraClip procedure may not be trivial and may significantly damage the mitral apparatus. A multidisciplinary approach is crucial in terms of MitraClip patient selection, procedure execution and problem solving.

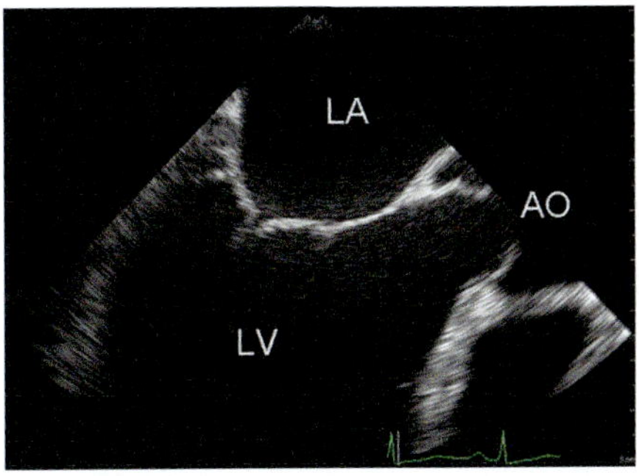

Fig. 3.32 In a mid-esophageal long-axis view, impaired left ventricular systolic function along with tenting mitral valve was revealed

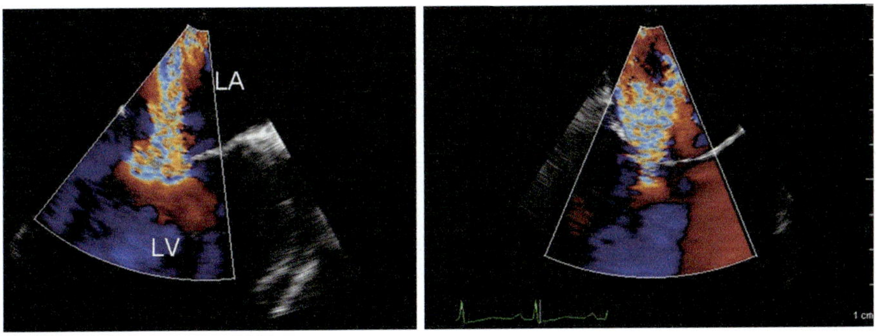

Fig. 3.33 X-plane view with color Doppler showed severe ischemic mitral regurgitation with a central jet in systole

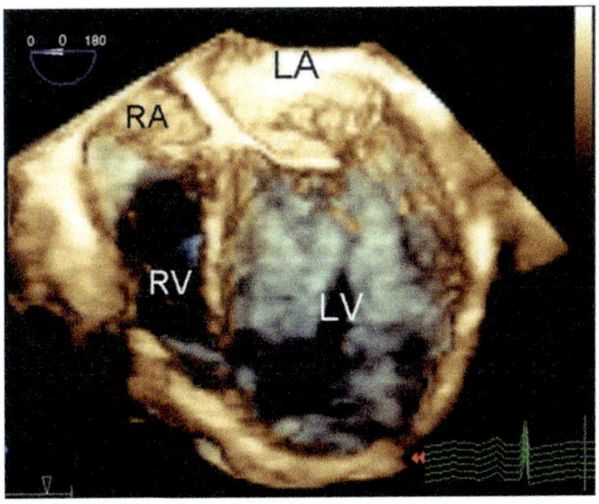

Fig. 3.34 In a three dimensional four-chamber view, dilated left ventricle with impaired systolic function was revealed

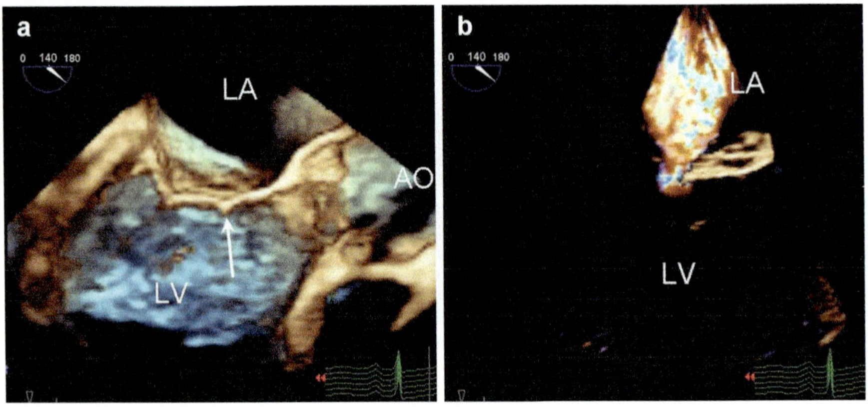

Fig. 3.35 (**a**) Three dimensional mid-esophageal long-axis view showed ischemic tethering of anterior mitral leaflet (arrow), which gives rise to the "sea gull" appearance. (**b**) Color Doppler presented severe ischemic mitral regurgitation

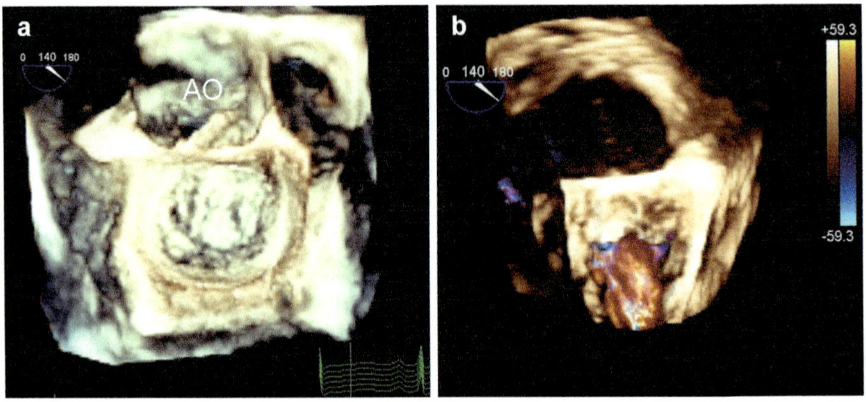

Fig. 3.36 Three dimensional surgical en-face view of the mitral leaflet tethering (**a**) which induced severe mitral regurgitation (**b**)

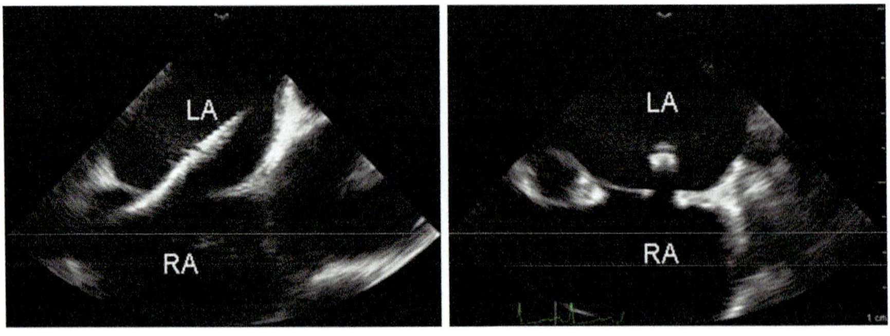

Fig. 3.37 During the MitraClip procedure, transseptal puncture was demonstrated in transesophageal echocardiography x-plane view. The guiding sheath advanced into left atrium through the atrial septum

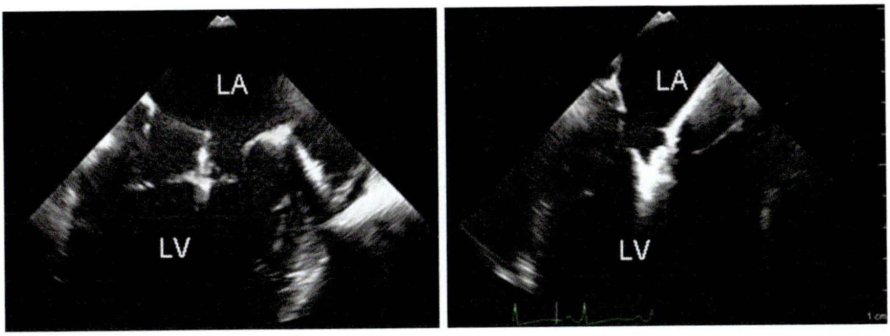

Fig. 3.38 In x-plane view (long-axis and two-chamber views) during MitraClip delivering, the mitral valve was used to orient the device in an anteroposterior direction

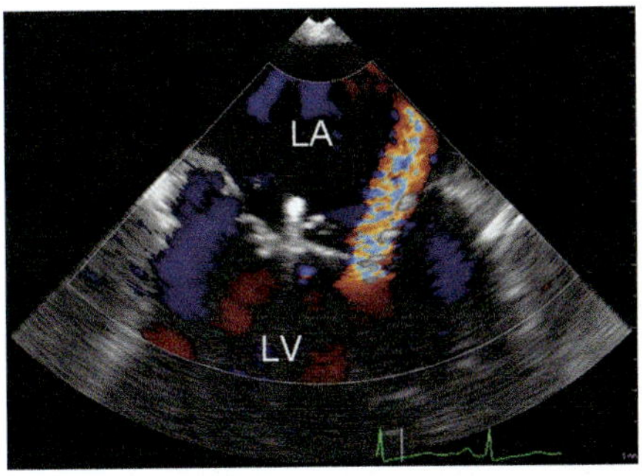

Fig. 3.39 Color Doppler in two dimensional long-axis view after the clip deployment. Moderate mitral regurgitation jet remained

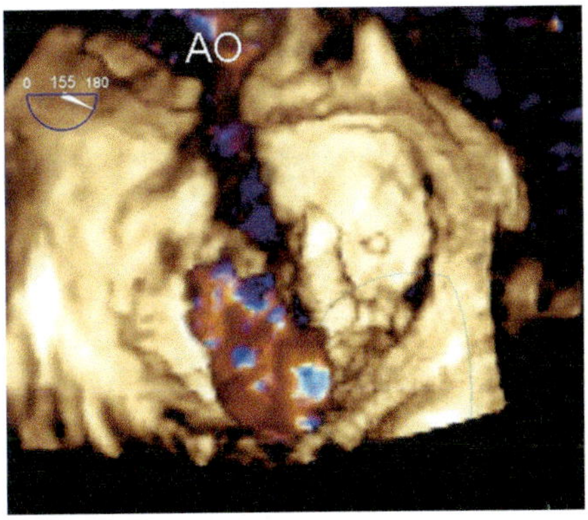

Fig. 3.40 Three dimensional surgical en-face color Doppler after the clip deployment. The MitraClip device was at the level of A2-P2. Moderate mitral regurgitation jet remained at the level of A1-P1

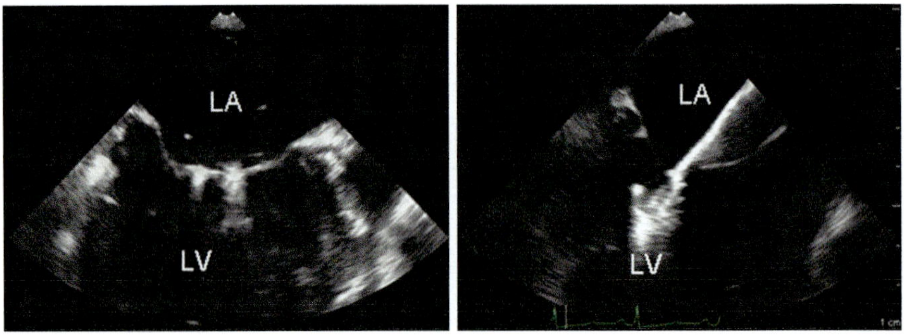

Fig. 3.41 To reduce the remained mitral regurgitation, a second MitraClip was indicated. The device advanced into the left ventricle through the origin of mitral regurgitation

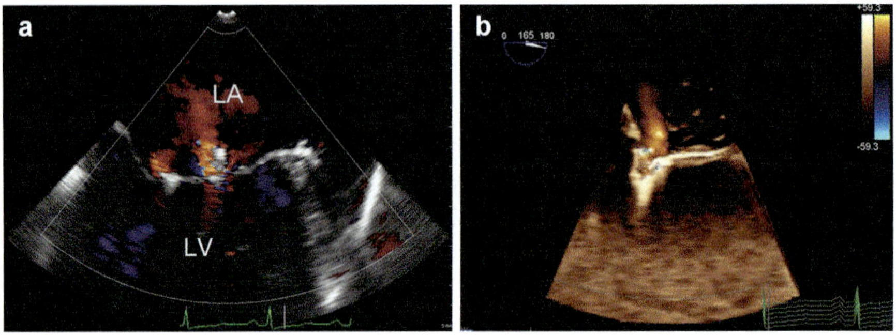

Fig. 3.42 Color Doppler in two (**a**) and three dimensional (**b**) mid-esophageal long-axis view right after the procedure showed merely mild mitral regurgitation in systole

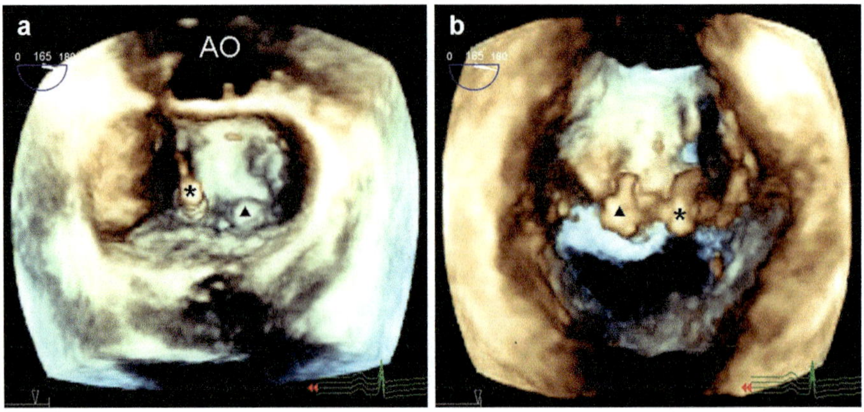

Fig. 3.43 Three dimensional en-face view of the mitral valve from the left atrium (**a**) and the left ventricle (**b**) aspect after the double MitraClip procedure. The first MitraClip (▲) grasped the A2 and the P2 segments and the second one (asterisk) gripped the A1 and P1 segments

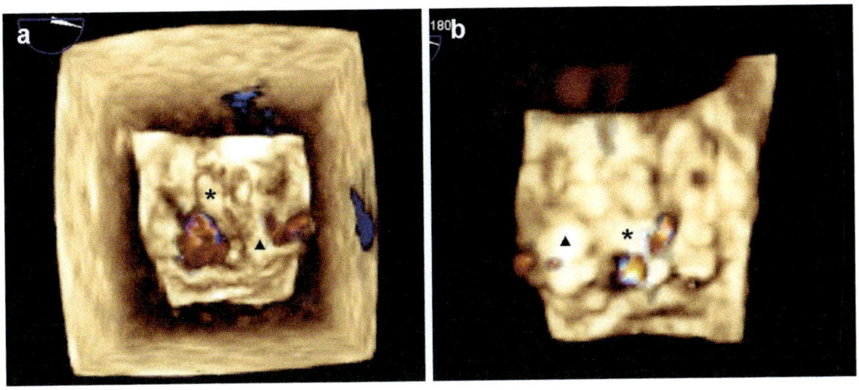

Fig. 3.44 Color Doppler of three dimensional en-face view of the mitral valve from the left atrium (**a**) and the left ventricle aspect (**b**) after the first (▲) and the second MitraClip (asterisk) implantation. Mild mitral regurgitation was presented

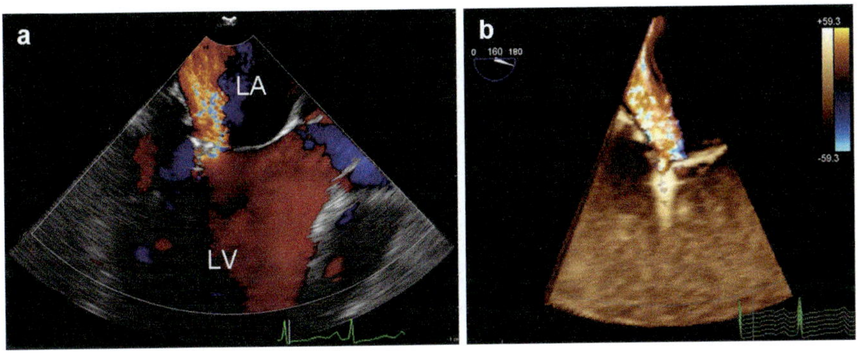

Fig. 3.45 Color Doppler in two (**a**) and three dimensional (**b**) mid-esophageal long-axis view. However, in a short while, the mitral regurgitation became moderate once again

Fig. 3.46 Three dimensional en-face view of the mitral valve showed tearing anterior mitral leaflet at the level of A1 (arrow). The first (▲) and the second MitraClip devices (asterisk) were also demonstrated

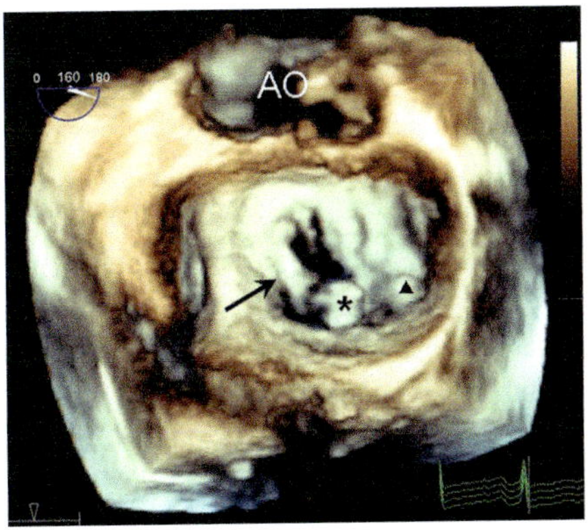

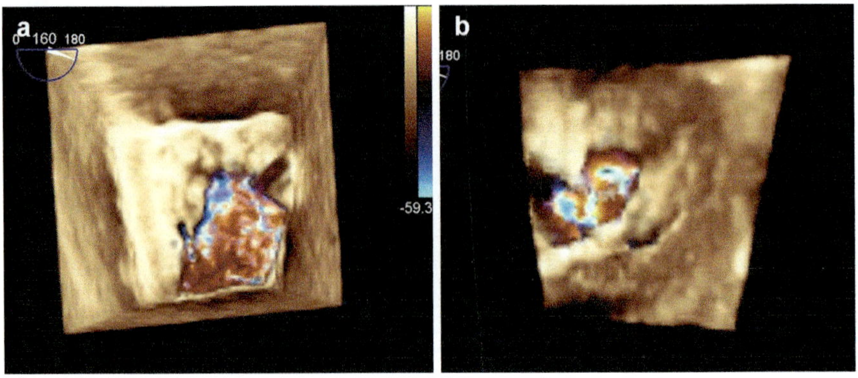

Fig. 3.47 Color Doppler of three dimensional en-face view of the mitral valve from the left atrium (**a**) and the left ventricle aspect (**b**). Moderate mitral regurgitation was presented

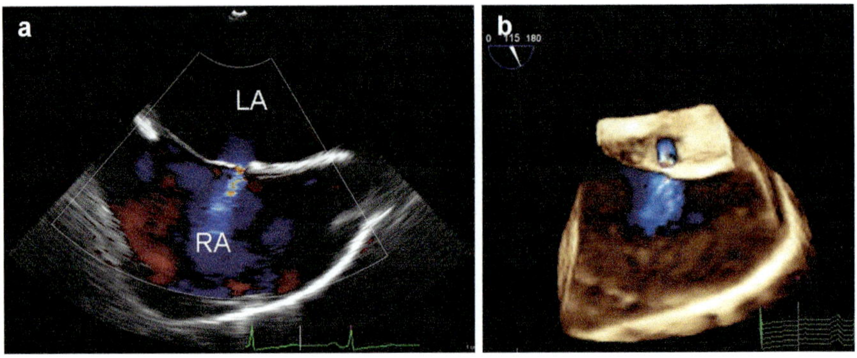

Fig. 3.48 Two (**a**) and three dimensional (**b**) color Doppler after the procedure, an iatrogenic atrial septal defect with a left-to-right shunt was demonstrated

Suggested Readings

1. Ong SH, Beucher H, Mueller R, et al. Percutaneous double-valve interventions for aortic stenosis and pure mitral regurgitation. Am J Cardiol. 2011;108:893–5.
2. John DC, John GW. Structural heart disease interventions. Philadelphia: Lippincott Williams & Wilkins; 2012. Chap. 23.
3. John ML, Jason HR. Interventional procedures for adult structural heart disease. Philadelphia: Elsevier; 2014. Chap. 11.
4. Fabio G, Rubia B, Baldassare F, et al. Transesophageal echocardiography during MitraClip procedure. Anesth Analg. 2014;118:1188–96.
5. Vicenzo D, Luigi F, Giuseppe M, et al. An intriguing case report of functional mitral regurgitation treated with MitraClip. Medicine. 2015;94(20):e608.
6. Rabie S, Reba AA. Anesthesia for high-risk patients undergoing percutaneous mitral valve repair with the MitraClip system in the catheterization laboratory. Egypt J Cardiothorac Anesth. 2015;9:33–8.

7. Zouhair R, Ben R, Frans O, et al. Mitral valve injury after MitraClip implantation. JACC Cardiovasc Interv. 2016;18:e185–6.
8. Saji M, Ailawadi G, Fowler DE, et al. Progressive mitral stenosis after MitraClip implantation in a patient with systemic inflammatory disease. Ann Thorac Surg. 2016;102:e89–91.

Check for updates

4 Percutaneous Closure of Congenital and Acquired Cardiac Defects

4.1 Introduction

Even if many transcatheter closure techniques are closely associated, atrial septal defects, ventricular septal defects, and patent ductus arteriosus each involve unique approaches. Similarly, aortic pseudoaneurysms and iatrogenic fistulas are discussed separately. Most closure techniques are improvisations of methods applied in more commonly encountered congenital defects. There is no standard approach to either of these conditions because the location and relation to surrounding structures varies significantly.

Consequently, respectively comprehensive assessments of the anatomic structures and the hemodynamic situations should be done carefully. Three dimensional transesophageal echocardiography provides attentive examination of morphology of the target defect from varies perspectives. In addition, along with fluoroscopy and computed tomography, it allows physicians to plan, monitor, and perform the procedure appropriately.

In this chapter, occluder implantations of cases with congenital heart diseases of atrial septal defects, ventricular septal defets, patent ductus arteriosus, and cases with iatrogenic cardiac defects are all involved.

4.2 Occluder Implantation of Secundum Atrial Septal Defect

A 59-year-old female patient had a history of hypertension, atrial septal defect and tri-vessel coronary artery disease received coronary artery bypass graft two years ago. This time, she was admitted for atrial septal defect closure (Figs. 4.1, 4.2, 4.3, 4.4, 4.5, 4.6, 4.7, 4.8, and 4.9; Videos 4.1a, 4.1b, 4.2a, 4.2b, 4.3, 4.4, 4.5, 4.6a, 4.6b, 4.7, 4.8, and 4.9).

Electronic supplementary material The online version of this chapter (https://doi.org/10.1007/978-981-10-6937-6_4) contains supplementary material, which is available to authorized users.

M.-C. Hsiung et al., *Atlas of 3D Transesophageal Echocardiography in Structural Heart Disease Interventions*, https://doi.org/10.1007/978-981-10-6937-6_4

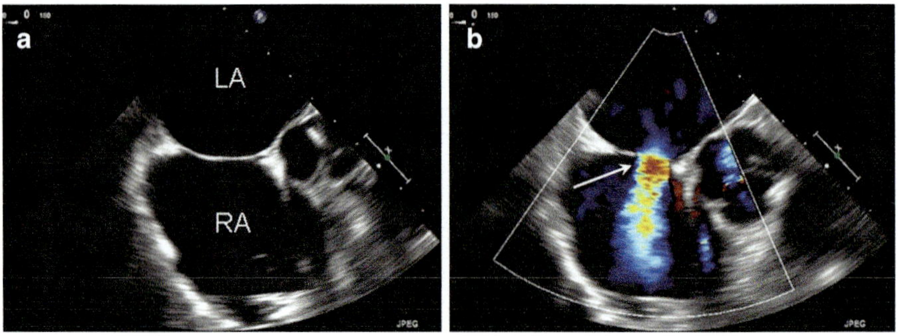

Fig. 4.1 In a transesophageal echocardiographic bicaval view, bubbles transit rapidly from the right to the left heart was demonstrated (**a**). A secundum atrial septal defect with a left-to-right shunt (arrow) was presented in color Doppler (**b**)

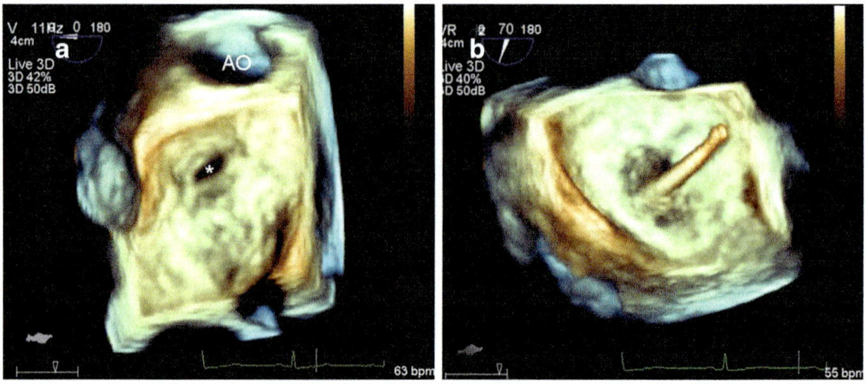

Fig. 4.2 Three dimensional transesophageal echocardiogram visualized from left atrial aspect showed the defect (asterisk) was located in the midsection of the atrial septum (**a**). During occluder implantation, a guidewire crossed the atrial septal defect (**b**)

Secundum septal defects are located in the central portion of the interatrial septum, which are the most amendable to transcatheter closure. A preprocedure transesophageal echocardiographic examination is essential to evaluate the size of the defects, the presence of septal rims, and the relationship to the adjacent structures and to ensure whether the patient is appropriate for occluder implantation. Furthermore, before device release, encroachment of the device of the surrounding structures and evidence of residual shunting must be confirmed.

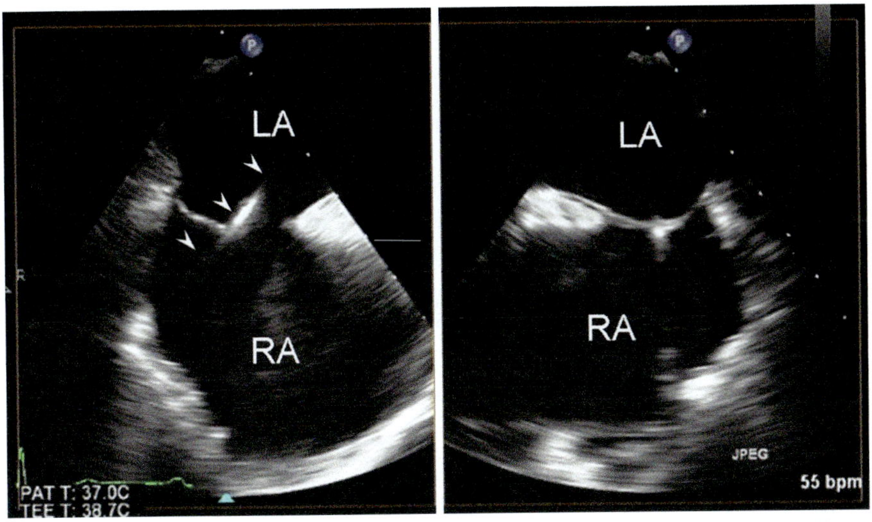

Fig. 4.3 X-plane view during percutaneous atrial septal defect closure showed a delivery cable (arrow heads) crossed the atrial septal defect

Fig. 4.4 Color Doppler during the occluder implantation, flow (arrow) across the defect along with the delivery cable was demonstrated

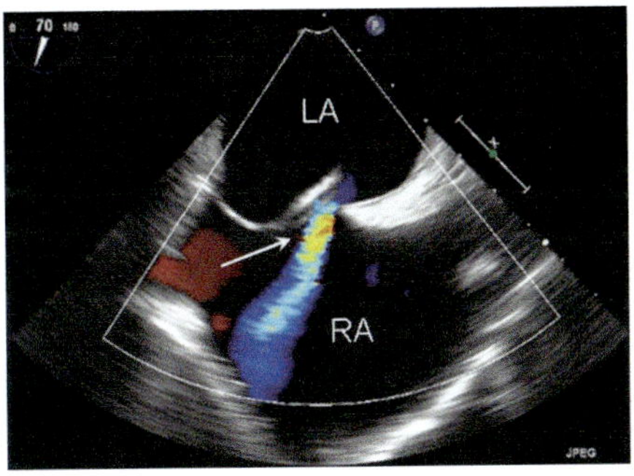

Fig. 4.5 During the procedure, a bicaval view showed an occluder (arrow) was advancing across the defect along the delivery sheath

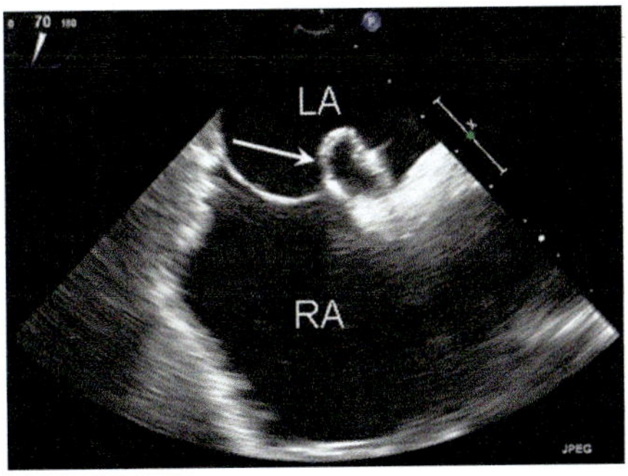

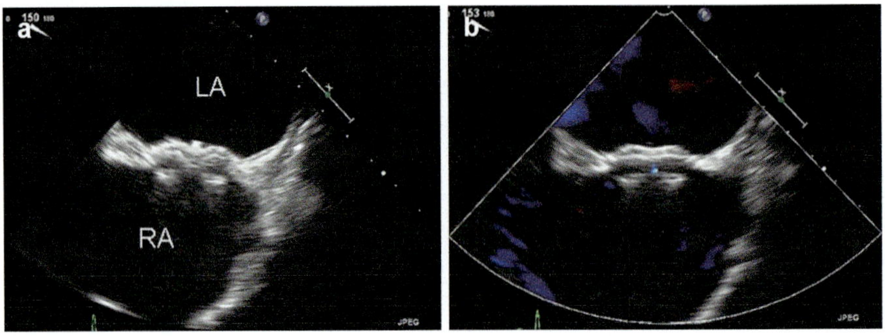

Fig. 4.6 After the occluder released, bicaval view showed good position of the device (**a**), and only minimal recurrent flow was demonstrated in color Doppler (**b**)

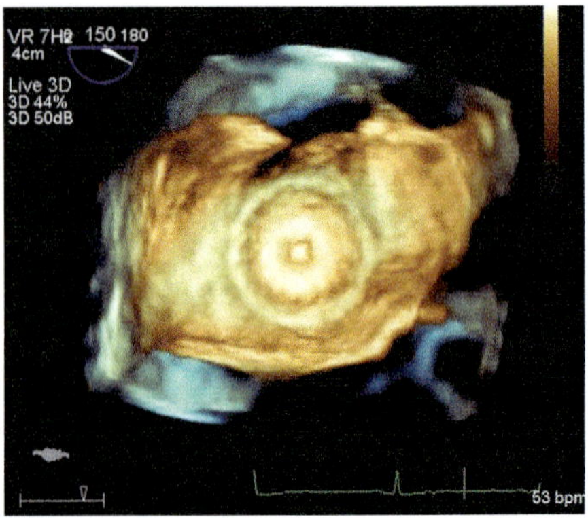

Fig. 4.7 Three dimensional transesophageal echocardiogram visualized from left atrial aspect after the occluder implantation showed full deployment of the device

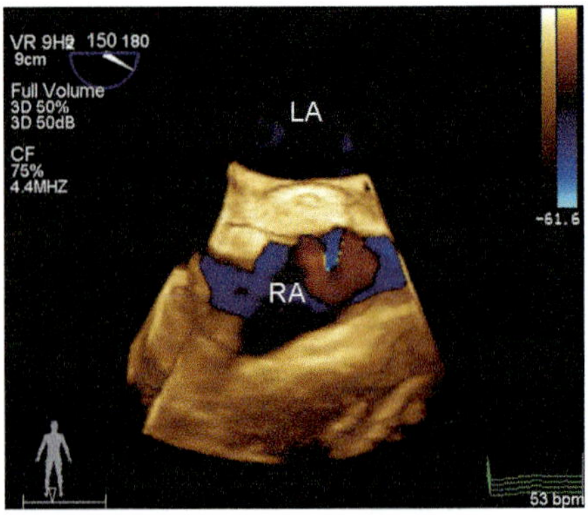

Fig. 4.8 Only minimal recurrent flow was demonstrated in color Doppler

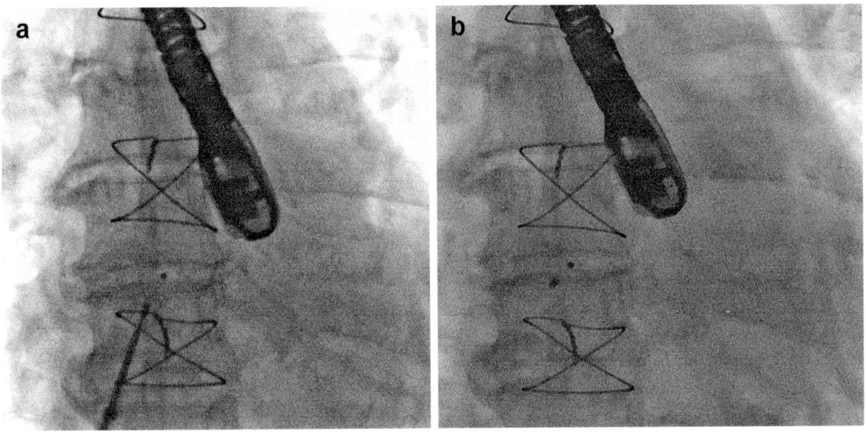

Fig. 4.9 Fluoroscopy during the procedure showed the occluder attached to the delivery sheath at first (**a**), and then released (**b**)

4.3 Occluder Implantation of Multiple Atrial Septal Defect

An 18-year-old female patient suffered from chest pain, shortness of breath, and severe palpitation. Grade 2/6 systolic murmurs over left sternal border and apex were noted and echocardiography showed multiple atrial septal defects. Therefore an occluder implantation was arranged (Figs. 4.10, 4.11, 4.12, 4.13, 4.14, and 4.15; Videos 4.10a, 4.10b, 4.11, 4.12, 4.13, 4.14a, 4.14b, and 4.15).

There was a similar case in our previous book, *Atlas of Perioperative 3D Transesophageal Echocardiography*. A 43-year-old male patient with Swiss cheese like secundum atrial septal defects received occluder implantation. During the procedure, after two occluders had been implanted, there were residual defects with significant shunting. Unfortunately, when the third device was attempted, the first one dropped into the left atrium, rapidly migrated to the right iliac artery and caused embolization. To tackle the emergency, the device was pushed back to proximal descending aorta intravascularly. In the end, sternotomy was done to remove the device and accomplish patch repair of atrial septal defects. We have learned a painful lesson from last time, so we just used a large device to cover the four defects. Transesophageal echocardiography demonstrated the procedure was done successfully.

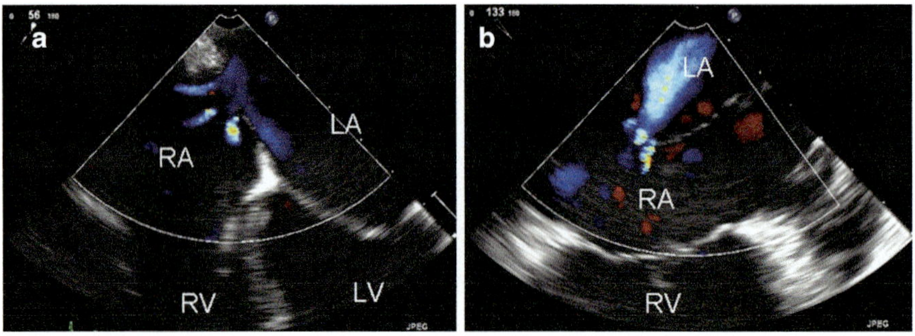

Fig. 4.10 In transesophageal echocardiographic color Doppler of four-chamber (**a**) and bicaval (**b**) views, multiple Swiss cheese like defects with left-to-right shunts were seen in the central portion of the atrial septum

Fig. 4.11 In three dimensional color Doppler of four-chamber view, four atrial septal defects with left-to-right shunts were seen

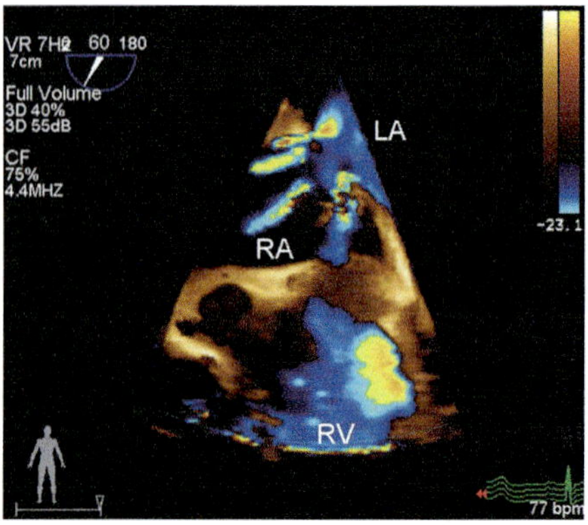

Fig. 4.12 Three dimensional transesophageal echocardiogram visualized from left atrial aspect revealed thin atrial septum with multiple defects on it

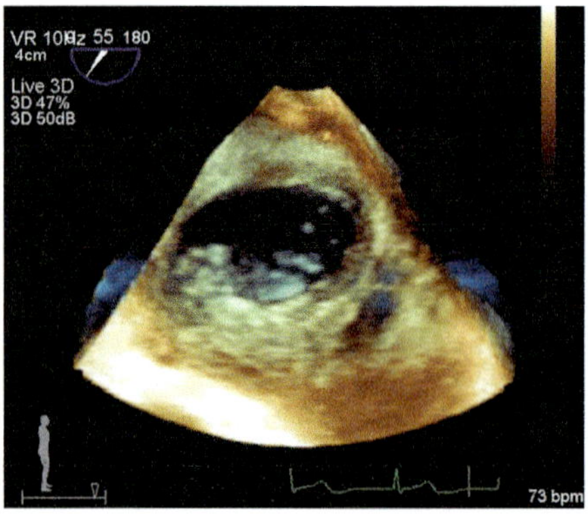

Fig. 4.13 Three dimensional transesophageal echocardiogram visualized from left atrial aspect during occluder implantation showed a guiding wire crossed the atrial septal defect

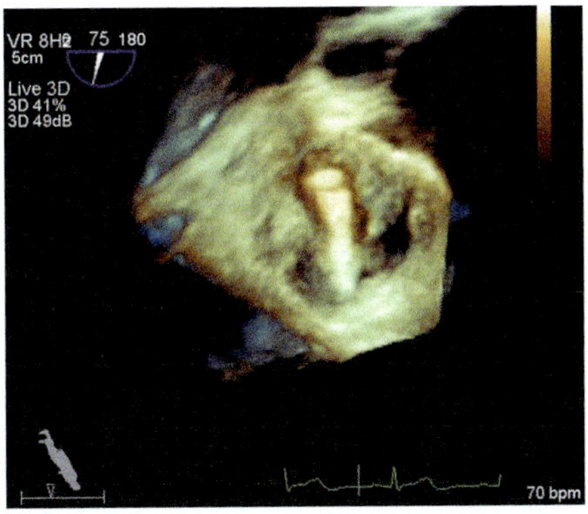

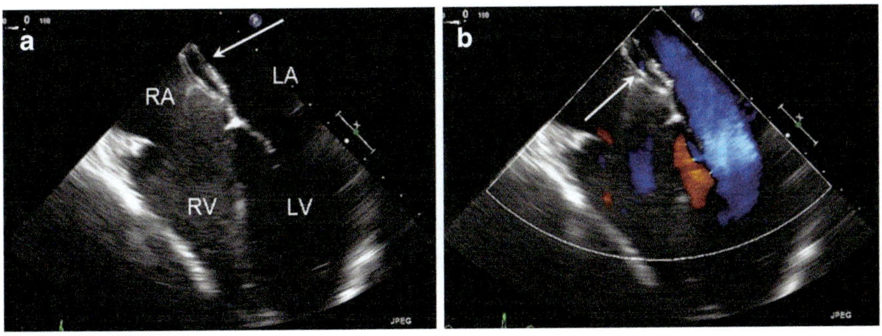

Fig. 4.14 After deployment of the occluder (arrow), four-chamber view showed the device was in good position (**a**). All of the defects are covered and only minimal residual flow was demonstrated in color Doppler (**b**)

Fig. 4.15 Three dimensional four-chamber view after the occluder (arrow) implantation showed good position of the device

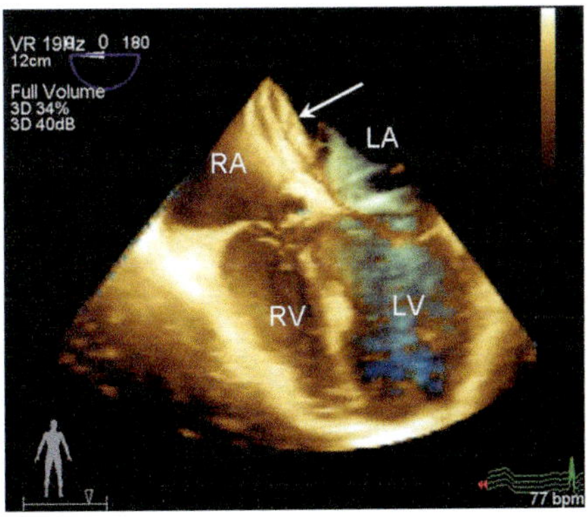

4.4 Occluder Implantation of Muscular Ventricular Septal Defect

A 38-year-old male patient with congenital heart disease of muscular type ventricular septal defect had an event of infective endocarditis last year. After antibiotic therapy, the patient remained stable. Unfortunately, he produced reduced intolerance recently. Auscultation showed regular rhythm with a grade 3/6 pan-systolic murmur over left sternal border and apex. According to doctor's advice, he decided to receive an occluder implantation (Figs. 4.16, 4.17, 4.18, 4.19, 4.20, 4.21, 4.22, 4.23, and 4.24; Videos 4.16a, 4.16b, 4.17, 4.18, 4.19a, 4.19b, 4.20, 4.21, 4.22a, 4.22b, 4.23a, 4.23b, and 4.24).

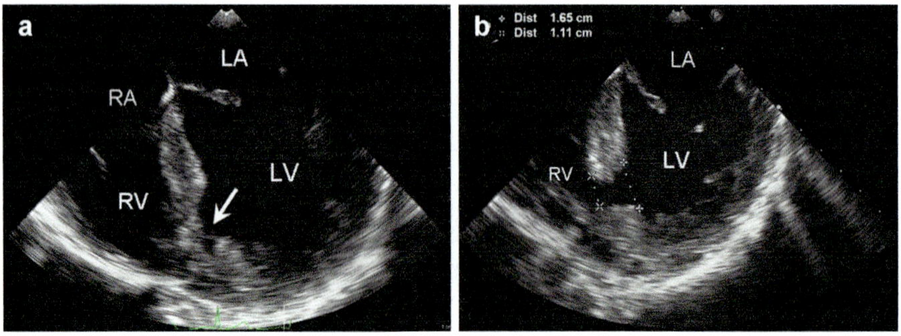

Fig. 4.16 Transesophageal echocardiographic four-chamber view of muscular ventricular septal defect. (**a**) the defect (arrow) was near the apex of the ventricular septum. (**b**) the diameter of the defect on the left and the right ventricular levels measured 1.65 cm and 1.11 cm respectively

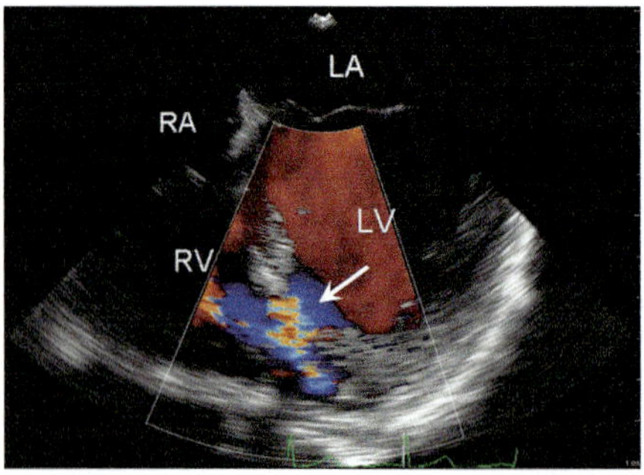

Fig. 4.17 Color Doppler showed a left-to-right shunt (arrows) crossed the muscular ventricular septal defect

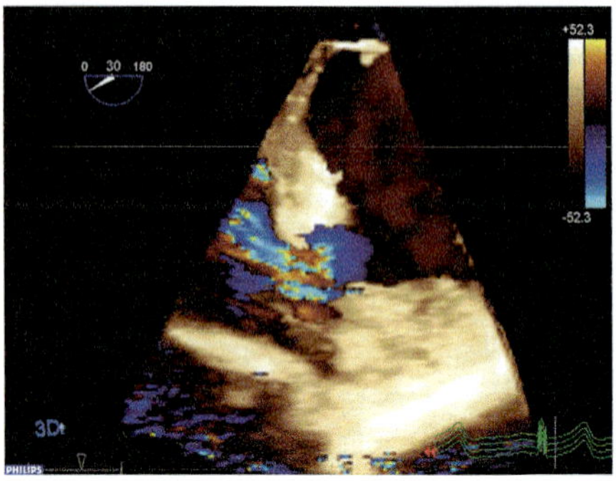

Fig. 4.18 Three dimensional color Doppler showed a left-to-right shunt (arrows) crossed the muscular ventricular septal defect

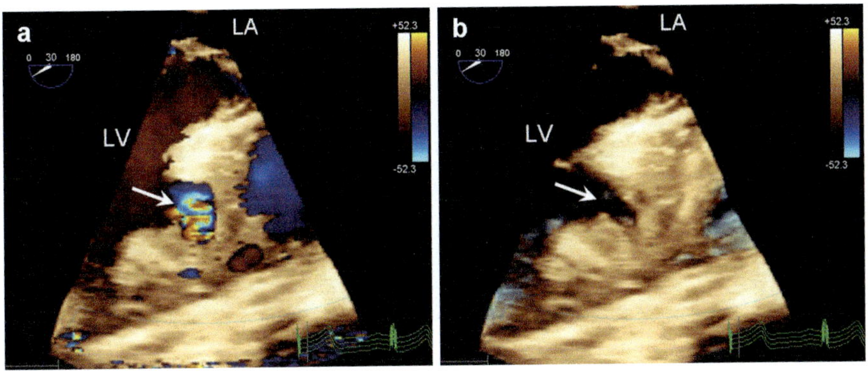

Fig. 4.19 Three dimensional color Doppler (**a**) and color suppressed (**b**) images in long-axis view. A left-to-right shunt (arrows) crossed the muscular ventricular septal defect

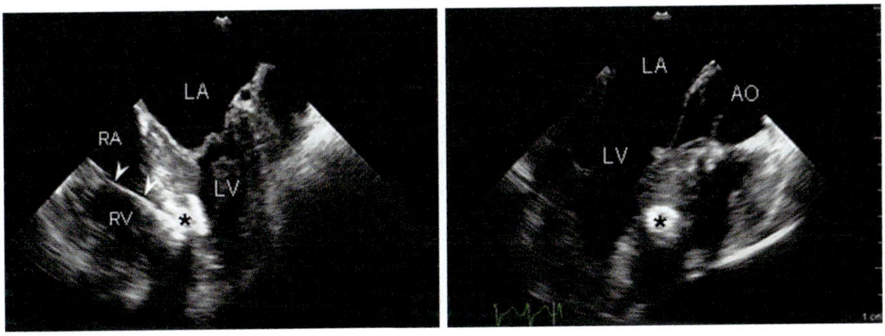

Fig. 4.20 X-plane view during percutaneous occluder implantation. A delivery cable (arrow) crossed the defect and the disks of the occluder (asterisk) deployed in both ventricles

Fig. 4.21 In three dimensional four-chamber view during the procedure. The delivery cable (arrow) crossed the defect and the occluder (asterisk) deployed

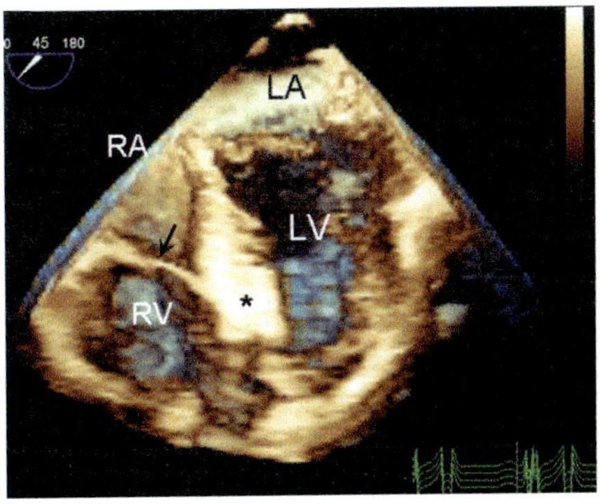

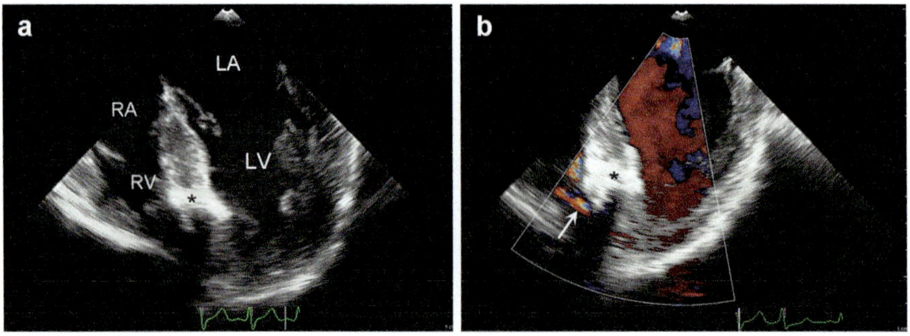

Fig. 4.22 The occluder (asterisk) was released (**a**). Color Doppler showed there was mild residual shunt (arrow) across the ventricular septal defect (**b**)

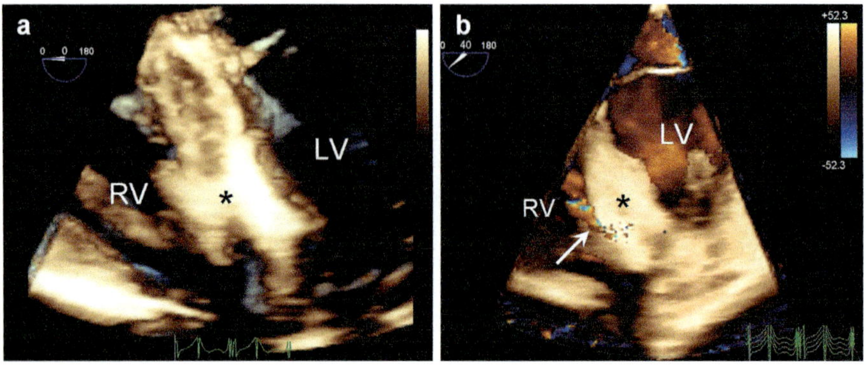

Fig. 4.23 In three dimensional images, the occluder (asterisk) was released from the delivery cable (**a**) and there was mild residual shunt (arrow) across the VSD by color Doppler (**b**)

This case has demonstrated excellent outcome and low mortality using the occluder to close a congenital muscular ventricular septal defect. The device appears to be safe and effective. The incidence of permanent morbidity after this procedure is low. However, patient selection and an experienced operator are very important for procedural success. Device closure should be considered an important alternative to the surgical approach in treating congenital muscular ventricular septal defects.

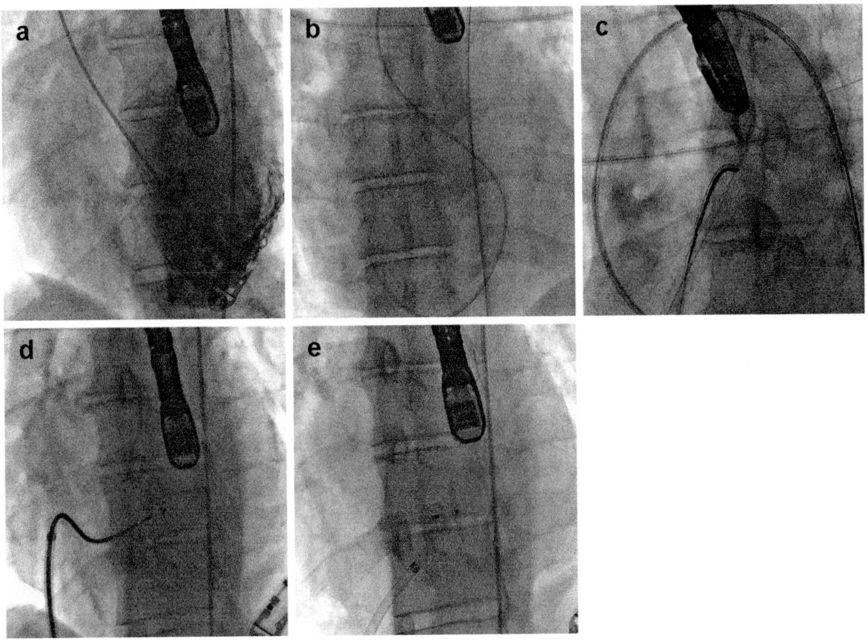

Fig. 4.24 Fluoroscopic angiographic steps in the closure of the muscular ventricular septal defect. (**a**) Left ventricle angiogram demonstrated the presence of a single apical muscular ventricular septal defect. (**b**) The wire was across the defect from the left ventricle. (**c**) The deliver sheath advanced. (**d**) The occluder was deployed. (**e**) After the device was released, the whole procedure was completed

4.5 Occluder Implantation of Patent Ductus Arteriosus

A 45-year-old female patient had no history before. Recently, she suffered from reduce exercise tolerance and shortness of breath. Auscultation showed a continuous murmur in left subclavicular region. After admission, cardiac catheterization was done and a patent ductus arteriosus was revealed. Therefore, occluder implantation was indicated (Figs. 4.25, 4.26, 4.27, 4.28, 4.29, 4.30, 4.31, 4.32, and 4.33; Videos 4.25, 4.26, 4.27, 4.28, 4.29, 4.30a, 4.30b, 4.30c, 4.30d, 4.31, 4.32, and 4.33).

The Amplatzer Duct Occluder should be approximately 2–3 mm larger than the narrowest portion of the patent ductus arteriosus.

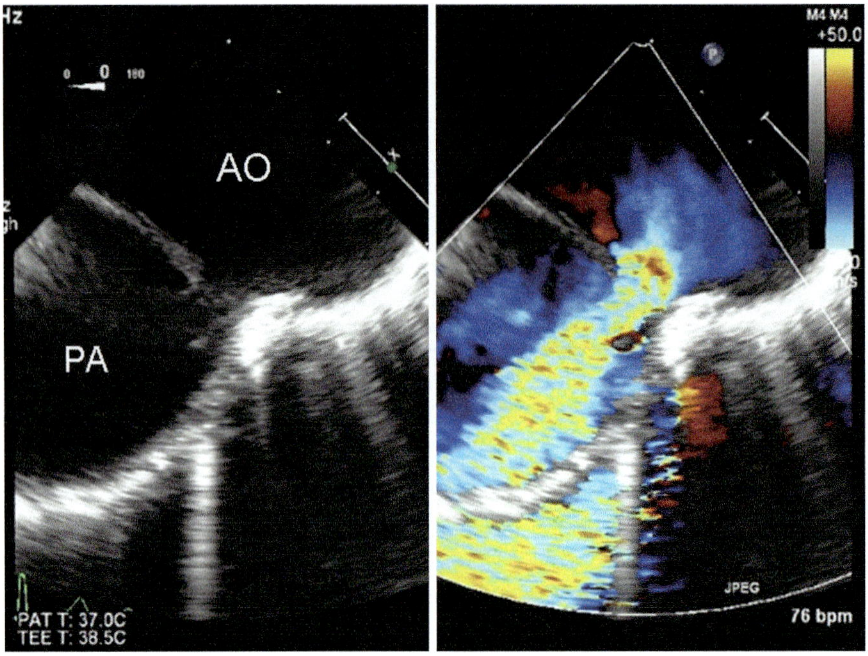

Fig. 4.25 In upper esophageal aortic arch short- axis view with color Doppler compare, continuous blood flow from *distal* aortic arch to pulmonary artery through patent ductus arteriosus was demonstrated

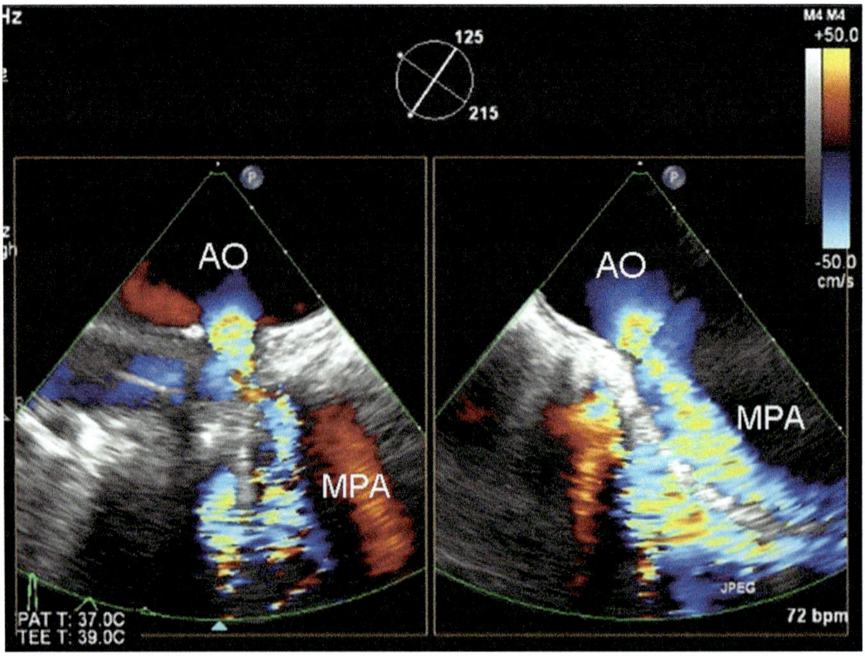

Fig. 4.26 In upper esophageal aortic arch x-plane color Doppler, continuous blood flow from aortic arch to pulmonary artery through patent ductus arteriosus was demonstrated

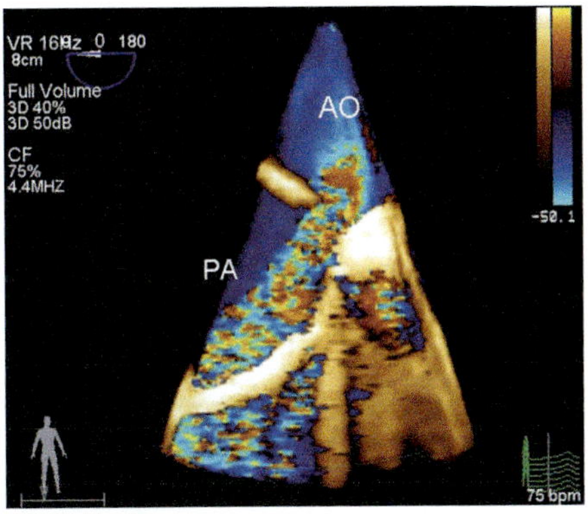

Fig. 4.27 In three dimensional echocardiography for patent ductus arteriosus, flow from aortic arch streams into the patent ductus arteriosus along the lateral wall of the pulmonary artery

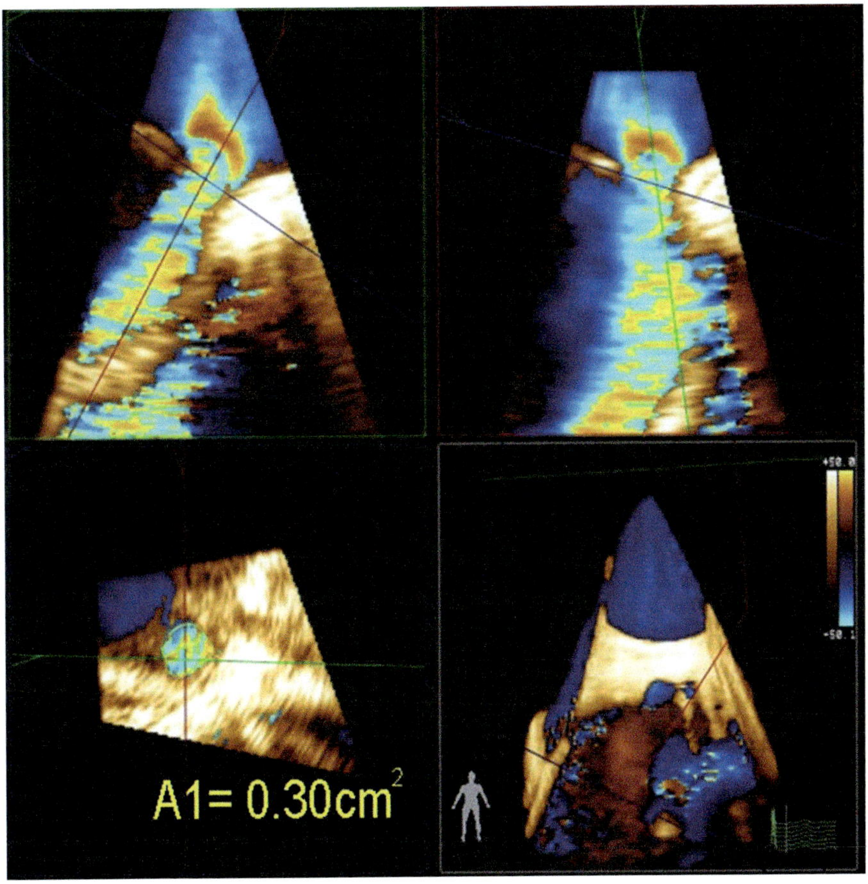

Fig. 4.28 In multi-plane reconstruction, the orifice of the patent ductus arteriosus was measured as 0.30 cm^2

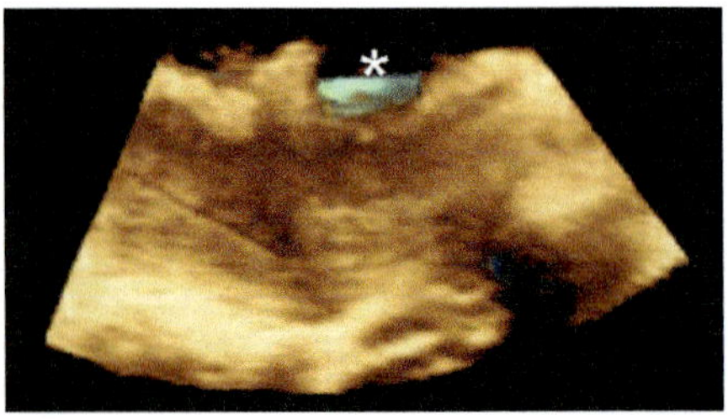

Fig. 4.29 Three dimensional transesophageal echocardiogram visualized from aortic arch shows the orifice of the patent ductus arteriosus (asterisk)

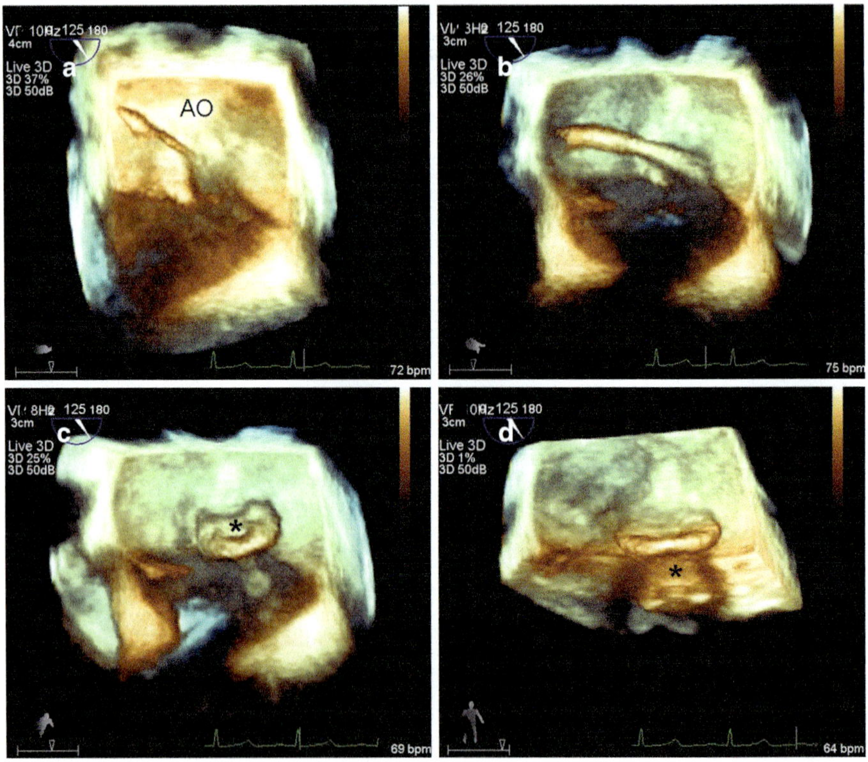

Fig. 4.30 During occluder implantation, a guiding wire (**a**) followed by a delivery cable (**b**) advances into the aorta from pulmonary artery through the patent ductus arteriosus, allowing the aortic retention skirt of an Amplatzer Duct Occluder (12.0 × 10.0 mm, asterisk) to open up in the aorta (**c**). Than the entire delivery system is brought back and the remainder of the device is deployed to block the patent ductus arteriosus (**d**)

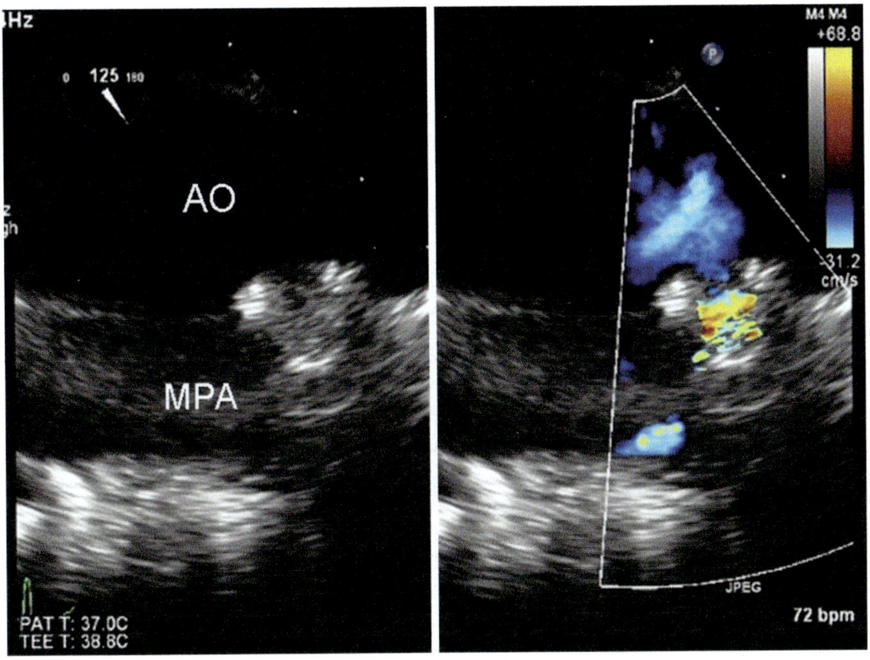

Fig. 4.31 After the device release, color Doppler shows mild residual flow across the patent ductus arteriosus occluder

Fig. 4.32 Three dimensional color Doppler shows mild residual flow across the patent ductus arteriosus occluder

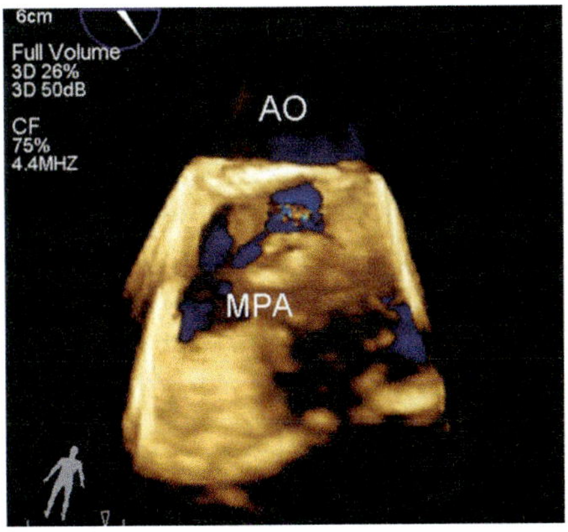

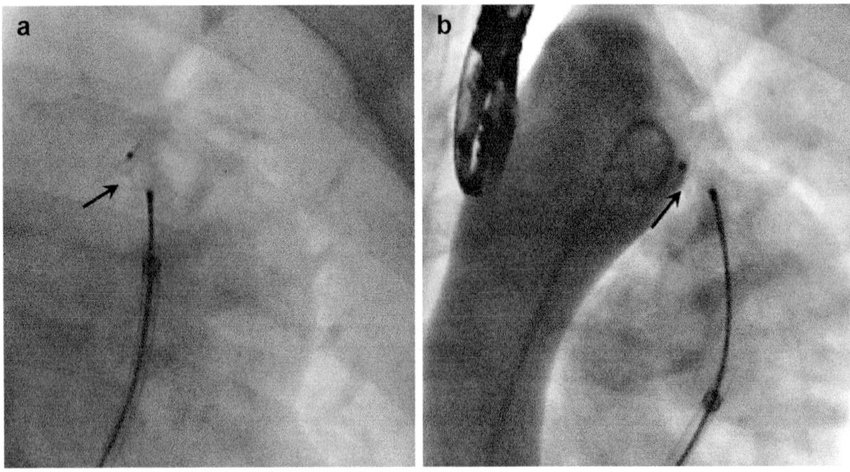

Fig. 4.33 In fluoroscopy, the Amplatzer Duct Occluder (arrow) was appropriately deployed (**a**) and it was still attached to the delivery cable while mild residual shunt flow through it (**b**)

The occluder is threaded on a flexible delivery cable and across the patent ductus arteriosus from the pulmonary artery side. The cable allowed the aortic retention skirt to open up in the descending aorta. The entire delivery system is brought back to snug the occluder into the patent ductus arteriosus. At this point, the delivery sheathe deployed the remainder of the device as it enters the main pulmonary artery. The occluder can be recaptured and reposition at any point prior to device release. After appropriate device position is confirmed by aortography, the device can be released.

4.6 Occluder Implantation of Aortic Annular Pseudoaneurysm After Aortic Valve Replacement

A 73-year-old male patient had a history of diabetes mellitus, coronary artery disease and chronic obstructive pulmonary disease. He presented to the emergency department for sternal pain and intermittent swelling after received aortic valve replacement, mitral valve repair and atrial fibrillation ablation 4 months ago. Chest computed tomography with contrast showed a huge pseudoaneurysm protruding from the ascending aorta of sternum, which might be induced by suture split of the heart-lung machine insertion during the prior operation. To block the tear, an occluder implantation was indicated (Figs. 4.34, 4.35, 4.36, 4.37, 4.38, 4.39, 4.40, 4.41, 4.42, 4.43, and 4.44; Videos 4.34, 4.35, 4.36, 4.37, 4.38a, 4.38b, 4.39, 4.40, 4.41, 4.42, 4.43, and 4.44).

Pseudoaneurysms are characterized by the rupture of the inner wall of a structure, such as the ascending aorta, with an intact outer layer or the rupture

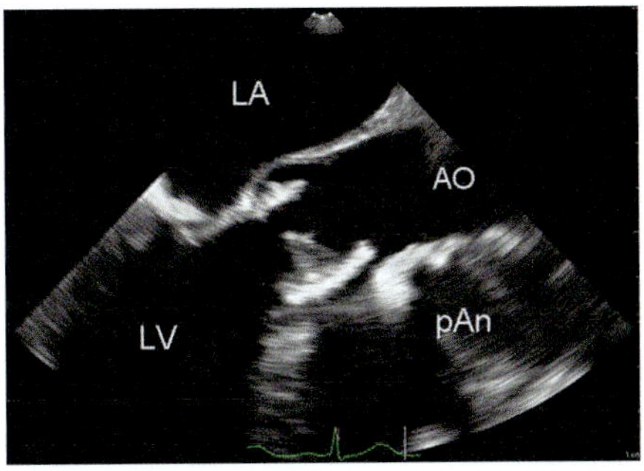

Fig. 4.34 In a mid-esophageal long-axis view, the bioprosthetic tissue aortic valve appeared to open normally and a pseudoaneurysm (pAn) adjacent to ascending aorta was demonstrated

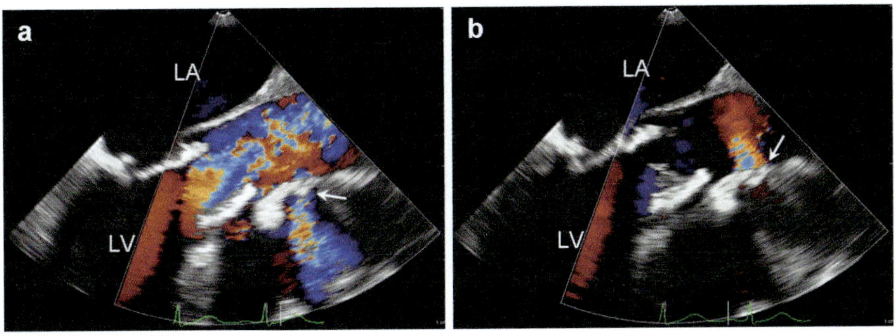

Fig. 4.35 Color Doppler demonstrated forward flow (arrows) into the pseudoaneurysm from the ascending aorta in systole (**a**) and retrograde flow into the aorta during diastole (**b**). The ruptured site was located superior to the aortic prosthesis about 1.5 cm, which may be induced by suture split of the heart-lung machine insertion during the prior operation

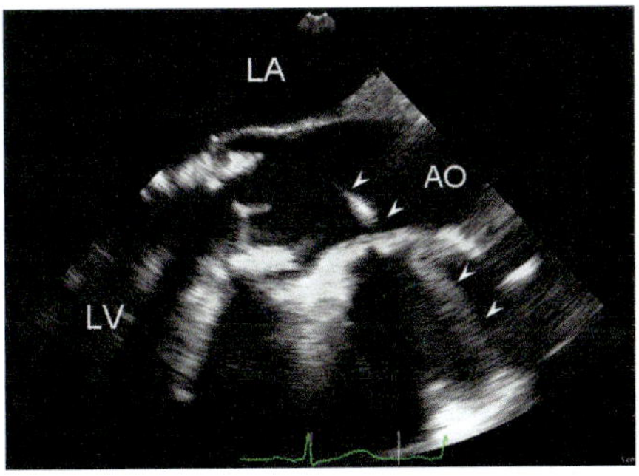

Fig. 4.36 During occluder implantation, a delivery cable (arrow heads) crossed the tear of ascending aorta

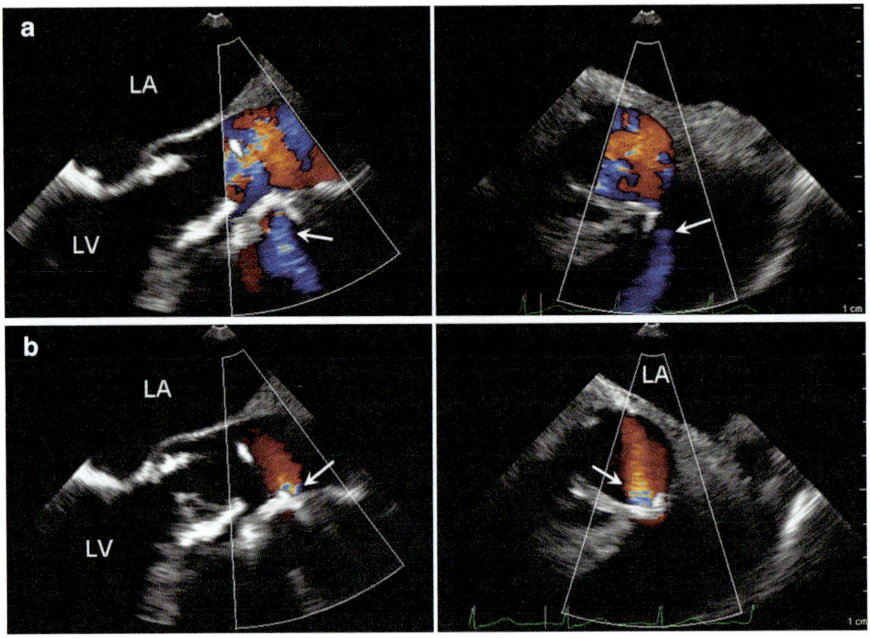

Fig. 4.37 Color Doppler of x-plane views during the procedure, showed bilateral shunt (arrows) crossed the tear of ascending aorta along with the delivery cable in systole (**a**) and diastole (**b**)

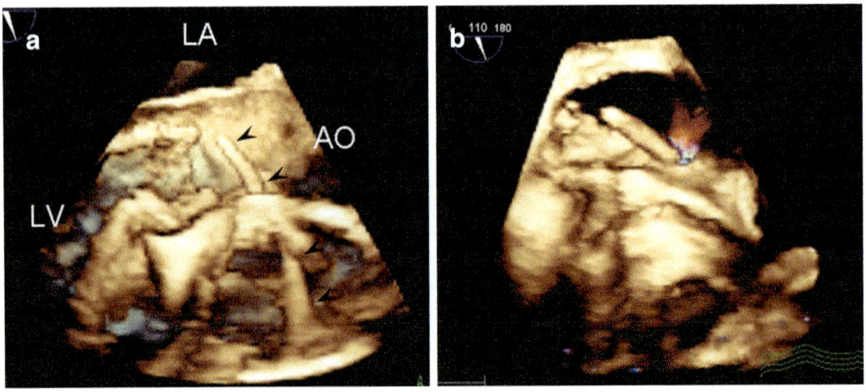

Fig. 4.38 Three dimensional mid-esophageal long-axis view (**a**) with color Doppler (**b**) during the occluder implantation, flow across the tear along with the delivery cable (arrow heads) was demonstrated

of all layers of a vessel with the resulting dilation contained by surrounding structures.

The most common cause of ascending aorta pseudoaneurysms is cardiac surgery. If left aorta pseudoaneurysms untreated, they will be complicated by a high rate of

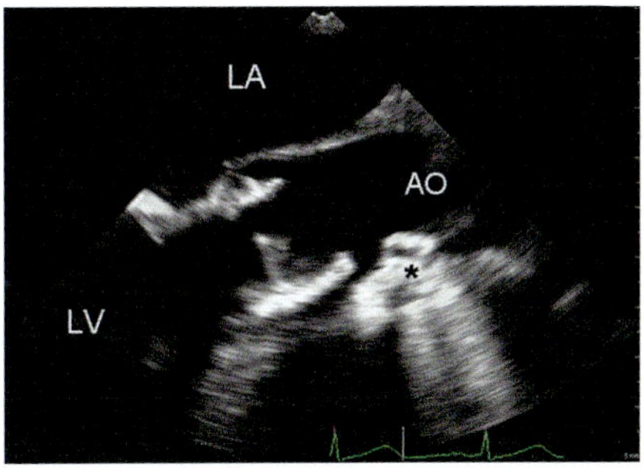

Fig. 4.39 The occluder (asterisk) was deployed and released. It was well implanted

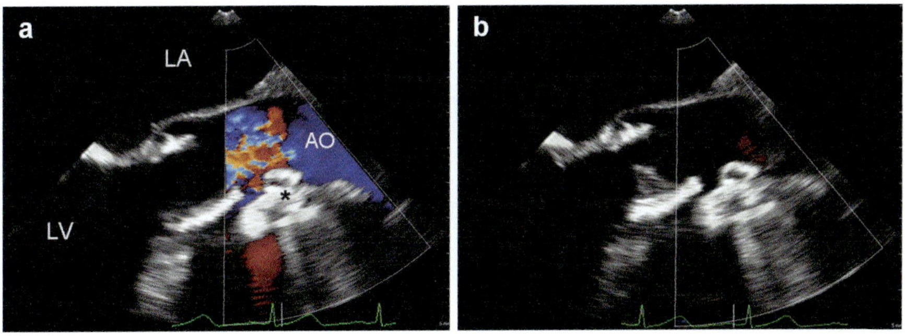

Fig. 4.40 After the occluder (asterisk) implantation, minimal residual shunting was seen in systole (**a**) and diastole (**b**)

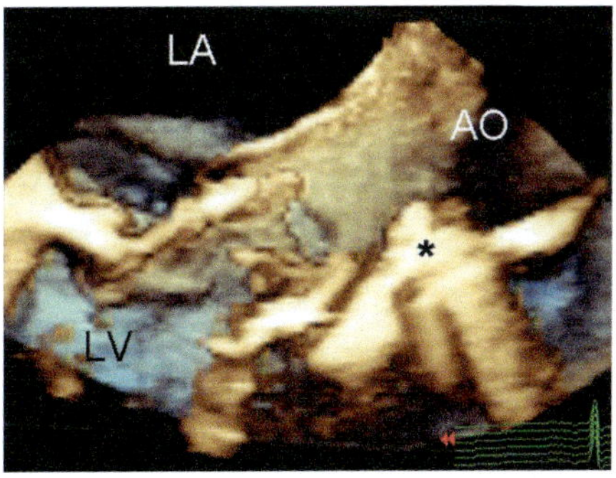

Fig. 4.41 Three dimensional long-axis view after the procedure, the occluder was implanted well

rupture resulting in significant morbidity and mortality. In the past, the ascending aorta pseudoaneurysms were exclusively repaired through open surgery, whereas the technique carries a high mortality rate. Percutaneous interventions have now been developed as a safe and viable alternative in patients unable to undergo surgery.

Still, percutaneous repair carries the risk of several complications, including residual leakage, device prolapse, and embolization of the device. Oversized devices may enlarge the opening of pseudoaneurysms and cause tearing and damage to

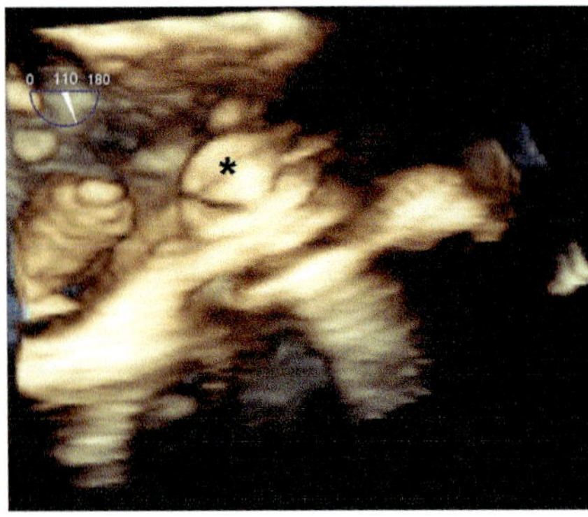

Fig. 4.42 In another three dimensional zoomed view, the closure device (asterisk) was situated at the mural of the ascending aorta

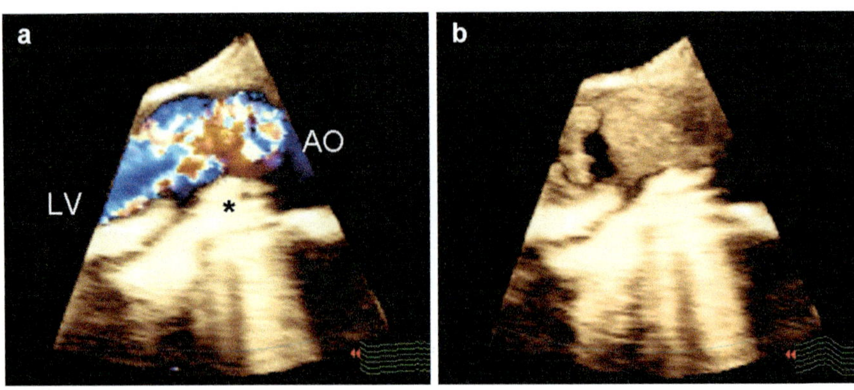

Fig. 4.43 In three dimensional color Doppler, there was scarcely no residual shunting cross through the closure device (asterisk) in systole (**a**) and diastole (**b**)

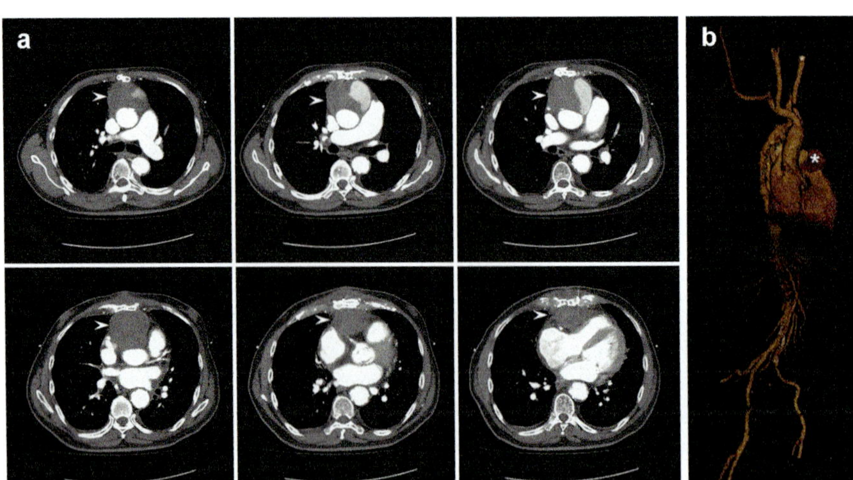

Fig. 4.44 Computed tomography in the axial dimension (**a**) and three dimensional reconstruction (**b**) showed a giant pseudoaneurysm (arrow heads, asterisk) protruding from the ascending aorta of sternum

aortic wall. Therefore, it becomes important to measure the size of the opening correctly prior the procedure and three dimensional transesophageal echocardiography is the first choice.

4.7 Occluder Implantation of Left Ventricle to Right Atrium Shunt

An 86-year-old male patient had prior aortic valve replacement, mitral and tricuspid valve repaired for valvular disease and coronary artery bypass graft for left anterior descending artery and left circumflex. During the previous surgery, an iatrogenic left ventricle to right atrium shunt was revealed by real time transesophageal echocardiography; however, owing to high rate of complications of prolonged operation, the iatrogenic defect was left untouched. Unfortunately, a month later, the patient suffered from headache and chest pain, and the symptoms exacerbated when he presented to hospital. After careful evaluation, an occluder implantation was indicated (Figs. 4.45, 4.46, 4.47, 4.48, 4.49, 4.50, 4.51, 4.52, 4.53, 4.54, 4.55, and 4.56; Videos 4.45, 4.46a, 4.46b, 4.47, 4.48, 4.49, 4.50, 4.51, 4.52a, 4.52b, 4.53, 4.54a, 4.54b, 4.55, and 4.56).

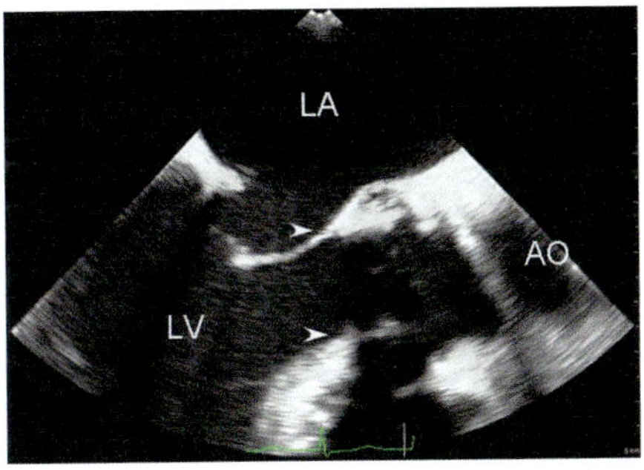

Fig. 4.45 In a mid-esophageal long-axis view, the patient had received mitral valve repaired and aortic valve replacement, the bioprosthetic valve (arrow heads) appeared to open normally

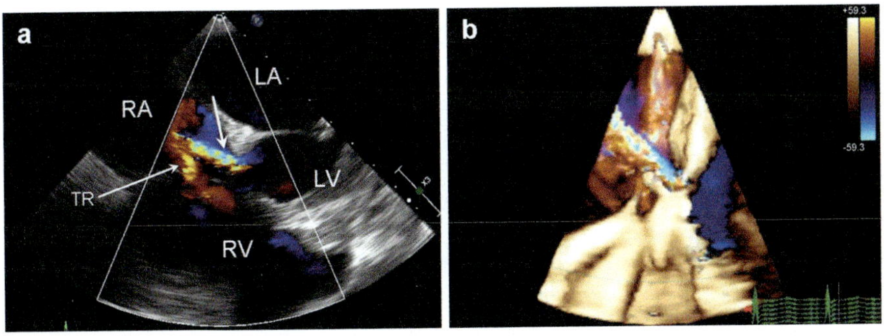

Fig. 4.46 In two and three dimensional (**a**, **b**) modified right ventricle inflow views with color Doppler, a left ventricle-to-right atrium shunt (arrow) was revealed between the repaired mitral and tricuspid annulus

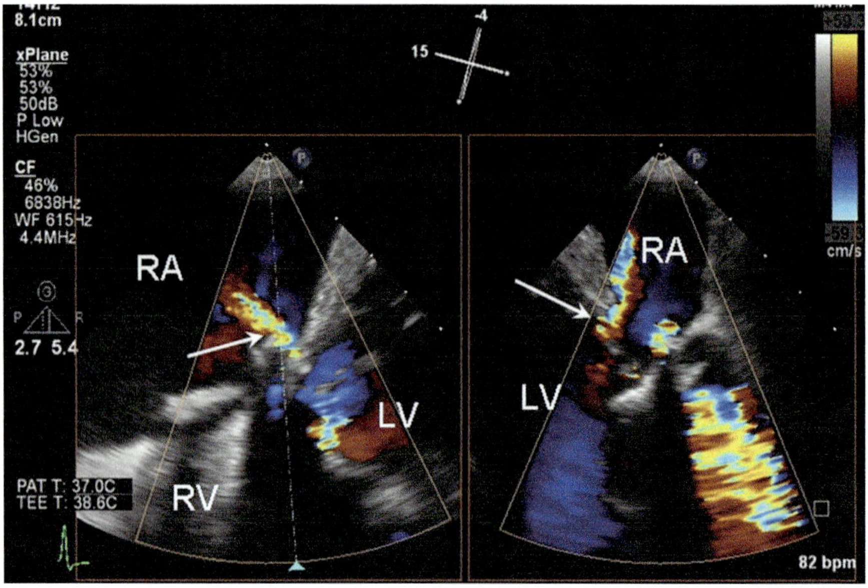

Fig. 4.47 In an x-plane view with color Doppler, a ventriculoatrial septum defect with a shunt from left ventricle to right atrium (arrow) was revealed

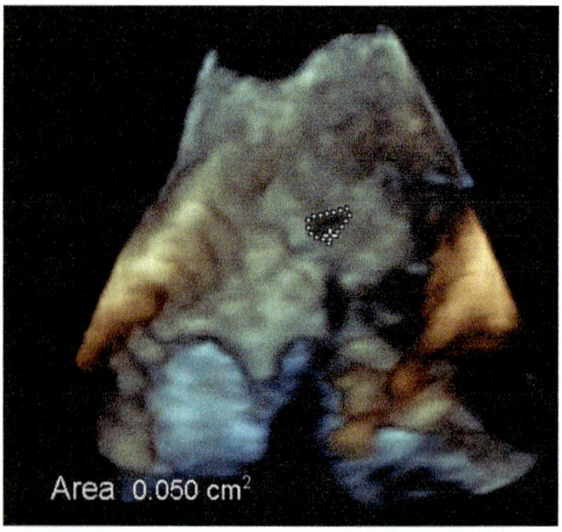

Fig. 4.48 The area of the ventriculoatrial septum defect is measured 0.05 cm^2 in a three dimensional view from the right atrium side

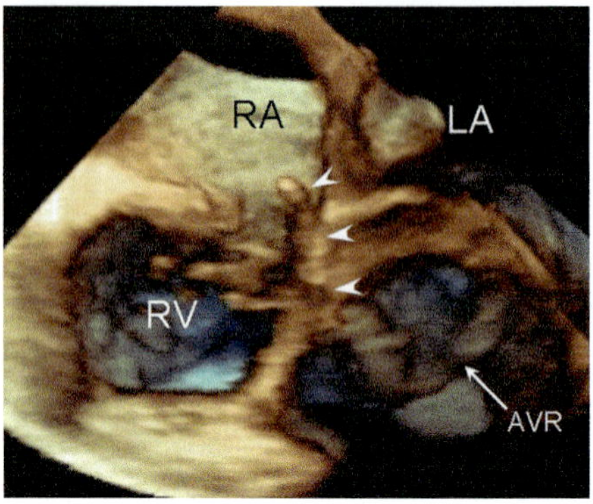

Fig. 4.49 During the occluder implantation, the guiding catheter (arrow heads) advanced across the defect

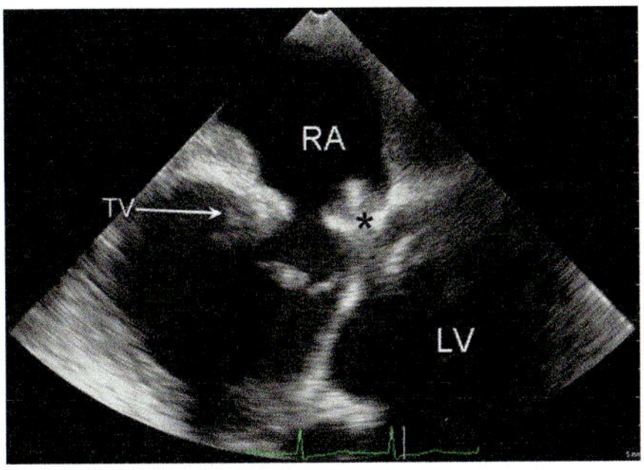

Fig. 4.50 The occluder (asterisk) was delivered across the ventriculoatrial septum defect and deployed

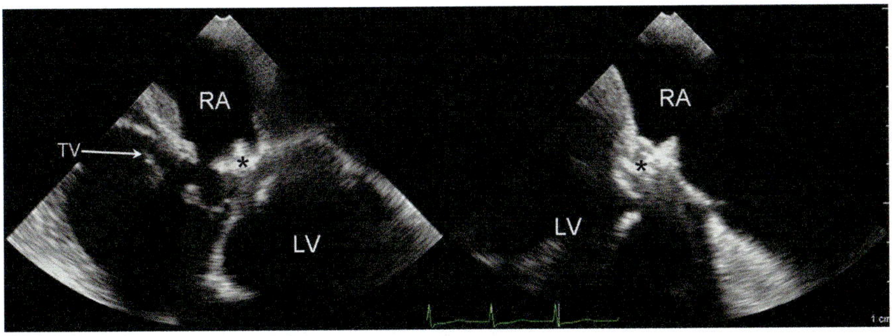

Fig. 4.51 In an x-plane view during the procedure, both disks of the occluder were deployed and the device (asterisk) was still attached to the delivery cable

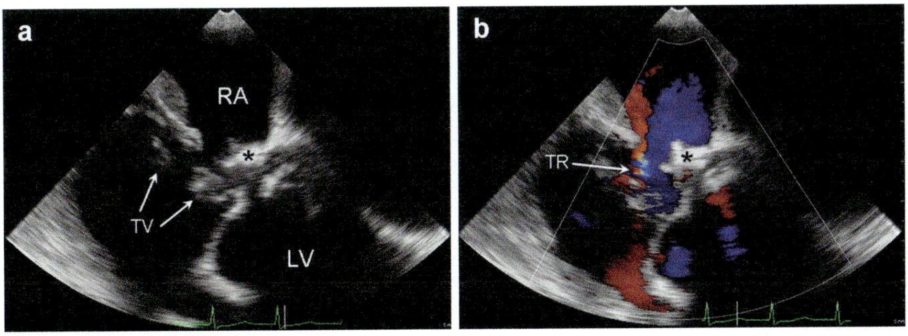

Fig. 4.52 Modified short-axis view after the occluder was released. (**a**) The device (asterisk) had no compromise to the tricuspid valve (TV). (**b**) There was no residual shunting across the defect in color Doppler

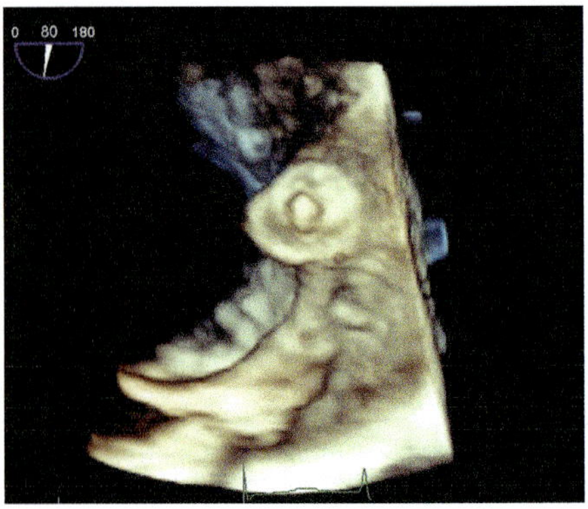

Fig. 4.53 A three dimensional view from right atrial aspect after the occluder implantation showed full deployment of the device

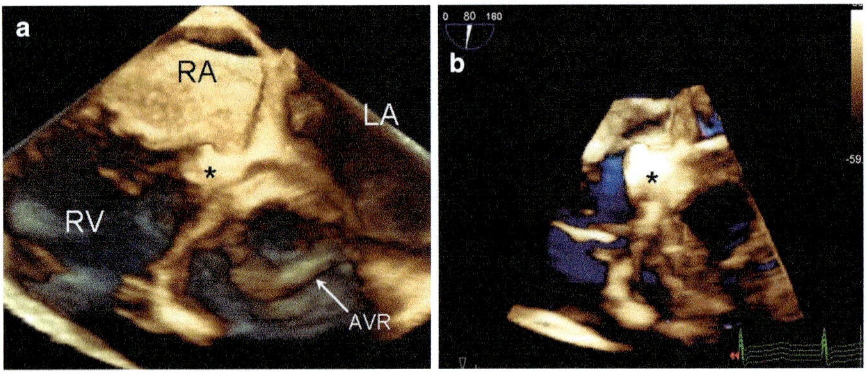

Fig. 4.54 Three dimensional modified short-axis views after the occluder (asterisk) implantation. (**a**) the device was away from the prosthetic aortic valve (AVR). (**b**) There was no residual shunting across the defect in color Doppler

Left ventricle-to-right atrium shunts are usually congenital defects, and acquired left ventricle-to-right atrium communications are rare. A ventriculoatrial septum is a thin membrane between the tricuspid valve and the mitral valve separate the left ventricle from the right atrium, which could be injured in case of cardiac surgery. A previous cardiac surgery involving aortic, mitral valve, or ventricular septal defect repair were the most common reasons of acquired left ventricle-to-right atrium defects.

Acquired left ventricle-to-right atrium shunt is traditionally fixed surgically, but surgical repair had risks of repeat thoracotomy and hazards of cardiopulmonary bypass. Recently, transcatheter closures with occluders in adults have been reported successfully, where trivial residual shunts and no major complications were noted. Therefore, to avoid repeat thoracotomy and bypass, transcatheter approach was a great alternative.

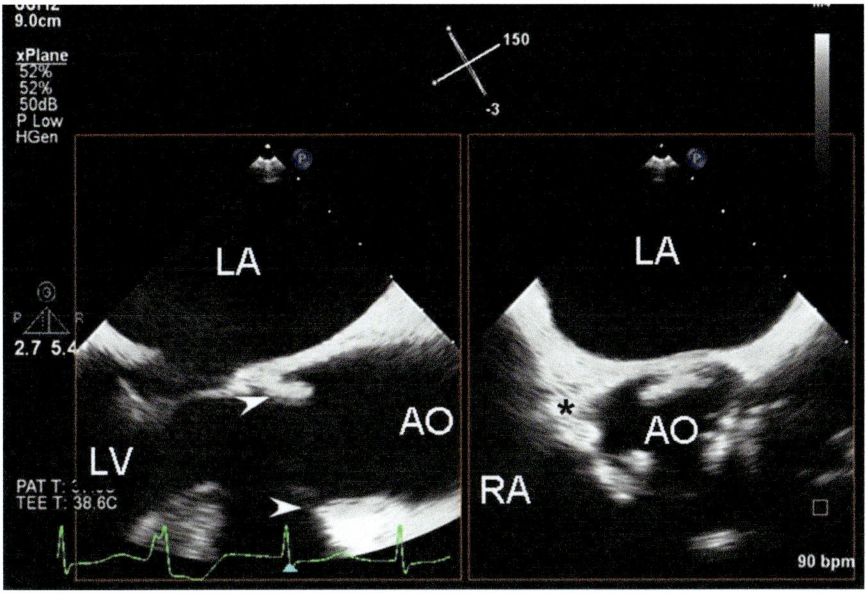

Fig. 4.55 In an x-plane view of long- and short-axis approach after the procedure, previously replaced bioprosthetic aortic valve (arrow heads) was demonstrated, and the occluder (asterisk) was revealed near it

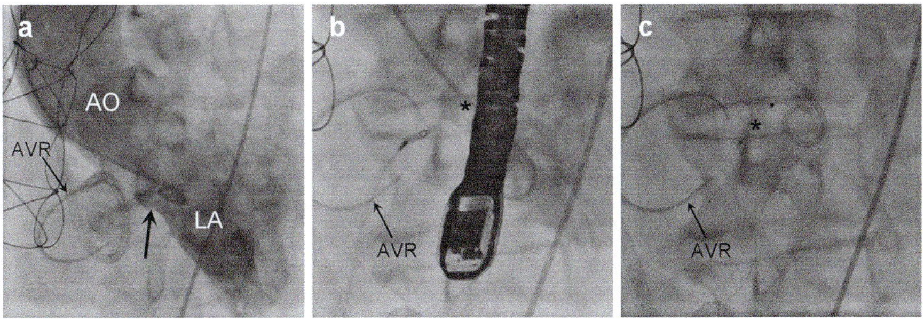

Fig. 4.56 Left-ventricular angiogram showed a left ventricle-to-right atrium shunt (arrow, **a**). (**b**) The left ventricular disk of the occluder (asterisk) was deployed and was still attached to the delivery cable. (**c**) After right disk was also deployed, the device (asterisk) was released

Suggested Readings

1. Amir D, Manish B, Yasser AK, et al. Transcatheter closure of acquired left ventricle-to-right atrium shunt: first case report in an infant and review of the literature. Pediatr Cardiol. 2013;34:1258–60.
2. Anna B, Emily G, Jacob G, et al. Percutaneous closure of a left ventricular pseudoaneurysm after Sapien XT transapical transcatheter aortic valve replacement. JACC Cardiovas Interv. 2012;5(12):e37–8.
3. Assaidi A, Sumian M, Mauri L, et al. Transcatheter closure of complex atrial septal defects is efficient under intracardiac echocardiographic guidance. Arch Cardiovasc Dis. 2014;107(12): 646–53.
4. Baruteau AE, Petit J, Lambert V, et al. Transcatheter closure of large atrial septal defects: feasibility and safety in a large adult and pediatric population. Circ Cardiovasc Interv. 2014;7(6): 837–43.
5. Bayar N, Arslan Ş, Çağırcı G, et al. Assessment of morphology of patent foramen ovale with transesophageal echocardiography in symptomatic and asymptomatic patients. J Stroke Cerebrovasc Dis. 2015;24(6):1282–6.
6. Chen HY, Pan CZ, Shu XH. Partially nroofed coronary sinus diagnosed by real-time dimensional transesophageal echocardiagraphy after operation of secundum atrial septal defect. Int J Cardiovasc Imaging. 2015;31(1):45–6.
7. Ho-Ping Y, An-Ning F, Shen-Kou T, et al. Transcatheter repair of iatrogenic aortic perforation complicating transseptal puncture for a catheter ablation of atrial arrhythmia. Acta Cardiol Sin. 2014;30:490492.
8. Jeng W, Ming CH, Shen KT, et al. Atrial septal occluder device embolization to an iliac artery: a case highlighting the utility of three-dimensional transesophageal echocardiography during percutaneous closure. Echocardiography. 2012;29(9):1128–31.
9. John ML, Jason HR. Interventional procedures for adult structural heart disease. Philadelphia: Elsevier; 2014. Ch. 12
10. John DC, John GW. Structural heart disease interventions. Philadelphia: Lippincott Williams & Wilkins; 2012. Ch. 12–15
11. Rajeev N, Prashant V, Martin G, et al. Percutaneous closure of left ventricular pseudoaneurysm. Ann Thorac Surg. 2012;94:e123–5.
12. Ralf H, David B, Qi LC, et al. Device closure of muscular ventricular septal defects using the Amplatzer muscular ventricular septal defect occluder immediate and mid-term results of a U.S. registry. JACC. 2004;43(7):1257–63.
13. Rodrigo EL, Jorge SF, Niclas VG, et al. Percutaneous closure of an aorto-atrial fistula after surgery for infective endocarditis. JACC Cardiovas Interv. 2012;2012:e15–7.
14. Ziyad MH, Fakhri H, Fadel AF, et al. Transcatheter closure of single muscular ventricular septal defects using the Amplatzer muscular VSD occluder: initial results and technical considerations. Cathet Cardiovasc Intervent. 2000;49:167–72.

Complications of Interventional Procedures

5

5.1 Introduction

Interventions serve an alternative to surgical replacements for severe, symptomatic structural heart disease in high risk patients. Intraprocedural transesophageal echocardiography provides real-time imaging guidance throughout the procedure and allows for instant and accurate assessment of complications and procedural results, which can significantly lower patients' morbidity and mortality.

Complications of interventions contain a great variety, transcatheter heart valve malposition, cardiac injury, central or paravalvular regurgitation, bleeding, stroke, coronary occlusion, and so on. In this chapter, almost every category mentioned above is discussed. At least one or more cases are presented in each topic, while some of the patients had complicated complications. Each case demonstrates occurrence of incident, severity of situation, management taken, and outcome.

It is our hope to share our experiences, not only the fancy ones, but also the unpleasant or even fatal ones, to all the readers, so that you can be inspired by them, recognizing, predicting, or effectively reacting to all complications accurately. After all, to improve the safety of interventions is important and necessary.

5.2 Stroke After Transcatheter Aortic Valve Implantation

An 84-year-old male patient had a history of tri-vessel coronary artery disease, critical aortic stenosis, chronic renal insufficient, and hyperlipidemia. He suffered from chest tightness and exertional dyspnea for days. Therefore transcatheter aortic valve

---

Electronic supplementary material The online version of this chapter (https://doi.org/10.1007/978-981-10-6937-6_5) contains supplementary material, which is available to authorized users.

M.-C. Hsiung et al., *Atlas of 3D Transesophageal Echocardiography in Structural Heart Disease Interventions*, https://doi.org/10.1007/978-981-10-6937-6_5

implantation was highly recommended by the heart team (Figs. 5.1, 5.2, 5.3, 5.4, 5.5, 5.6, 5.7, 5.8, and 5.9; Videos 5.1, 5.2, 5.3a, 5.3b, 5.4, 5.5, 5.6, 5.7a, 5.7b, 5.8, and 5.9).

The occurrence of stroke may occur at various times during the procedure, possibly linked to several factors: manipulation of a bulky catheter through the artery,

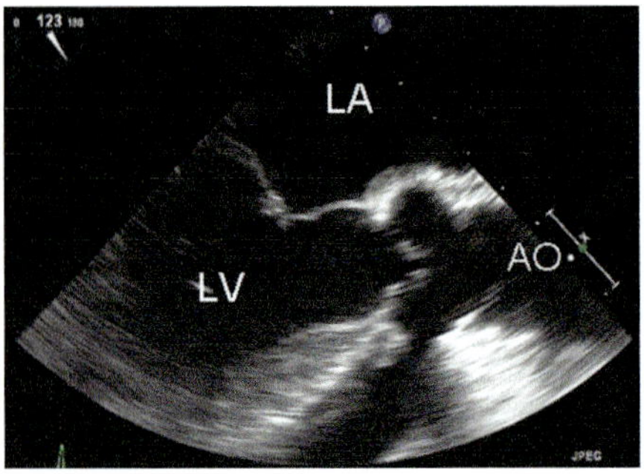

Fig. 5.1 In transesophageal echocardiographic midesophageal long-axis approach, thickened aortic valve with restricted cusp mobility reduced cusp separation

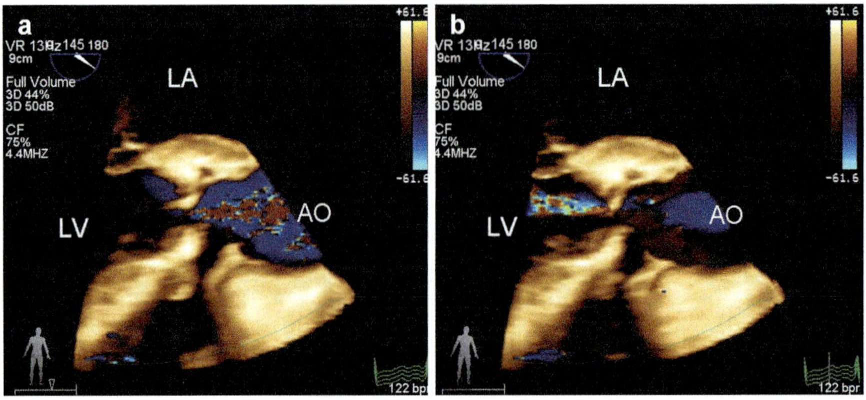

Fig. 5.2 Three dimensional color Doppler showed turbulent flow across the thickened aortic valve in systole (**a**) and mild regurgitation in diastole (**b**)

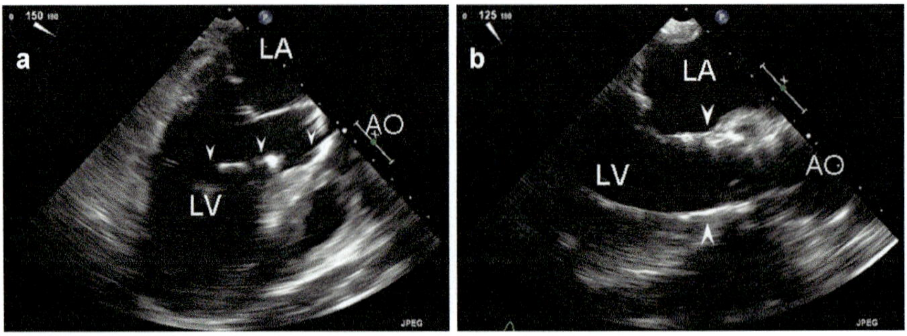

Fig. 5.3 During the transcatheter aortic valve implantation, the guiding wire (arrow heads, **a**) advanced across the calcified native aortic valve, then the CoreValve (29 mm, arrow heads, **b**) was delivered and deployed

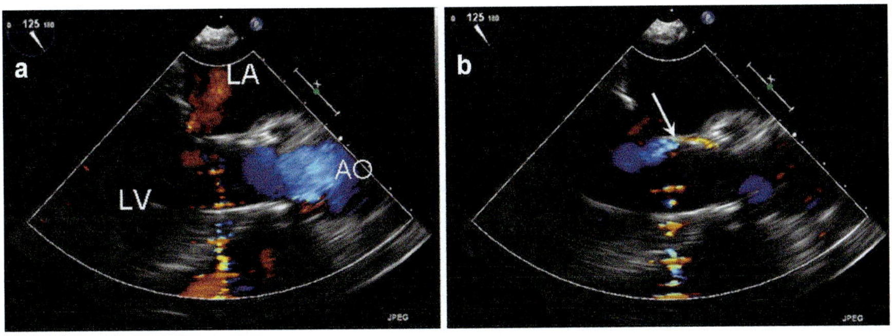

Fig. 5.4 In long-axis views after the implantation. The CoreValve was well positioned without accelerated flow across it in systole (**a**), and mild paravalvular leakage was present in diastole (arrow, **b**)

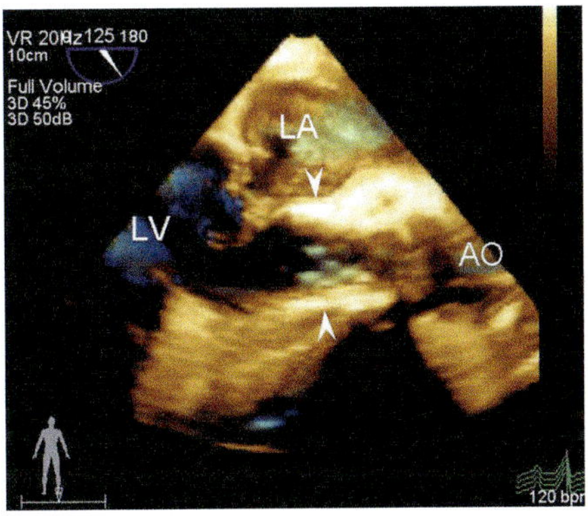

Fig. 5.5 In three dimensional long-axis view after the implantation, the CoreValve was well positioned and deployed (arrow heads)

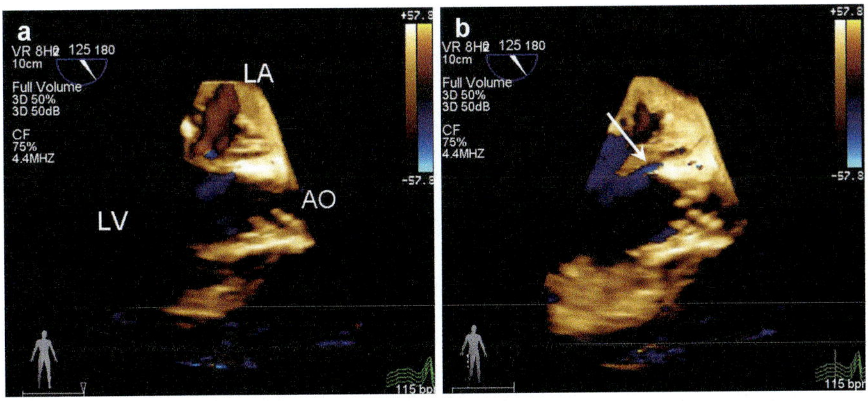

Fig. 5.6 Three dimensional color Doppler showed the CoreValve was well positioned without accelerated flow across it in systole (**a**), and mild paravalvular leakage in diastole (arrow, **b**)

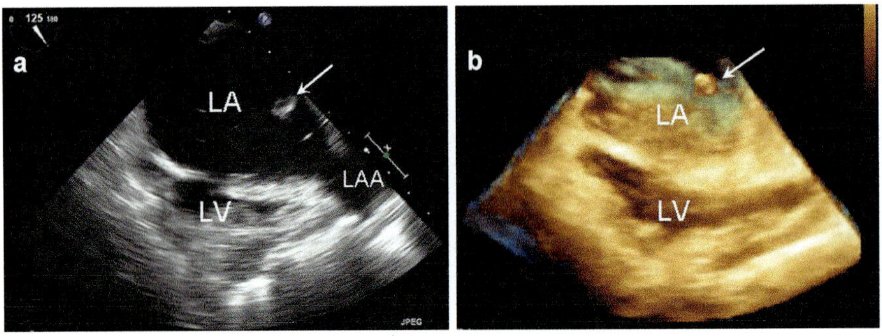

Fig. 5.7 Two (**a**) and three dimensional (**b**) transesophageal echocardiogram during the procedure, a thrombus-like echodensity (arrows) floated rapidly through the left atrium

Fig. 5.8 Another perspective from the left atrium toward the ventricular also demonstrated a thrombus-like echodensity (asterisk) floating rapidly through the left atrium. After procedure, the thrombus was gone and the patient never woke up afterward

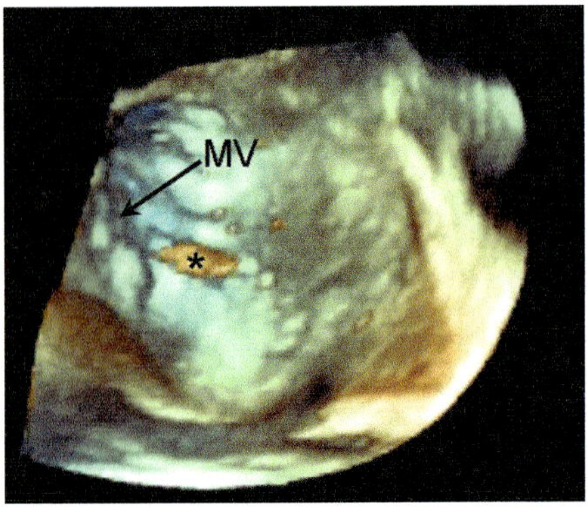

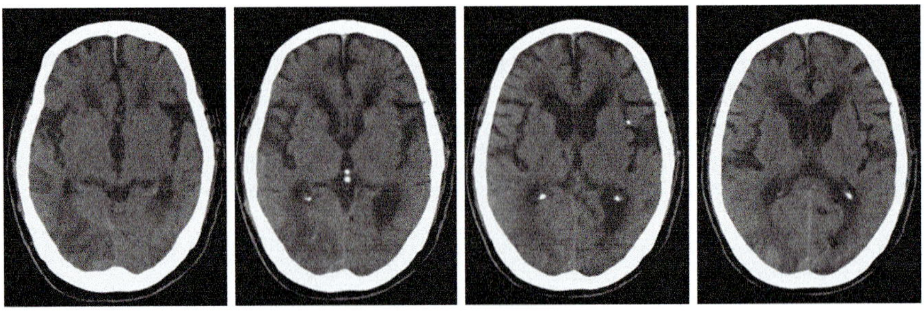

Fig. 5.9 Brain computed tomography was done to confirm thrombotic status, where multiple cerebral infarctions in bilateral frontal, parietal, occipital lobes were found

retrograde crossing of a severely diseased native aortic valve, and the hemodynamic insult to the brain during rapid pacing and device deployment. Besides, the incidence of atrial fibrillation and atherosclerotic disease has higher risk of cerebrovascular events. Lately, several novel embolic protection devices have been developed to lessen the incidence of stroke and cerebral perfusion abnormalities after transcatheter aortic valve implantation.

5.3 Aortic Valve-in-Valve Implantation of Lotus Valve for Paravalvular Leakage

An 85-year-old female patient had received transcatheter aortic valve implantation (Boston Lotus, 27 mm) 5 months ago due to severe aortic stenosis and moderate aortic regurgitation. Although moderate paravalvular leakage occurred right after the procedure, the patient tolerated it well. Therefore, she was discharged and received regular follow-up. However, recently, she developed worsening symptoms of cough and shortness of breath. Echocardiography revealed persisted paravalvular regurgitation. Redo valve-in-valve implantation was arranged as a result (Figs. 5.10, 5.11, 5.12, 5.13, 5.14, 5.15, 5.16, 5.17, 5.18, 5.19, 5.20, 5.21, and 5.22; Videos 5.10, 5.11, 5.12, 5.13a, 5.13b, 5.14a, 5.14b, 5.15, 5.16a, 5.16b, 5.17, 5.18a, 5.18b, 5.19, 5.20, 5.21, and 5.22).

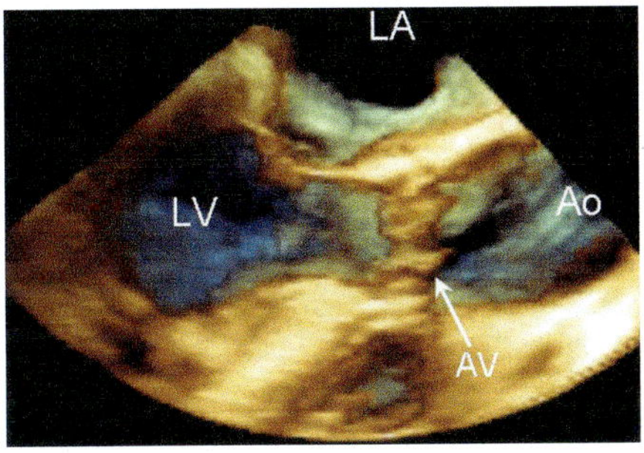

Fig. 5.10 Severe calcification of aortic valve with restricted cusp mobility is demonstrated from a three dimensional midesophageal long-axis approach

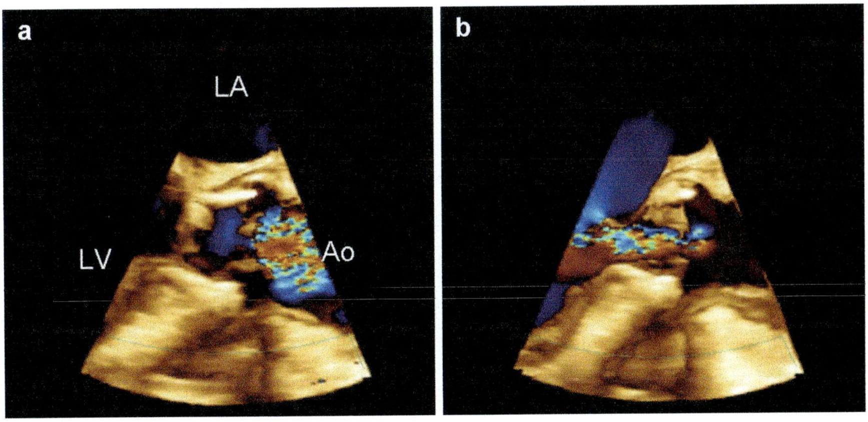

Fig. 5.11 In color Doppler, turbulence flow proximal to the aortic valve and moderate regurgitation occurred in systole (**a**) and diastole (**b**)

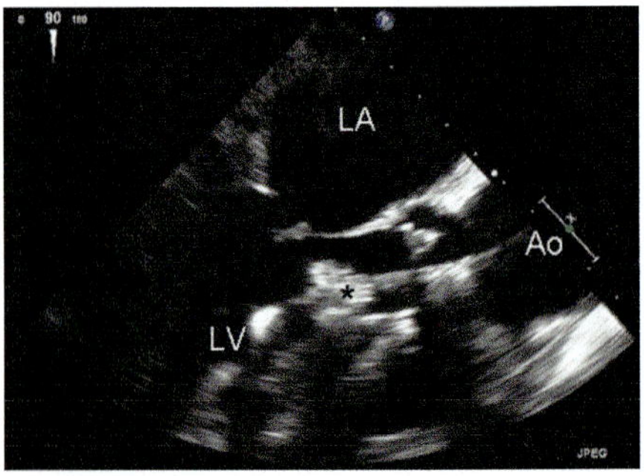

Fig. 5.12 During the transcatheter aortic valve implantation, the first crimped Lotus valve (asterisk, 27 mm) was delivered

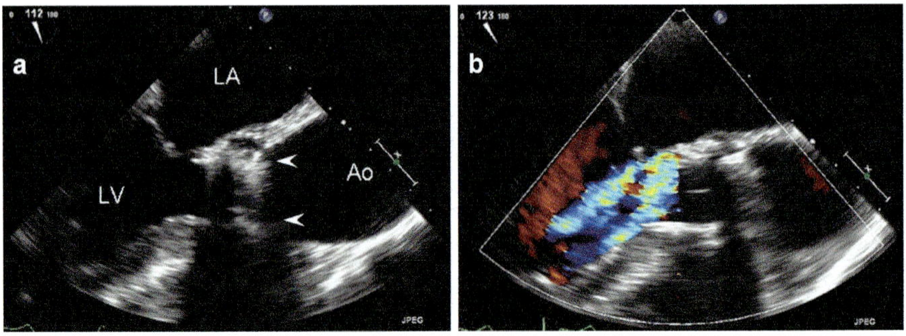

Fig. 5.13 After deployment of the Lotus valve (arrow heads, **a**), moderate paravalvular regurgitation was noted by color Doppler (**b**)

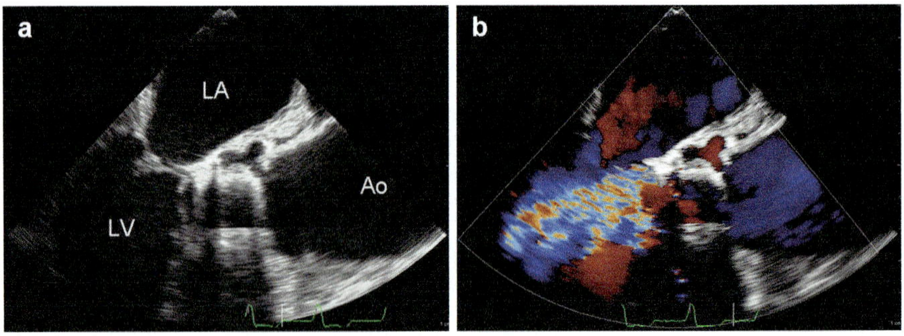

Fig. 5.14 A five-month follow-up (**a**) showed persist moderate to severe paravalvular regurgitation (**b**)

Accurate positioning of the transcatheter heart valve with respect to the native aortic annulus is critical to ensure a successful procedure, while suboptimal deployment can result in incomplete apposition of the valve and annulus letting a significant diastolic backflow into the left ventricle. For malpositioned transcatheter heart valves with too shallow or too deep implantation of the prosthesis, valve-in-valve implantation is a feasible treatment strategy to reduce significant paravalvular aortic

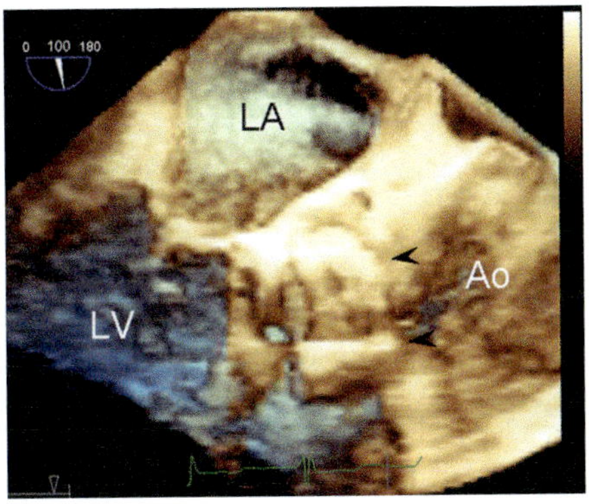

Fig. 5.15 Three dimensional long-axis view showed the Lotus valve (arrow heads) was within the aortic root

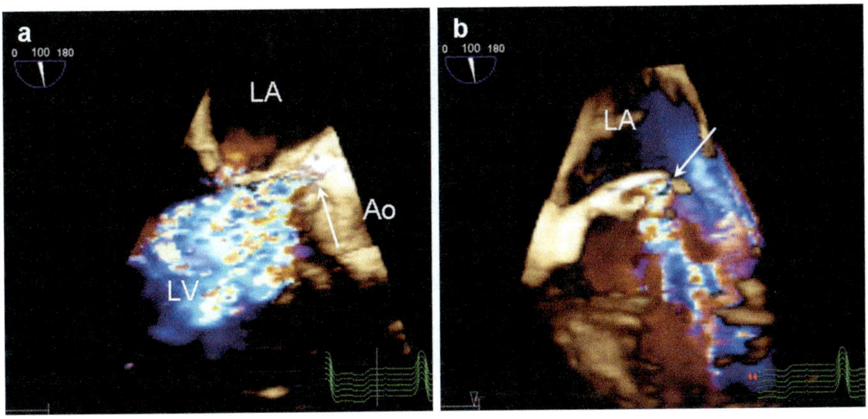

Fig. 5.16 In three dimensional color Doppler, long- (**a**) and modified short-axis view (**b**), the origin of the paravalvular regurgitation was at 12 o'clock position (arrow)

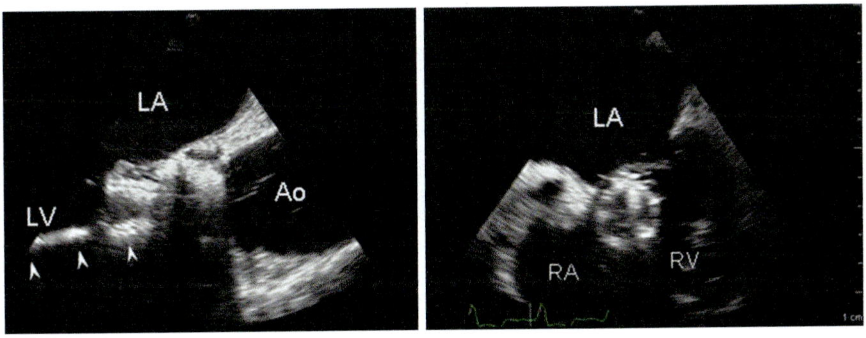

Fig. 5.17 In x-plane view during the redo valve-in-valve implantation, the second crimped Lotus valve was advanced into the first one by the delivery system (arrow heads)

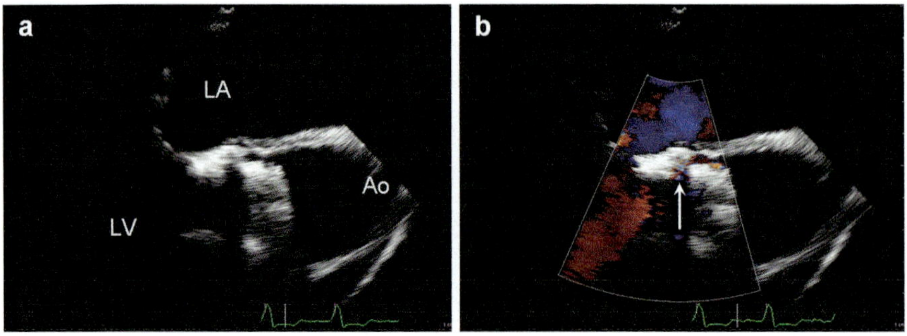

Fig. 5.18 After deployment, the Lotus valve was well positioned (**a**), only trivial paravalvular leakage (arrow, **b**) was demonstrated in color Doppler

Fig. 5.19 In three dimensional long-axis view after the valve-in-valve implantation, the second Lotus valve was well positioned and worked normally within the first one

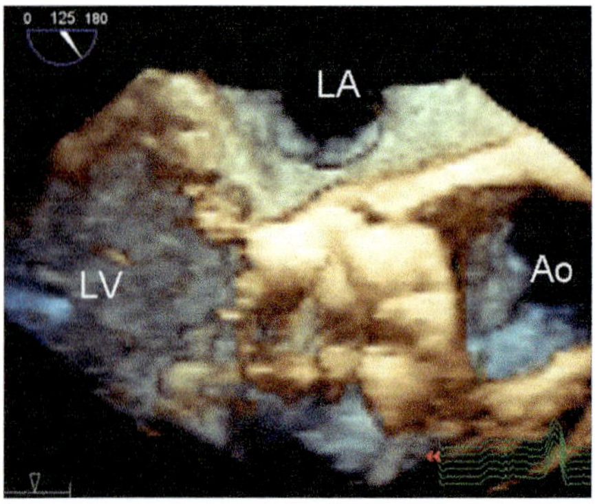

Fig. 5.20 In three dimensional long-axis view with color Doppler after the procedure, there was trivial paravalvular leakage remaining

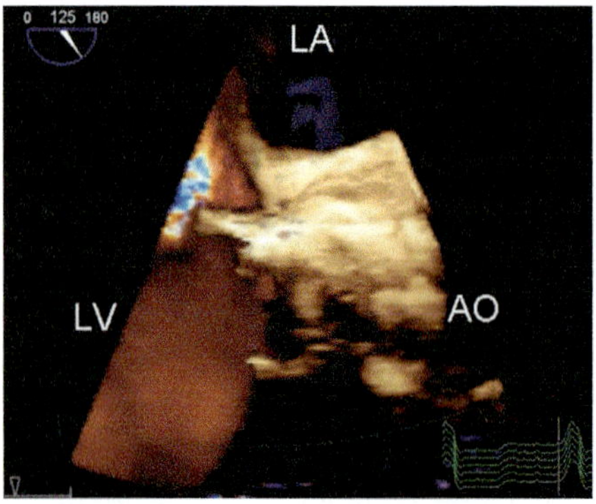

regurgitation. The second valve can be deployed to overlap both valves and seal the annulus. Consequently, initial procedural failure can be converted into procedural success

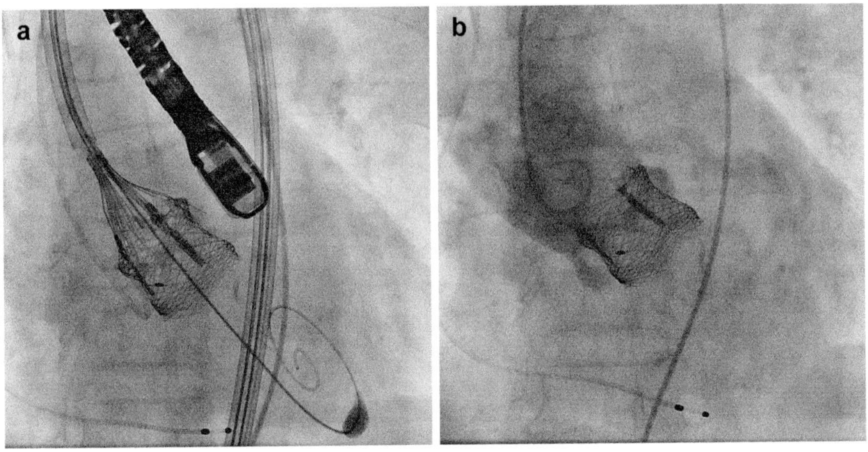

Fig. 5.21 Fluoroscopic images during the first transcatheter Lotus valve positioning. (**a**) The Lotus valve was delivered and expanded. (**b**) The position of the valve was confirmed then it was detached from the delivery system

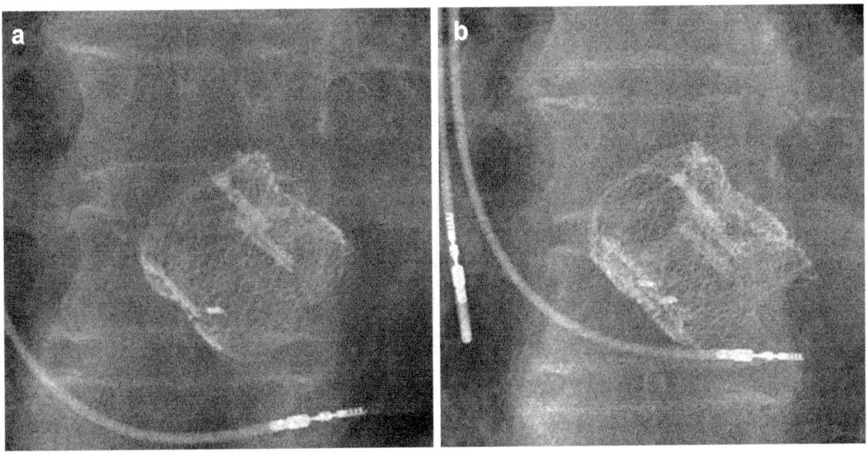

Fig. 5.22 Chest X ray after the first Lotus implantation (**a**) and the valve-in-valve procedure (**b**). The second Lotus valve was within the first one and deeper into the ascending aorta

5.4 Implantation of SAPIEN Valve in CoreValve for Paravalvular Leakage

A 67-year-old male patient had received transcatheter aortic valve implantation with CoreValve 31 mm for severe aortic stenosis. Severe paravalvular leakage was revealed right after the procedure; however, patient refused to tolerated further interventional treatment at that time. A half year later, the patient developed dyspnea and dizziness. Echocardiography showed severe paravalvular leakage persisting. According to the condition, a transcatheter aortic valve-in-valve implantation was indicated (Figs. 5.23, 5.24, 5.25, 5.26, 5.27, 5.28, 5.29, 5.30, 5.31, 5.32, 5.33, 5.34, 5.35, 5.36, 5.37, 5.38, and 5.39; Videos 5.23, 5.24, 5.25, 5.26, 5.27, 5.28, 5.29, 5.30, 5.31a, 5.31b, 5.32, 5.33, 5.34, 5.35a, 5.35b, 5.36a, 5.36b, 5.37a, 5.37b, 5.38, and 5.39).

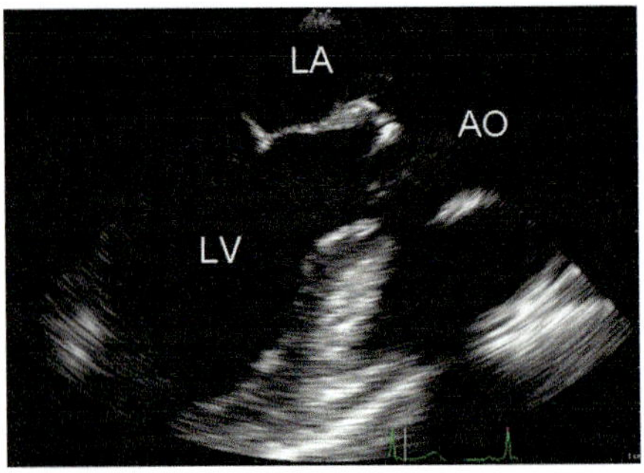

Fig. 5.23 In transesophageal echocardiographic mid-esophageal long-axis view, calcified native aortic valve with reduced cusp separation was demonstrated

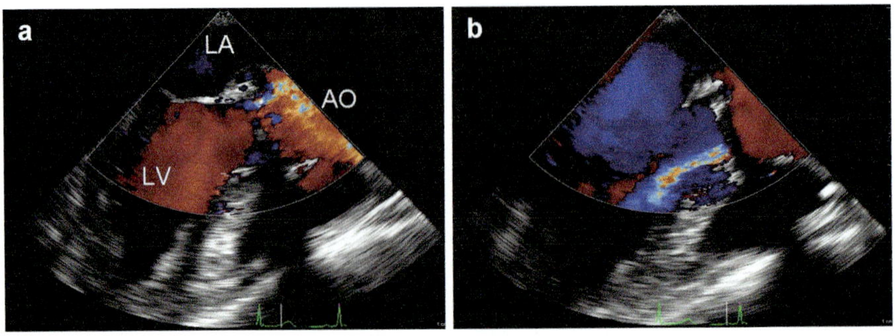

Fig. 5.24 With color Doppler, the calcified aortic valve induced turbulent left ventricular outflow in systole (**a**) and moderate regurgitation in diastole (**b**)

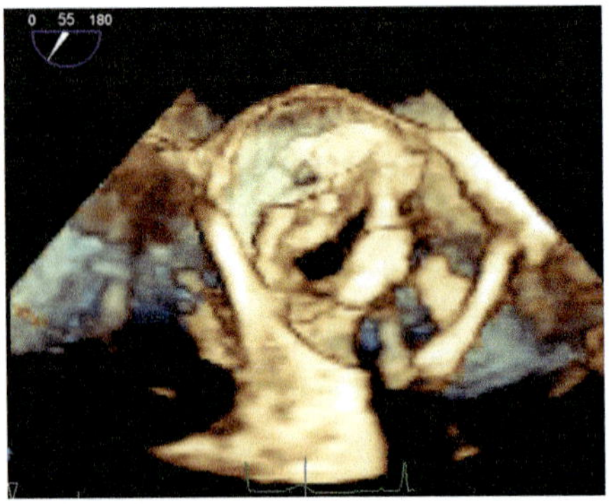

Fig. 5.25 Three dimensional short-axis view showed severe calcified bicuspid aortic valve with stenotic aortic orifice

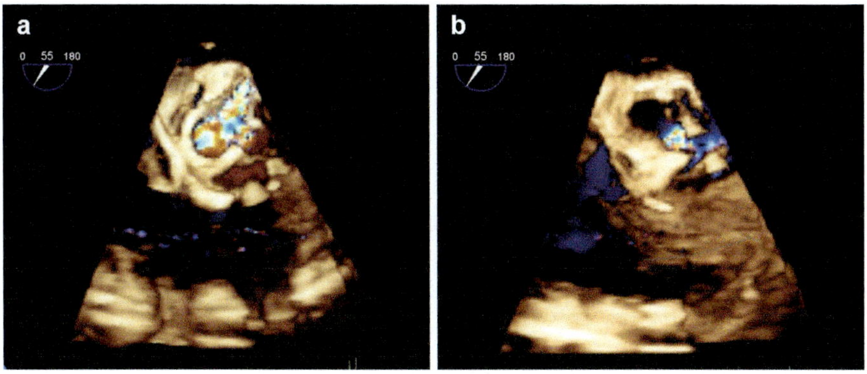

Fig. 5.26 Three dimensional short-axis color Doppler showed turbulent left ventricular outflow in systole (**a**) and moderate aortic regurgitation in diastole (**b**)

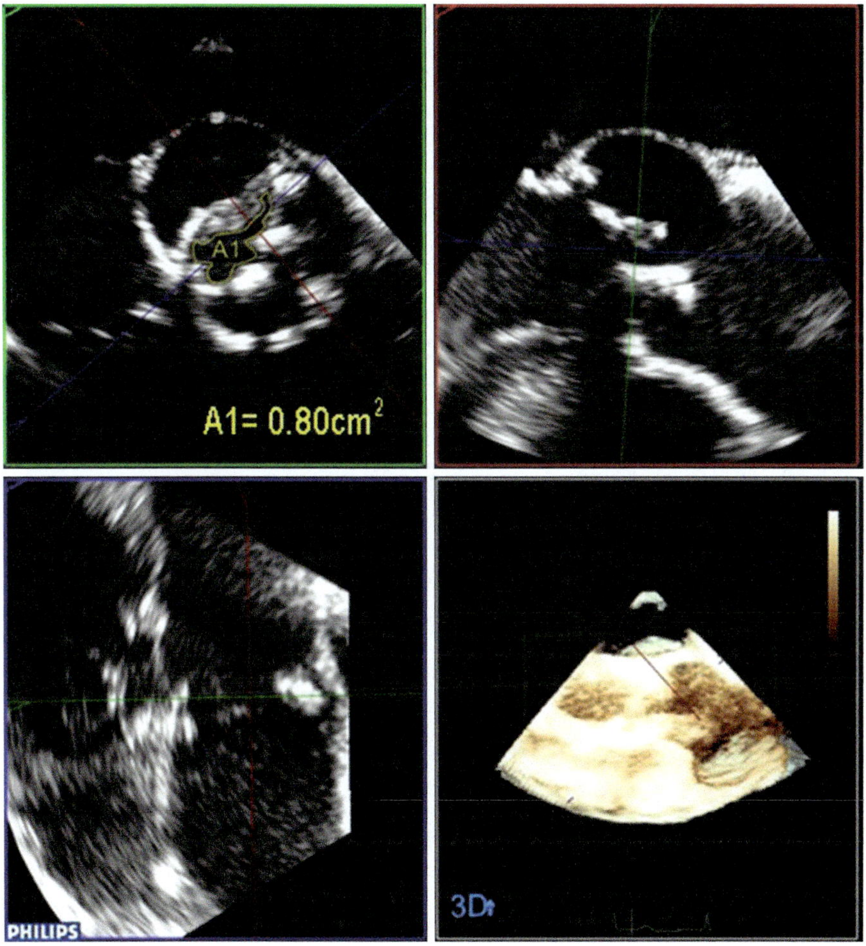

Fig. 5.27 Through multi-planar reconstruction of the three dimensional image, the orifice of the bicuspid aortic valve was measured 0.80 cm^2

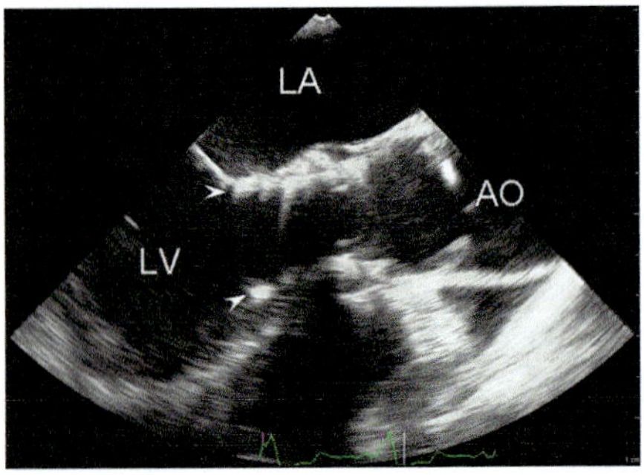

Fig. 5.28 After the first interventional treatment, the CoreValve (31 mm, arrow heads) was deployed within the aortic root

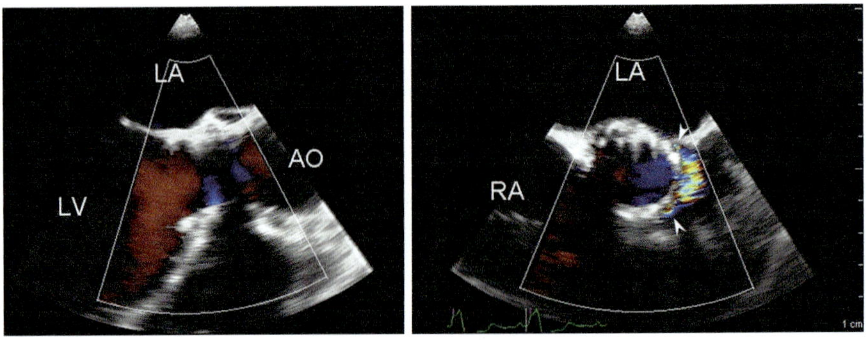

Fig. 5.29 In x-plane color Doppler, the right panel showed severe paravalvular leakage, whose origin ranged from one to four o'clock position (between arrow heads)

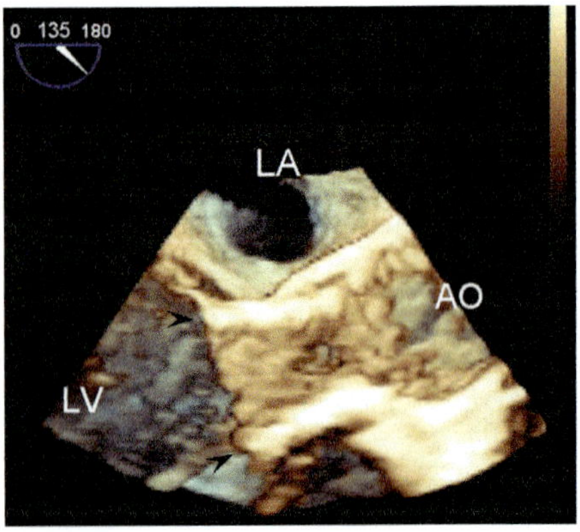

Fig. 5.30 Three dimensional long-axis view showed the CoreValve (arrow heads) was within the aortic root

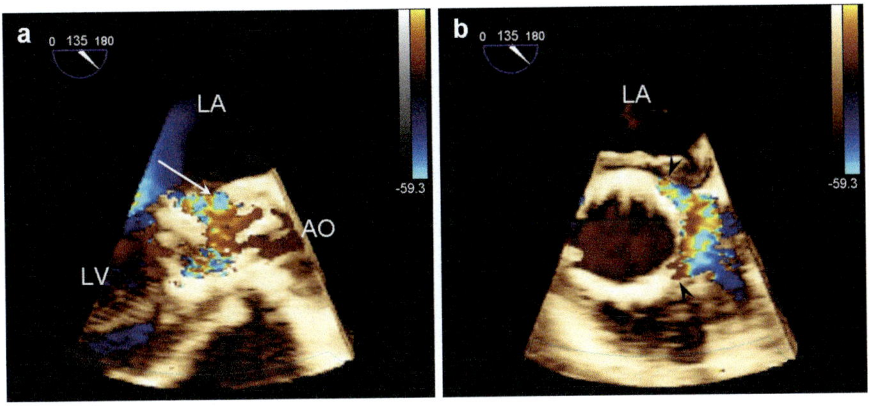

Fig. 5.31 In three dimensional color Doppler, long-axis view showed severe paravalvular leakage (arrow, **a**). In short-axis view, the origin of the paravalvular regurgitation ranged from one to four o'clock position (arrow heads, **b**)

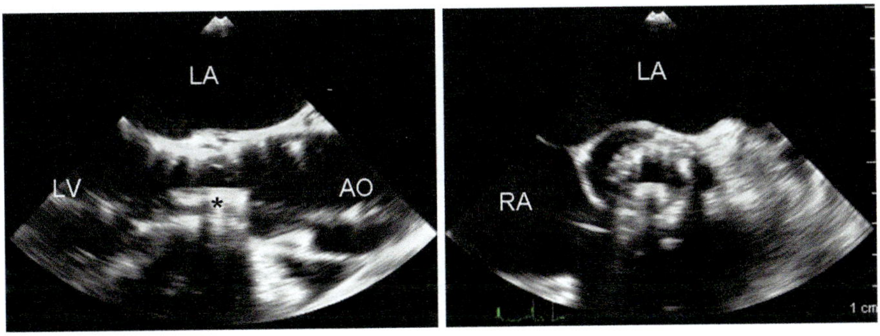

Fig. 5.32 In x-plane view during the redo valve-in-valve implantation, the crimped SAPIEN valve (29 mm, asterisk) was advanced into the previous implanted CoreValve by the delivery system (arrow heads)

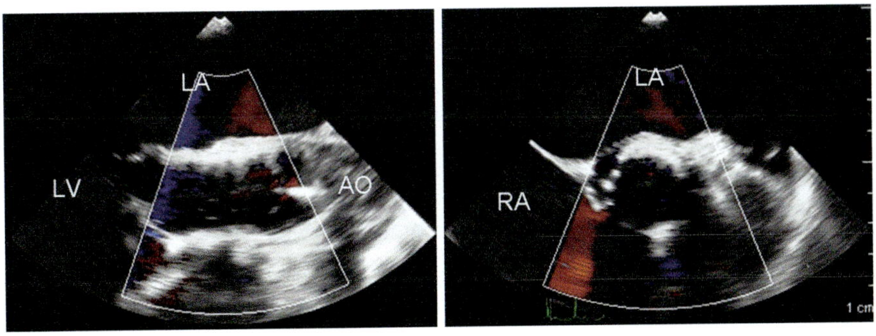

Fig. 5.33 In color Doppler during the procedure, the balloon was inflated to extend the SAPINE valve. There was trivial paravalvular leakage remaining

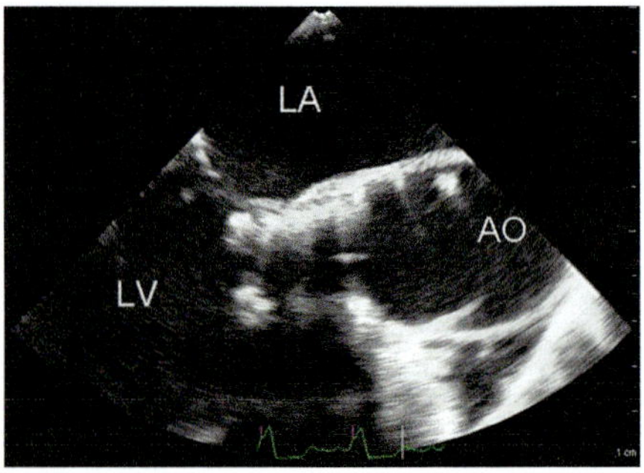

Fig. 5.34 After the valve-in-valve implantation, the SAPIEN valve was well positioned and worked normally within the CoreValve

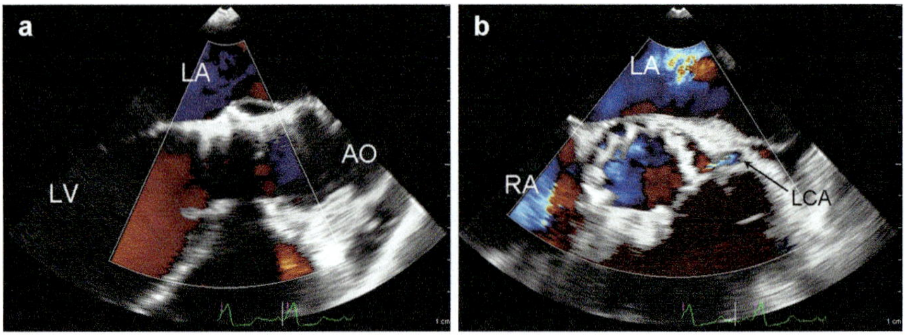

Fig. 5.35 In long- (**a**) and short-axis view (**b**) with color Doppler after the procedure, there was trivial paravalvular leakage remaining and the left coronary artery (LCA) with flow was also demonstrated in the short axis view

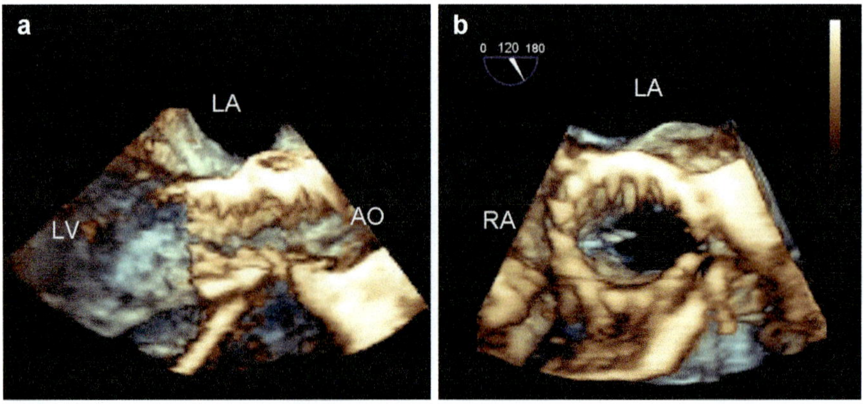

Fig. 5.36 In three dimensional long- (**a**) and short-axis view (**b**) after the valve-in-valve implantation, the SAPIEN valve was well positioned and worked normally within the CoreValve

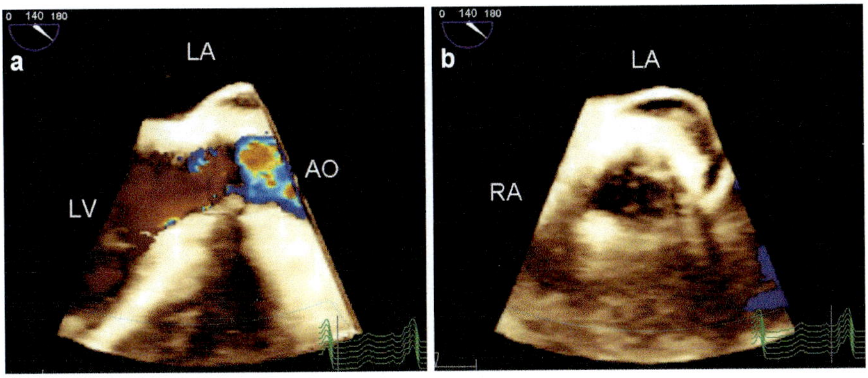

Fig. 5.37 In three dimensional long- (**a**) and short-axis view (**b**) with color Doppler after the procedure, there was trivial paravalvular leakage remaining

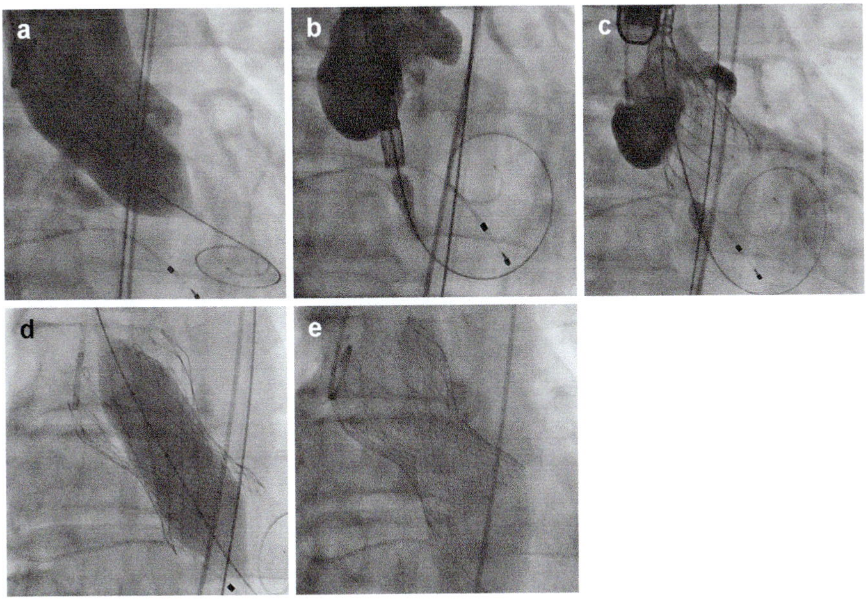

Fig. 5.38 Aortic root angiography during the first transcatheter aortic valve implantation of the CoreValve. (**a**) Contrast injection during valvuloplasty showed the position of cusps. (**b**) The crimped CoreValve aligned within the native aortic valve. (**c**) Then the CoreValve started to deploy from the proximal part of the frame to the distal. (**d**) Post-dilation was performed to reduce paravalvular leakage. (**e**) The CoreValve was detached form the catheter and the pigtail was withdrawn

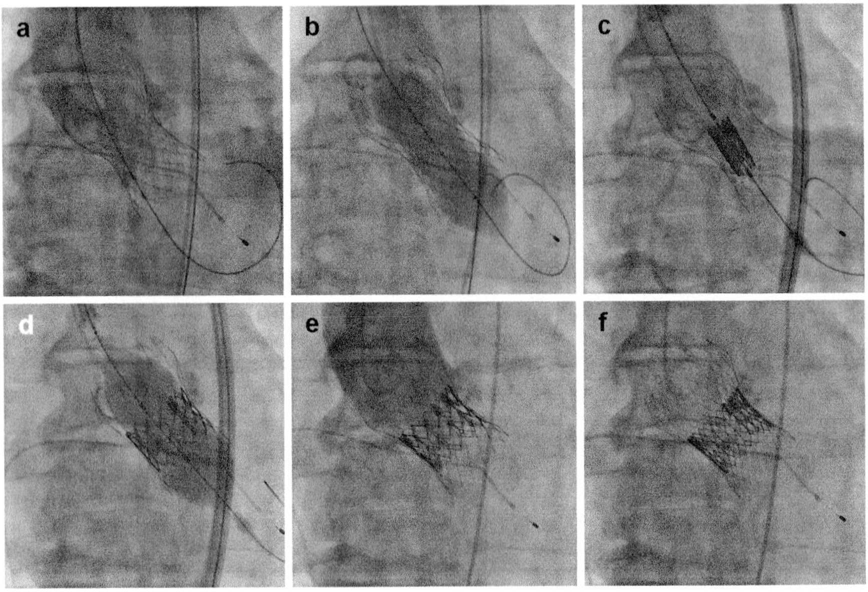

Fig. 5.39 Aortic root angiography during the second transcatheter aortic valve implantation of the SAPIEN valve. (**a**) The guiding wire advanced across the previous implanted CoreValve. (**b**) The balloon valvuloplasty was performed. (**c**) The SAPIEN valve was advanced into the CoreValve to its appropriate position. (**d**) The SAPIEN valve was expanded. (**e**, **f**) The deliver sheath was removed, the position of the valve was confirmed, and no coronary obstruction was revealed

Paravalvular leak happens more often after transcatheter aortic valve implantation than after surgical replacement. Paravalvular leak may be caused by prosthesis undersizing, underexpansion, incorrect positioning, or impingement of calcifications interfering with stent expansion. Even mild paravalvular leak is associated with increased late mortality. Clinical experience with percutaneous closure of paravalvular leak after transcatheter aortic valve implantation is limited, but valve-in-valve implantation could be a reasonable strategy in these high-risk patients.

In this patient, the native aortic valve was bicuspid with bulky calcification, which interfered with the CoreValve expansion, therefore induced severe paravalvular leakage. The SAPIEN valve has a frame shorter and denser than the CoreValve's which allowed controlled deployment and provided better annulus sealing. Thus, a SAPIEN valve was chosen to serve for the valve-in-valve implantation. In the end, the paravalvular leakage reduced significantly.

5.5 CoreValve Embolized to Ascending Aorta

An 86-year-old male patient had a history of hypertension, gouty arthritis, dyslipidemia, and dementia. He suffered from exertional dyspnea and general weakness for several months. Auscultation showed a grade 2/6 systolic murmur over right sternal border. Echocardiography showed moderate to severe aortic regurgitation and mild stenosis. Therefore he was scheduled for a transcastheter aortic valve implantation (Figs. 5.40, 5.41, 5.42, 5.43, 5.44, 5.45, 5.46, and 5.47; Videos 5.40a, 5.40b, 5.41a, 5.41b, 5.42a, 5.42b, 5.43, 5.44a, 5.44b, 5.45a, 5.45b, 5.46a, 5.46b, and 5.47).

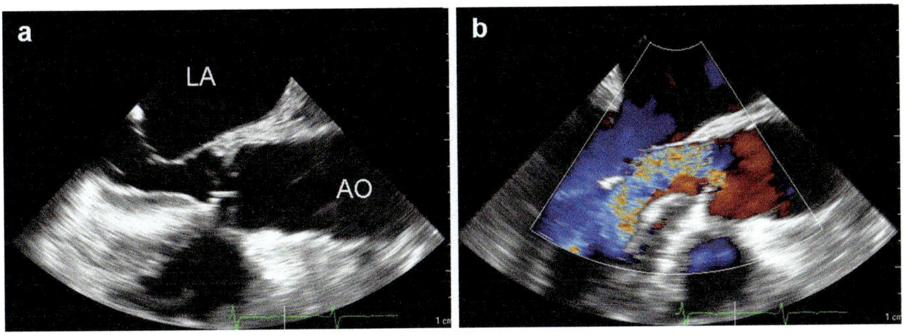

Fig. 5.40 In transesophageal echocardiography, midesophageal long-axis approach (**a**) with color Doppler (**b**), the thickened aortic valve with prolapse leaflet induced mild stenosis and moderate to severe regurgitation

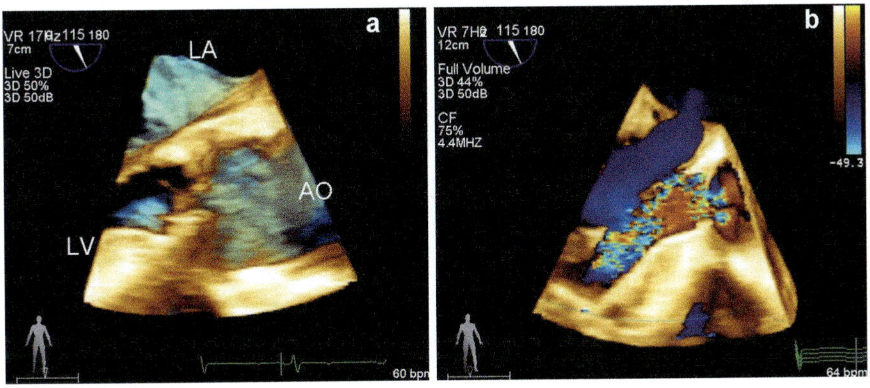

Fig. 5.41 Three dimensional midesophageal long-axis approach (**a**) with color Doppler (**b**) showed thickened aortic valve with prolapse leaflet induced mild stenosis and moderate to severe regurgitation

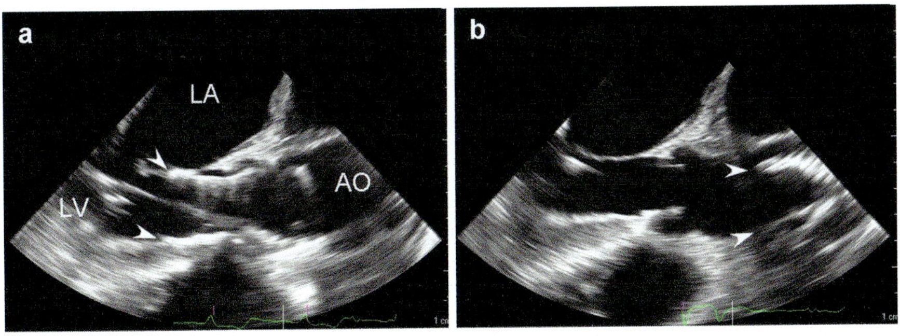

Fig. 5.42 During the transcatheter aortic valve implantation, the CoreValve (arrow heads) deployed (**a**); however, during detachment, it migrated upward into the ascending aorta (**b**)

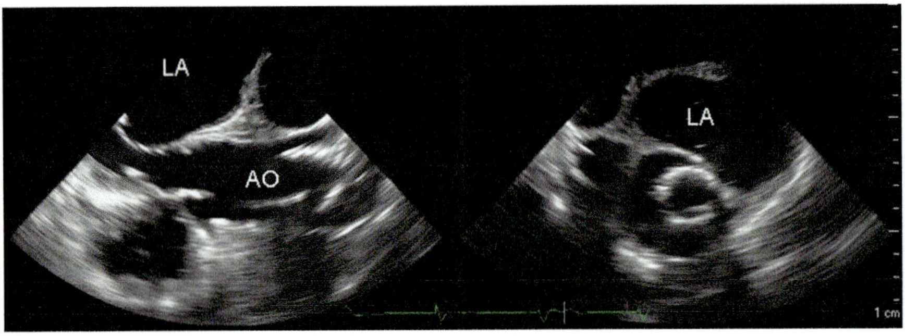

Fig. 5.43 In x-plane view, the CoreValve migrated upward into the ascending aorta without full deployment

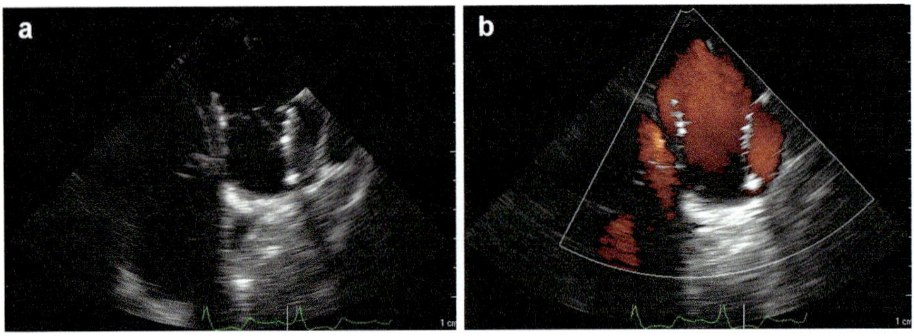

Fig. 5.44 The first implanted CoreValve slipped into ascending aorta after implantation in just few minutes. The device, which was in good shape, opened and closed fully with cardiac cycle (**a**) without significant mosaic flow (**b**)

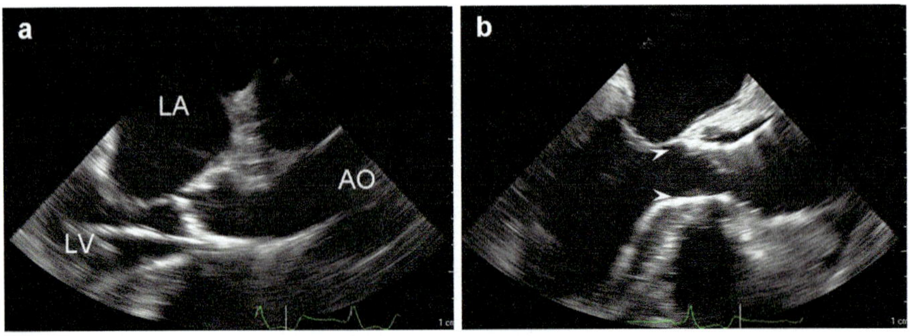

Fig. 5.45 The second CoreValve was implanted (**a**). This time, the device (arrow heads) was well deployed and positioned (**b**)

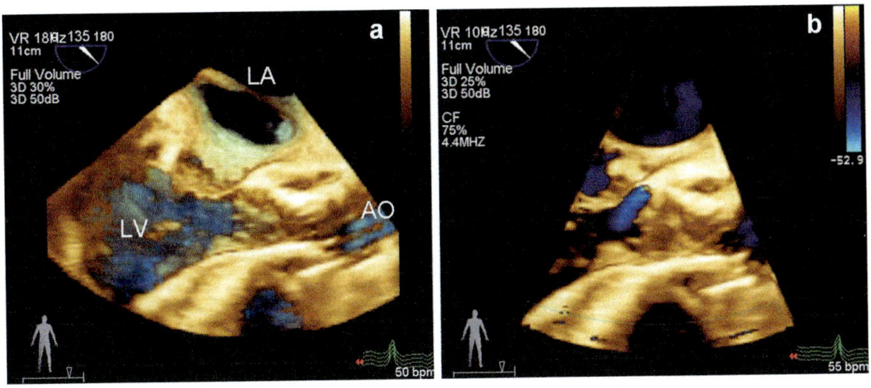

Fig. 5.46 Three dimensional long-axis views after the implantation. The newly implanted CoreValve was well positioned and deployed (**a**), and only trivial paravalvular leakage was present in color Doppler (**b**)

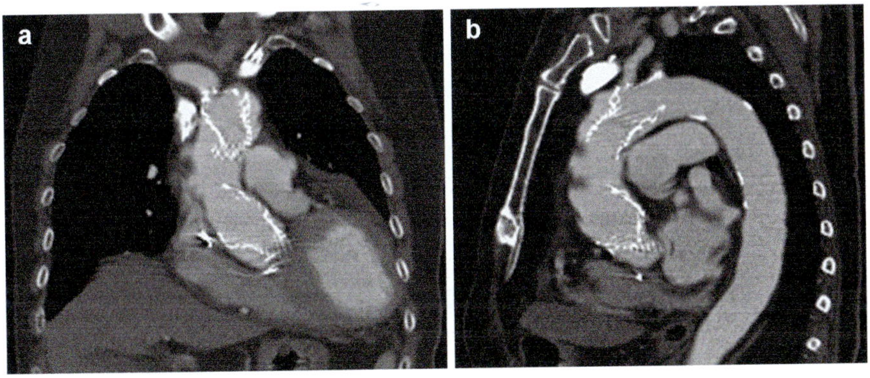

Fig. 5.47 Coronary (**a**) and sagittal slice (**b**) of computed tomography with contrast showed the position of the valves at the end of the procedure. The migrated CoreValve was seen in ascending aorta, the zone around the innominate artery and left common carotid artery. The other CoreValve was within the aortic root

Transcatheter heart valve migration is a largely but not entirely preventable complication with transcatheter heart valves. The absence of calcification of the native annulus, which is usually seen in stenosis degenerative valve disease, may increase the risk of prosthesis migration.

In this patient, to treat the aortic regurgitation due to leaflet prolapse was the major purpose of the transcatheter aortic valve implantation. Therefore, the non-calcified aortic annulus failed to block the CoreValve. Fortunately, owing to the self-expanding property, the CoreValve was stable within the ascending aorta without aortic injury or strut fracture.

5.6 SAPIEN Valve Embolized to Abdominal Aorta

An 86-year-old patient had a history of coronary artery disease, hypertension, and peripheral arterial occlusive disease. He had suffered from occasional chest pain and dyspnea of exertion for two years. He visited our outpatient department due to intolerable symptoms, where grade three murmurs over all auscultation areas were detected. Transthoracic echocardiography revealed severe aortic stenosis. Consequently, transcatheter aortic valve implantation was indicated (Figs. 5.48, 5.49, 5.50, 5.51, 5.52, 5.53, 5.54, 5.55, 5.56, 5.57, 5.58, 5.59, 5.60, and 5.61; Videos 5.48, 5.49, 5.50, 5.51, 5.52, 5.53, 5.54a, 5.54b, 5.55, 5.56, 5.57, 5.58, 5.59, 5.60, and 5.61).

The most common reason of transcatheter heart valve embolization was placing the valve too high into the ascending aorta. The migrated device can embolize in any portion of the aorta. Maintaining a coaxial wire within the prosthesis prevents it from becoming inverted and obstructing aortic flow. Repositioning can be accomplished by withdrawing the transcatheter heart valve on an inflated valvuloplasty balloon to a secure position in the more distal aorta while avoiding aortic injury.

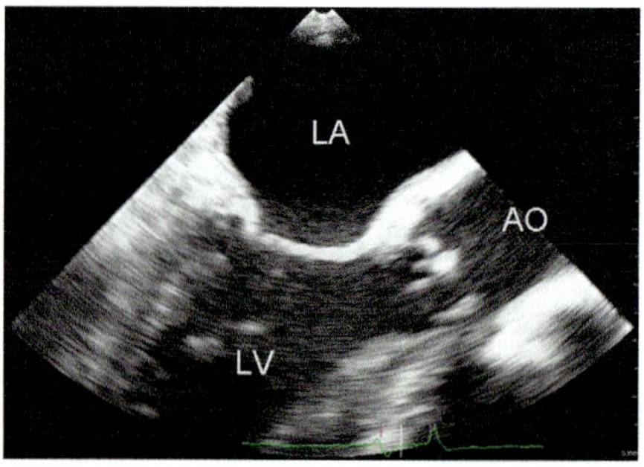

Fig. 5.48 In transesophageal echocardiographic mid-esophageal long-axis views, the calcified aortic valve reduced cusp separation

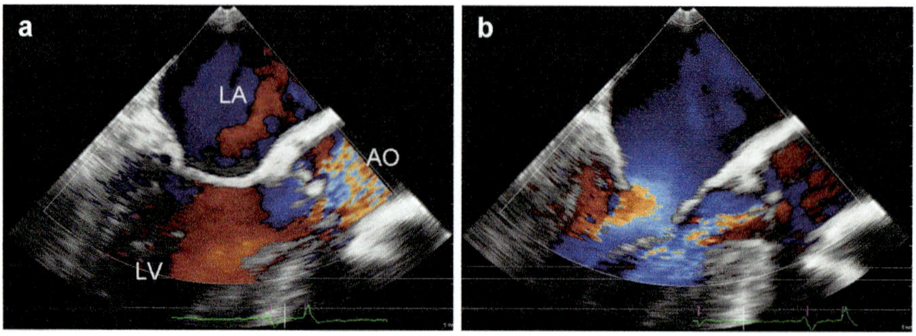

Fig. 5.49 In mid-esophageal long-axis views with color Doppler, the calcified aortic valve reduced cusp separation, which caused turbulent left ventricular outflow in systole (**a**) and mild to moderate regurgitation in diastole (**b**)

Fig. 5.50 In three dimensional mid-esophageal long-axis views, the calcified aortic valve reduced cusp separation

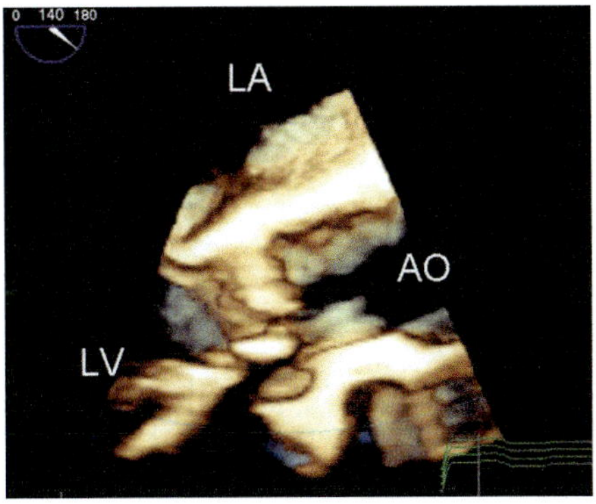

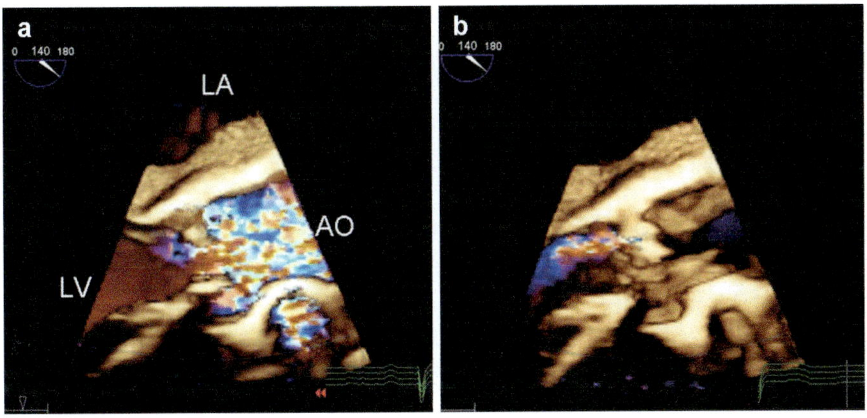

Fig. 5.51 Three dimensional color Doppler showed turbulent outflow across calcified aortic valve in systole (**a**) and mild to moderate aortic regurgitation in diastole (**b**)

Fig. 5.52 During transcatheter aortic valve implantation, the guiding wire advanced through the calcified aortic valve and the prosthetic SAPHINE valve (arrow heads) was deployed

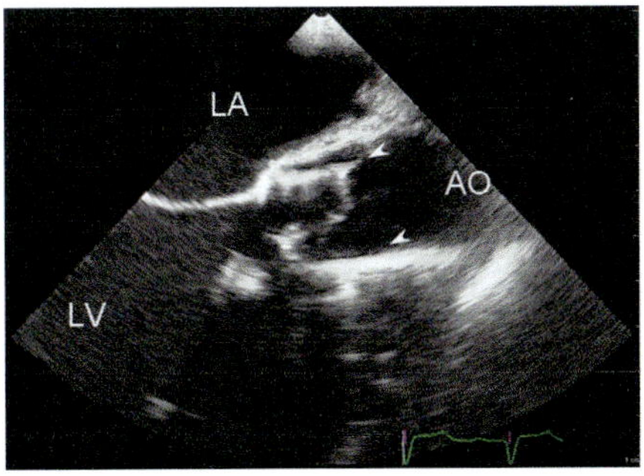

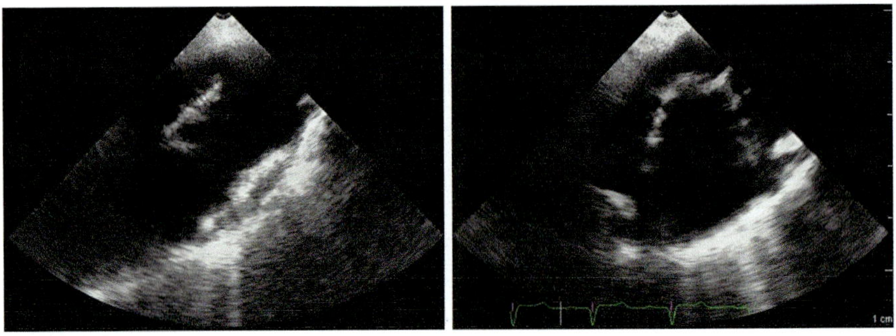

Fig. 5.53 In x-plane view, the SAPHINE valve migrated upward into the ascending aorta immediately after it was released

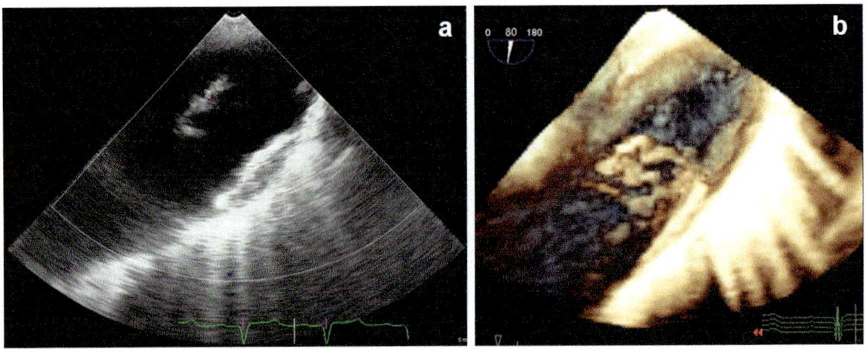

Fig. 5.54 In two (**a**) and three dimensional views (**b**) of ascending aorta, the migrated SARHINE valve stayed unstably and rocked in ascending aorta

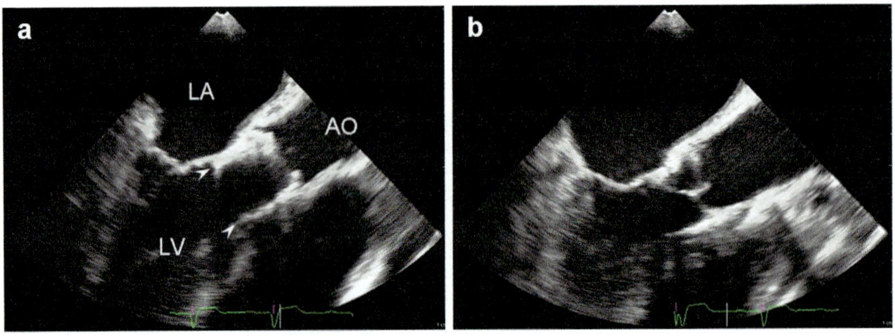

Fig. 5.55 The second SAPHINE valve (arrow heads) was implanted afterward. This time, the device was well positioned with in the aortic annulus and presented normal function in systole (**a**) and diastole (**b**)

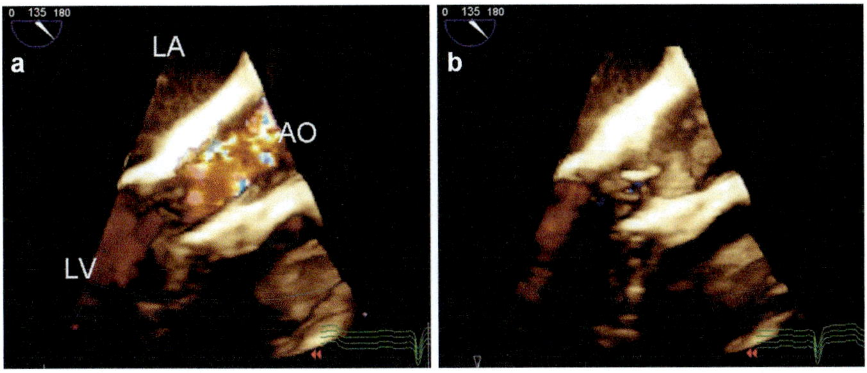

Fig. 5.56 Three dimensional color Doppler after the second SAPHINE valve implantation. There were normal left ventricular outflow in systole (**a**) and minimal valvular regurgitation in diastole (**b**)

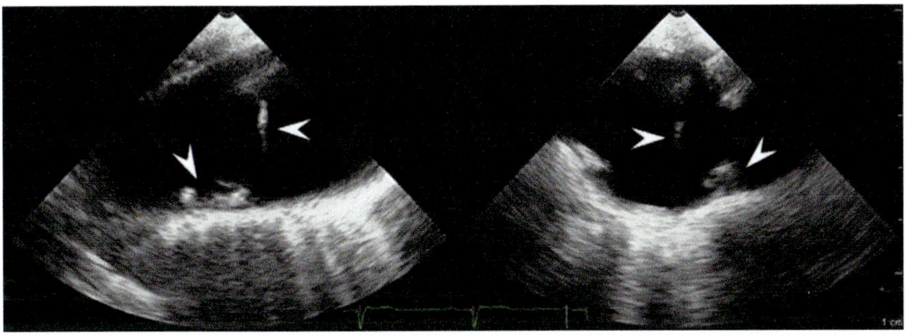

Fig. 5.57 Two dimensional transesophageal echocardiogram of ascending aorta during the procedure, several thrombus-like echodensitis (arrow heads) were floating in the ascending aorta

Fig. 5.58 Three dimensional view of ascending aorta during the procedure, several echodensitis (arrow heads) were floating in the ascending aorta

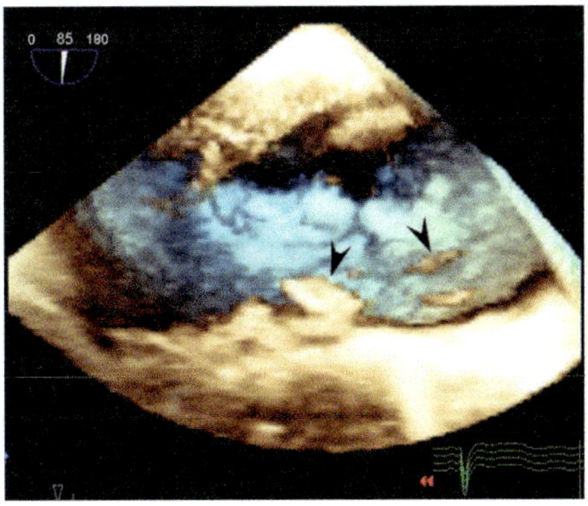

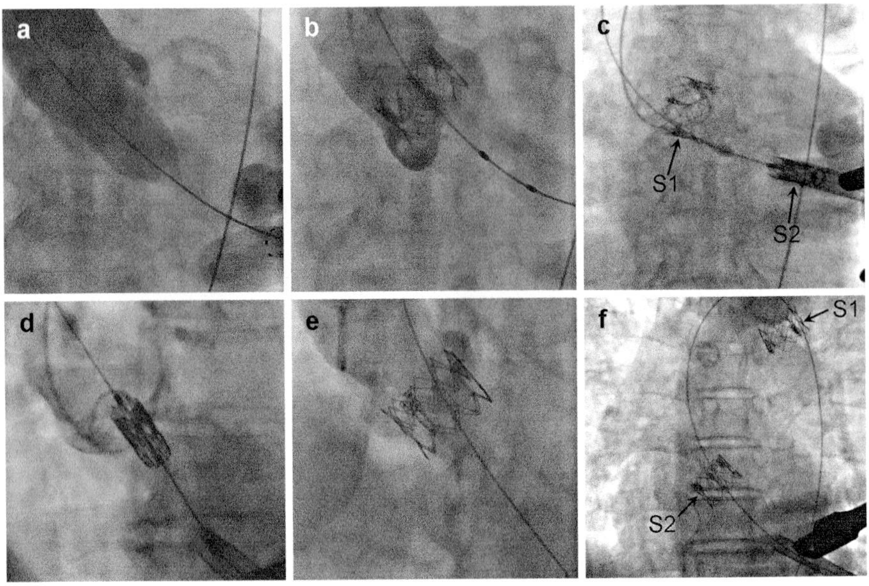

Fig. 5.59 Aortic root angiography during implantation of the SAPIEN valve. (**a**) Contrast injection ensured the position of the cusps, and the guiding catheter advanced across and aligned within the aortic annulus. (**b**) The SAPIEN valve was deployed, whose position was too high into the ascending aorta. (**c**) First implanted SAPIEN valve (S1) migrated upward to the ascending and the crimped following SAPINE (S2) valve was advanced. (**d**, **e**) The position of the transcatheter aortic valve was confirmed then it was deployed. (**f**) The relative position of the first and the following implanted SAPIEN valve was demonstrated

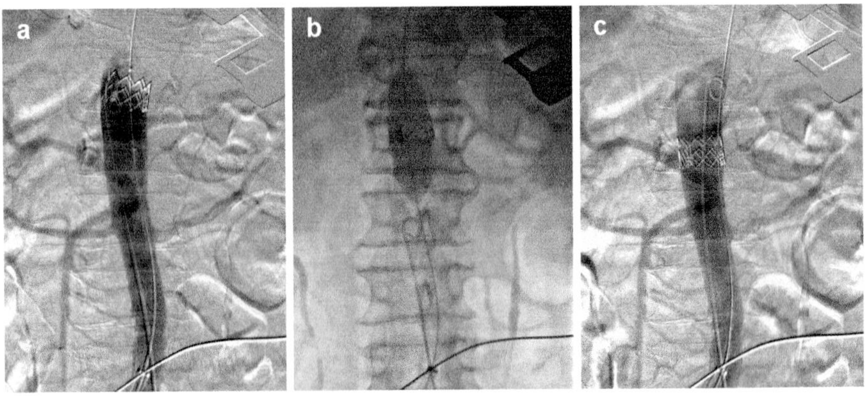

Fig. 5.60 Angiography of abdominal aorta with and without digital substraction. (**a**) The first implanted SAPIEN valve migrated to the abdominal aorta with the coaxial wire within it. (**b**) The valvuloplasty balloon was inflated to secure the position of the SAPIEN valve. (**c**) The final position the device anchored was revealed. There was no significant evidence of aortic injury or obstruction

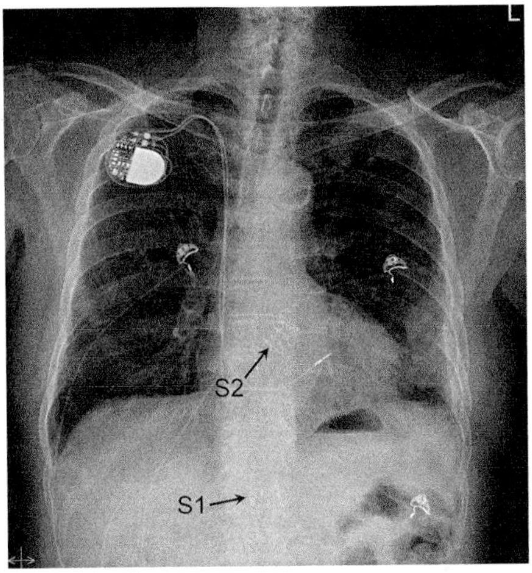

Fig. 5.61 Chest X-ray after the transcatheter aortic valve implantation. The migrated SAPIEN valve (S1), which was implanted first, was seen in the abdominal aorta. The other SAPIEN valve (S2) was seen in the aortic portion

5.7 Coronary Obstruction After Transcatheter Aortic Valve Implantation

An 84-year-old female patient had a past history of diabetes mellitus and hypertension. She suffered chest tightness recently. Echocardiography and cardiac catheterization showed severe aortic stenosis and double vessel coronary artery disease. Therefore, transcatheter aortic valve impanation and percutaneous coronary intervention were suggested by the heart team (Figs. 5.62, 5.63, 5.64, 5.65, 5.66, 5.67, 5.68, 5.69, 5.70, 5.71, and 5.72; Videos 5.62a, 5.62b, 5.63, 5.64, 5.65a, 5.65b, 5.66, 5.67a, 5.67b, 5.68, 5.69, 5.70, 5.71, and 5.72).

The majority of occlusions occurred immediately after valve implantation due to displacement of the calcified native cusp over the coronary ostium. Coronary obstruction occurred more frequently in the left coronary artery. Risk factors appeared to be female sex and no previous bypass surgery. A narrow aortic root with shallow sinuses of Valsalva (leaving little room to accommodate the calcified native aortic leaflets after valve deployment) may also be an important factor

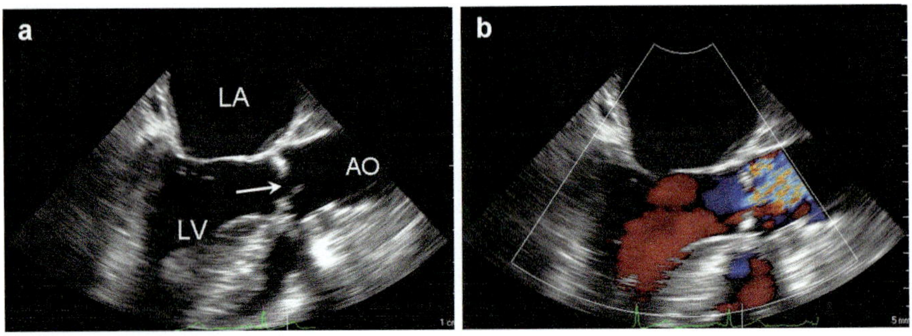

Fig. 5.62 In transesophageal echocardiographic midesophageal long-axis approach with color Doppler, thickened aortic valve reduced cusp separation (arrow, **a**) and caused turbulent left ventricular outflow (**b**)

Fig. 5.63 Three dimensional long-axis approach showed thickened aortic valve reduced cusp separation

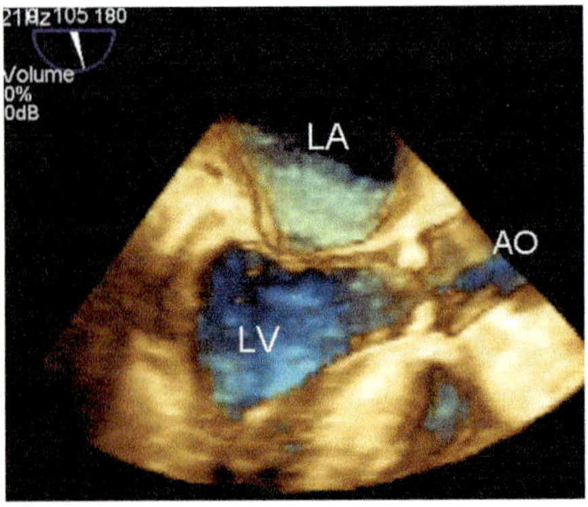

Fig. 5.64 During the transcatheter aortic valve implantation, the guiding wire advanced through the aortic valve and the CoreValve (26 mm) was delivered

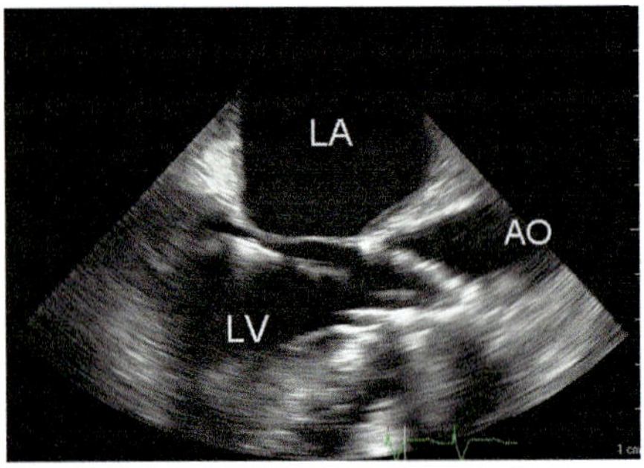

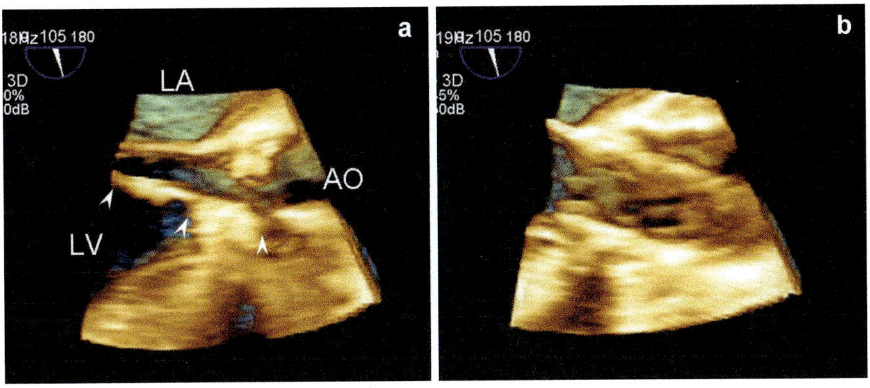

Fig. 5.65 In three dimensional views during the procedure, the guiding wire (arrow heads, **a**) advanced through the aortic valve, then the CoreValve was delivered and deployed (**b**)

Fig. 5.66 In three dimensional long-axis approach after the transcatheter aortic valve implantation, the aortic valve was well positioned

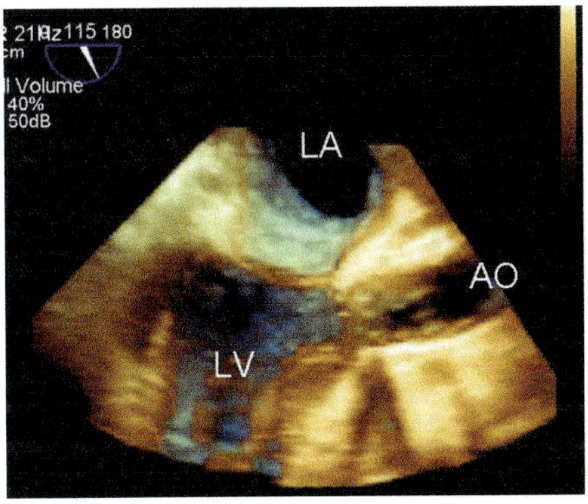

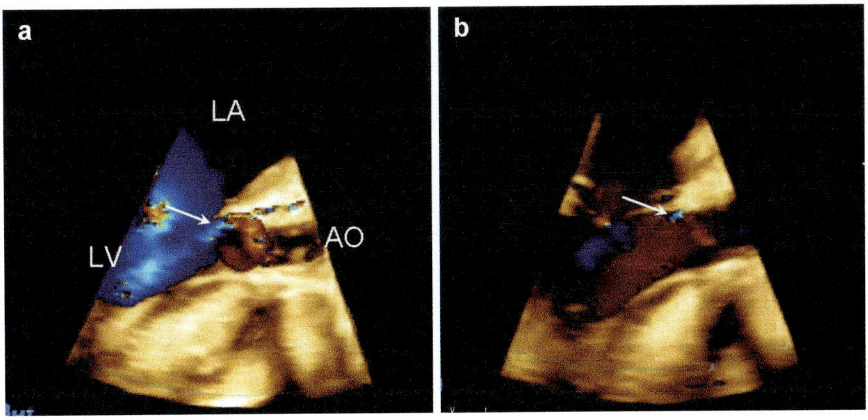

Fig. 5.67 In three dimensional color Doppler after the CoreValve detachment, mild paravalvular leakage (arrow, **a**) was presented initially, while the device kept self-expanding and reduced the leakage (**b**)

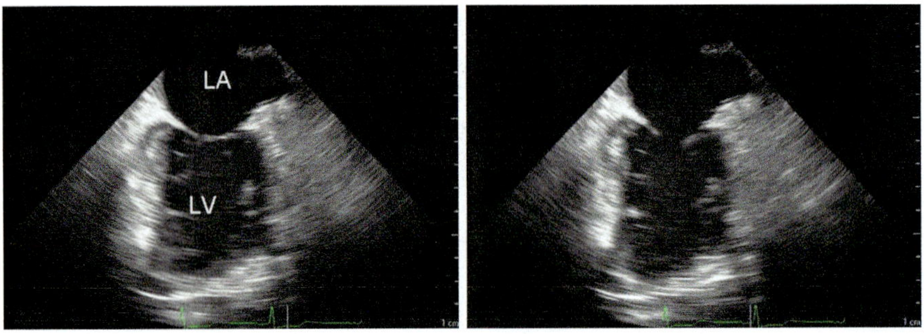

Fig. 5.68 However, severe left ventricle dysfunction presented immediately after the CoreValve full expansion

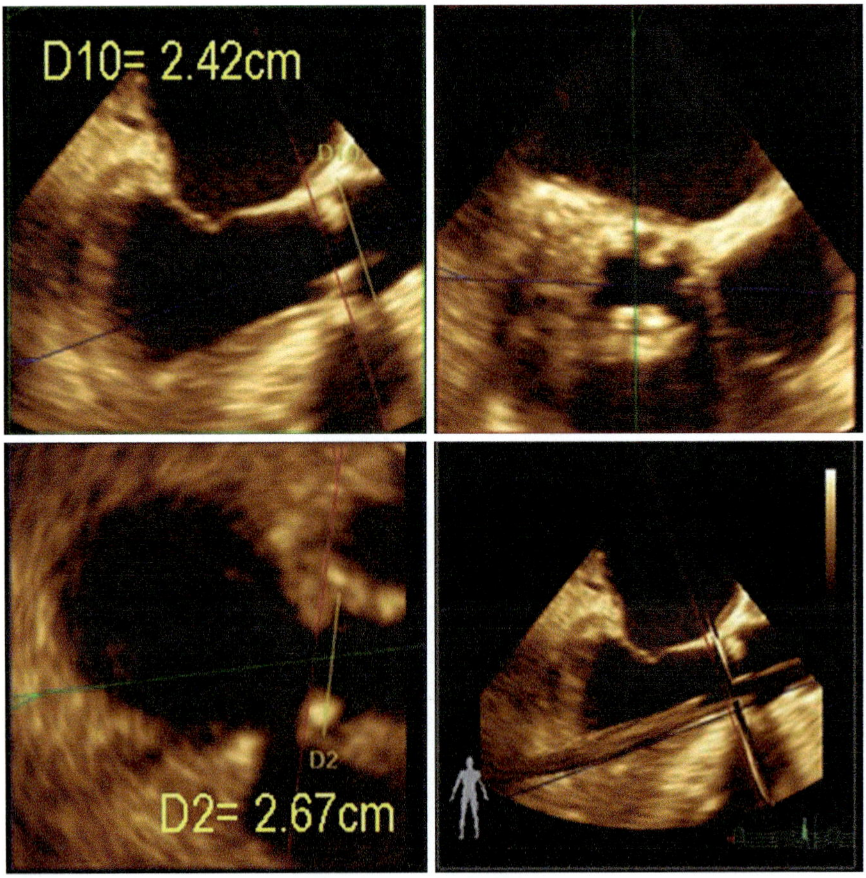

Fig. 5.69 To analyze the reason of the incident, multi-planer reconstruction of the three dimensional image was reviewed. The sinus of Valsalva diameter measured 2.42 cm (D1) and 2.67 cm (D2) in sagittal and coronal planes, which left little room to accommodate the native aortic leaflets after CoreValve deployment, therefore occluded the coronary ostium

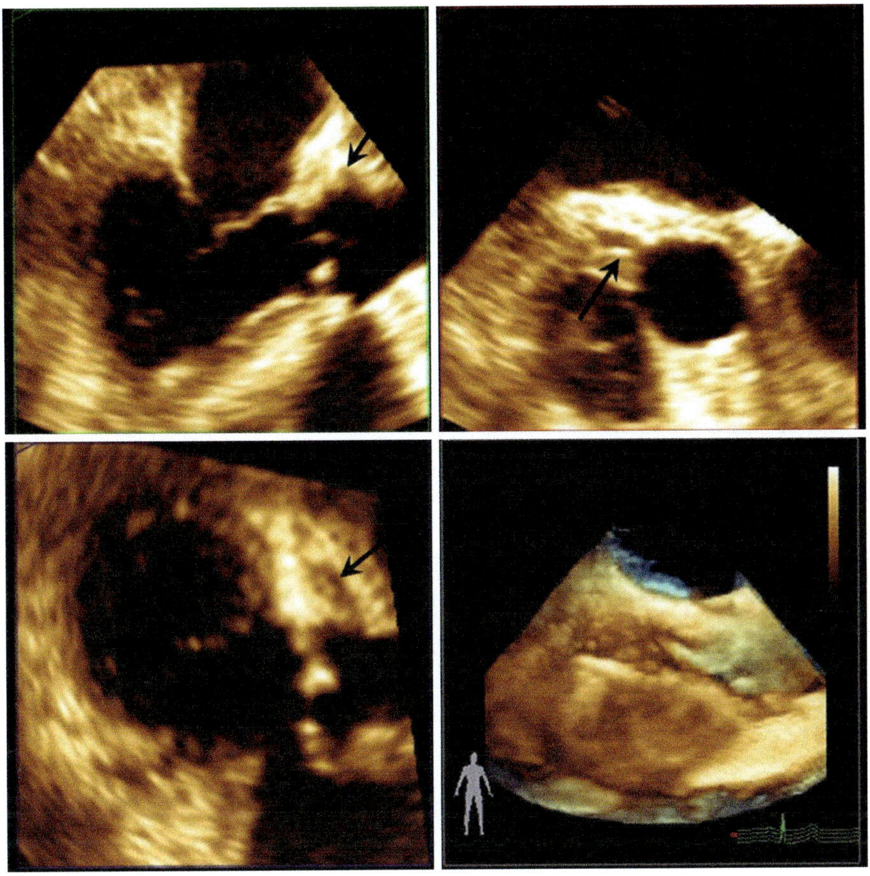

Fig. 5.70 The location of the patent of left main coronary artery (arrow) was demonstrated in multi-planar reconstruction

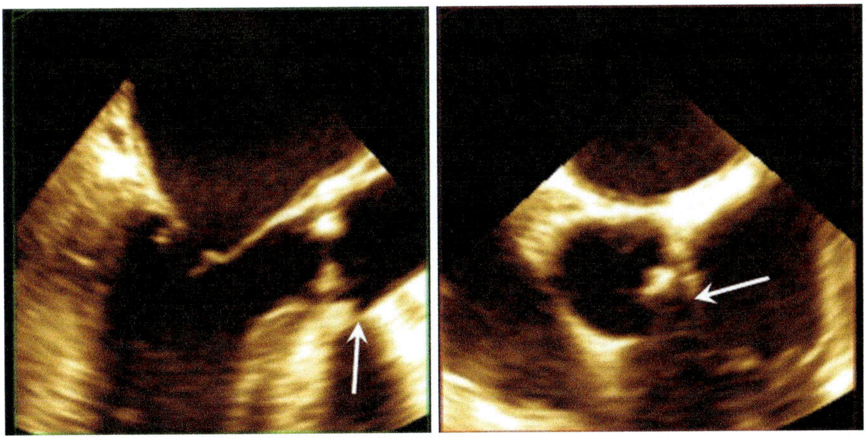

Fig. 5.71 The location of the patent of right coronary artery (arrow) was also demonstrated

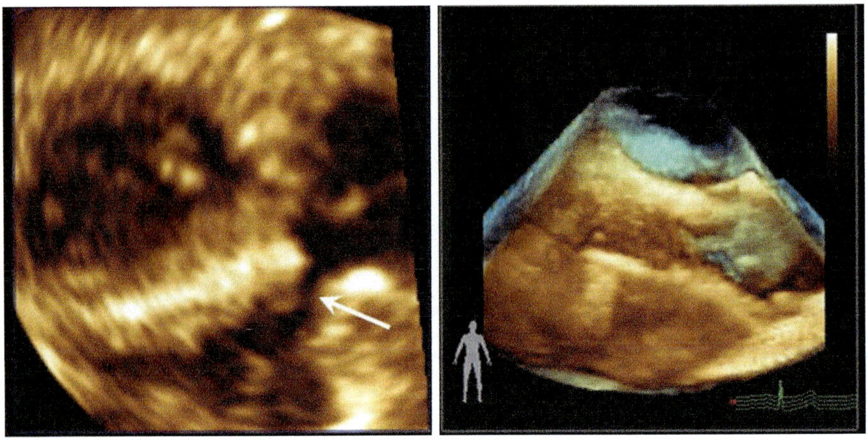

Fig. 5.71 (continued)

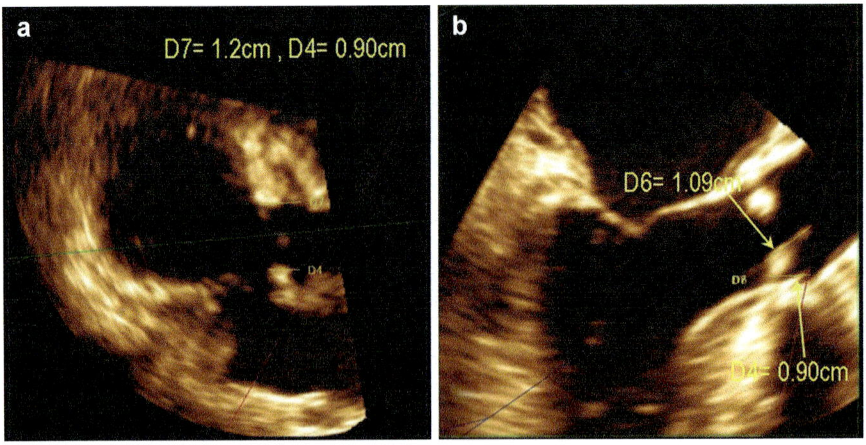

Fig. 5.72 The height of the left main coronary artery (D7) and right coronary artery (D4) was 1.2 and 0.90 cm (**a**). The right coronary cusp length (D6) was 1.09 cm, which was longer than the right coronary height (D4), the risk of occlusion was significant (**b**)

5.8 Iatrogenic Coronary Damage After Mitral Valve-in-Valve Implantation

A 42-year-old female patient with a history of infective endocarditis received mitral and aortic replacement 15 years ago. In spite of regular follow up with medical treatment, she developed dyspnea on exertion several months ago. The echocardiography showed failure of the mitral prosthesis along with severe regurgitation and moderate stenosis. Therefore, transcatheter mitral valve-in-valve replacement was arranged and done (Figs. 5.73, 5.74, 5.75, 5.76, 5.77, 5.78, 5.79, 5.80, 5.81, and 5.82; Videos 5.73, 5.74, 5.75, 5.76, 5.77, 5.78, 5.79a, 5.79b, 5.80a, 5.80b, 5.81, 5.82a, and 5.82b).

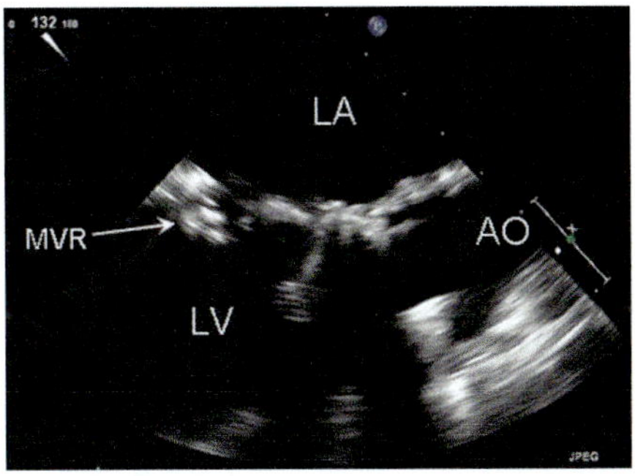

Fig. 5.73 Transesophageal echocardiography, mid-esophageal long-axis view. The patient had received mitral valve replacement (MVR) with porcine valve before. The bioprosthetic valve failed to open and close properly

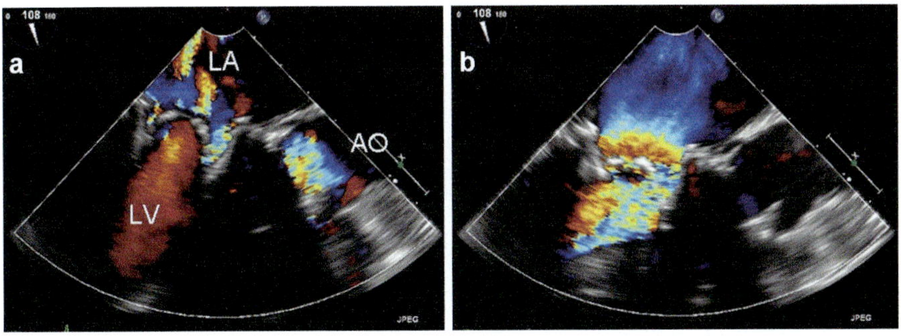

Fig. 5.74 In mid-esophageal long-axis color Doppler, severe mitral regurgitation was demonstrated in systole (**a**), and flow across the mitral prosthesis was mosaic in diastole (**b**)

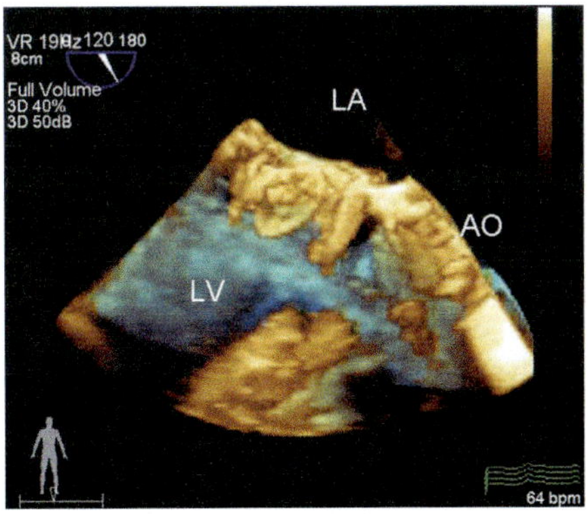

Fig. 5.75 In three dimensional long-axis view, the bioprosthetic mitral valve failed to open and close properly

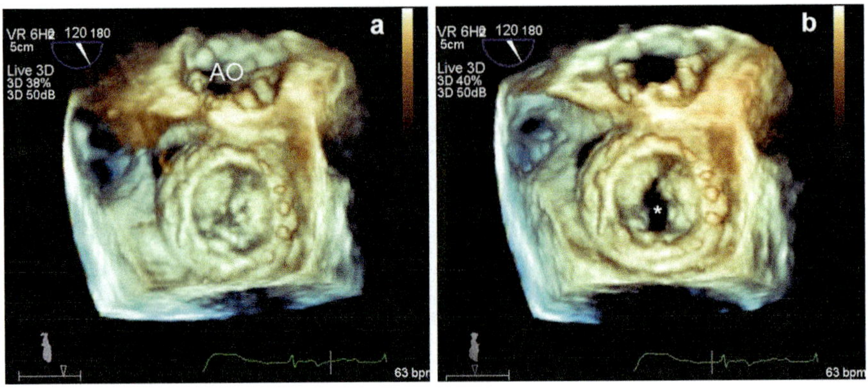

Fig. 5.76 Three-dimensional en face view showed thickened bioprosthetic mitral valve prolapsed into the left atrium in diastole (**a**) Restrictive mobility of the prosthetic leaflets reduced the orifice was also demonstrated (asterisk, **b**)

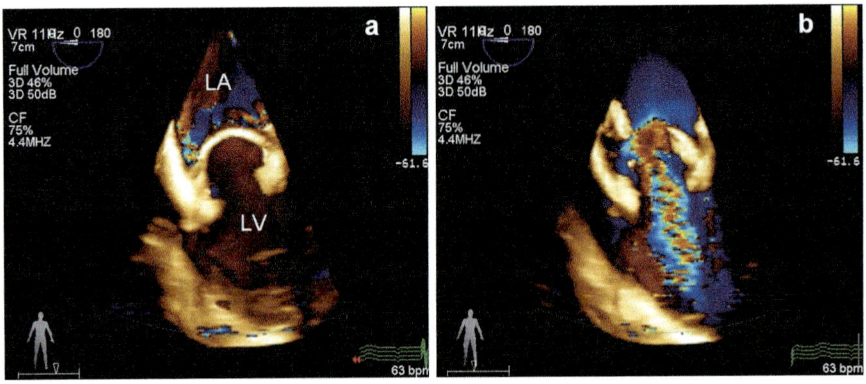

Fig. 5.77 In three-dimensional color Doppler, (**a**) severe mitral regurgitation was demonstrated in systole. (**b**) Flow across the mitral prosthesis was mosaic in diastole

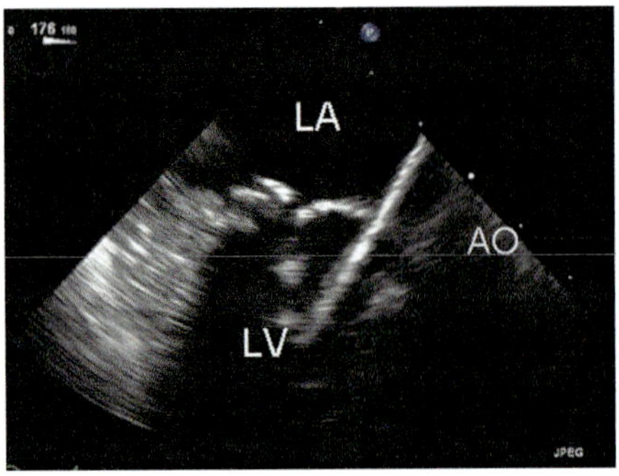

Fig. 5.78 During the transcatheter valve-in-valve implantation, after several times attempted try to find the left ventricular apex, the guiding catheter advanced across the mitral bioprosthesis

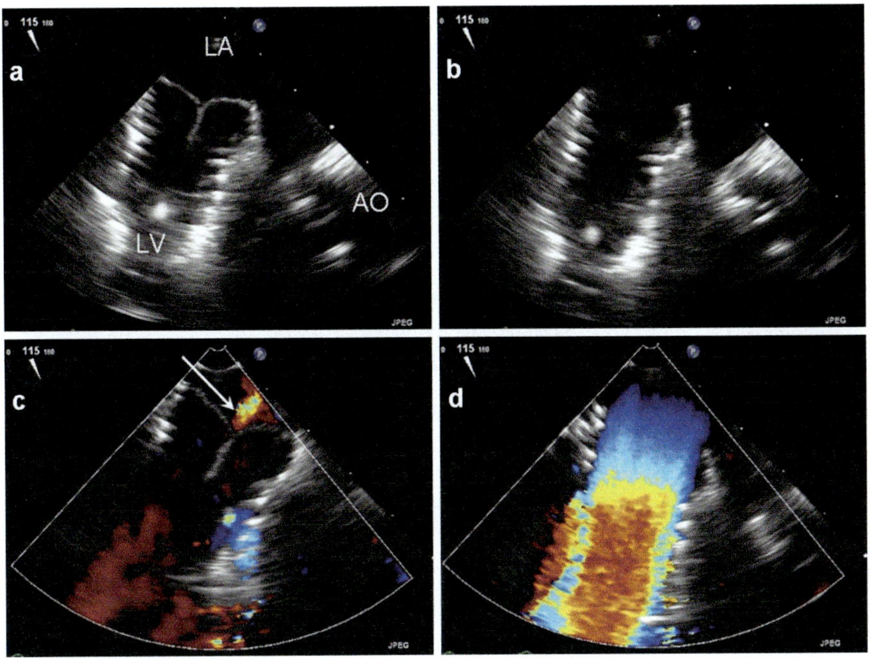

Fig. 5.79 After the Lotus valve (27 mm) was deployed, the valve closed (**a**) and opened (**b**) well with cardiac cycle. Color Doppler after the procedure showed trivial leakage (arrow, **c**) in systole and steady flow across the valve-in-valve mitral prosthesis in diastole (**d**)

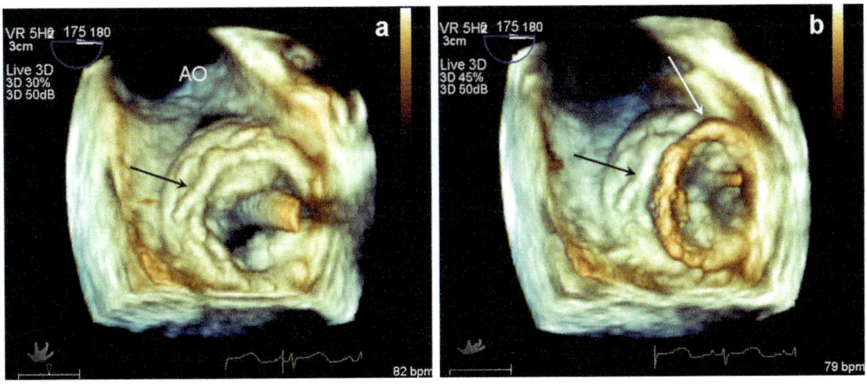

Fig. 5.80 Three-dimensional en face view during the procedure. The guiding catheter advanced across the mitral bioprosthesis (black arrow, **a**), and the Lotus valve (white arrow) was extended within it (**b**)

During the transapical mitral valve-in-valve procedure, a small left lateral thoracotomy to visualize the left ventricular apex was performed. Then a direct puncture of the left ventricle was made and a sheath was inserted into the chamber. However,

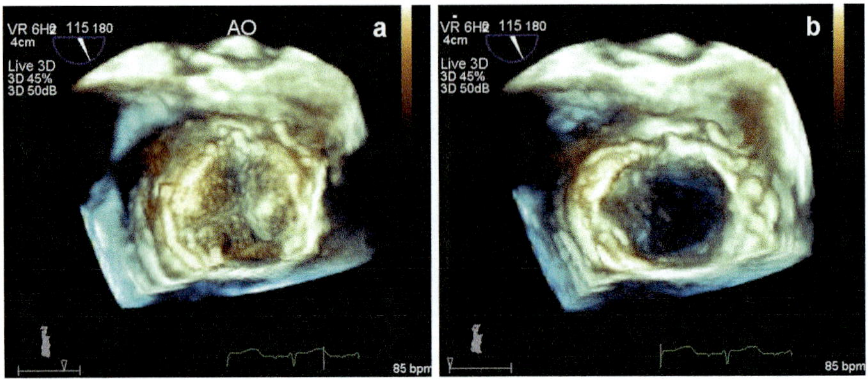

Fig. 5.81 In three-dimensional en face view after the procedure, the Lotus valve closed (**a**) and opened (**b**) well with cardiac cycle

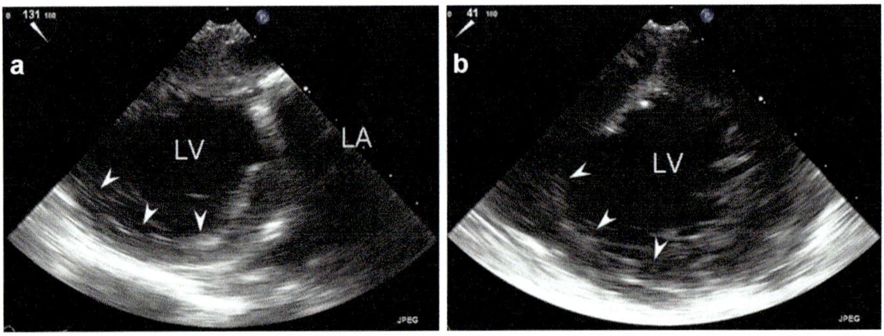

Fig. 5.82 Transgastric two-chamber (**a**) and short-axis (**b**) views after the closure of the thoracotomy for the transapical assessment, left ventricular anterior wall akinesis with aneurysm formation (arrow heads) was demonstrated

in this case, the patient received several times of direct punctures to find the most feasible position to advance the sheath. Therefore, closures of the punctured sites with patches were also done many times. Owing to the repeated sewing, the coronary arteries might be injured in the meanwhile. Finally, sadly, the patient turned out to have impaired heart function.

5.9 Periaortic Hematoma Formation and Coronary Injury After Transcatheter Aortic Valve Implantation

An 86-year-old male patient with a history of type two diabetes mellitus and chronic renal failure suffered exertional dyspnea and chest tightness for a month. Critical aortic stenosis was diagnosed by other hospital. Due persisted symptoms, he was admitted for further management (Figs. 5.83, 5.84, 5.85, 5.86, 5.87, 5.88, 5.89, 5.90, 5.91, 5.92, 5.93, 5.94, 5.95, 5.96, 5.97, 5.98, and 5.99; Videos 5.83, 5.84, 5.85, 5.86, 5.87, 5.88, 5.89, 5.90a, 5.90b, 5.91, 5.92a, 5.92b, 5.93, 5.94, 5.95, 5.96, 5.97, 5.98, and 5.99).

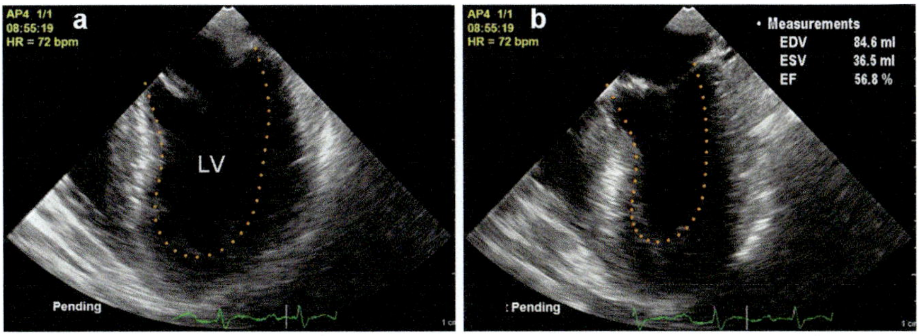

Fig. 5.83 In transesophageal echocardiographic midesophageal four-chamber approach in diastole (**a**) and systole (**b**), normal baseline ventricular function was demonstrated (*EDV* end diastolic volume, *ESV* end systolic volume, *EF* ejection fraction)

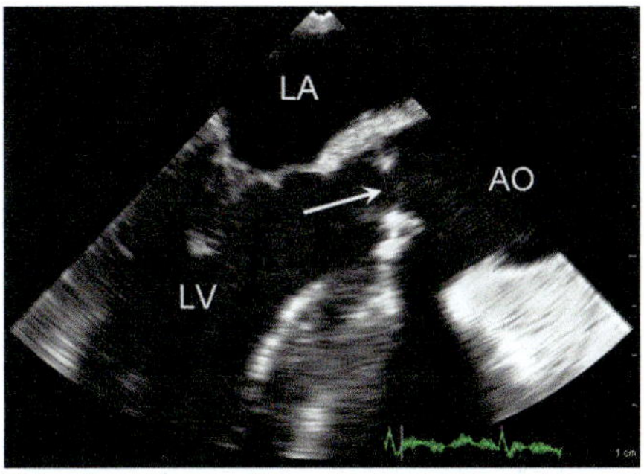

Fig. 5.84 In transesophageal echocardiographic midesophageal long-axis approach, thickened and calcified aortic valve (arrow) reduced its mobility

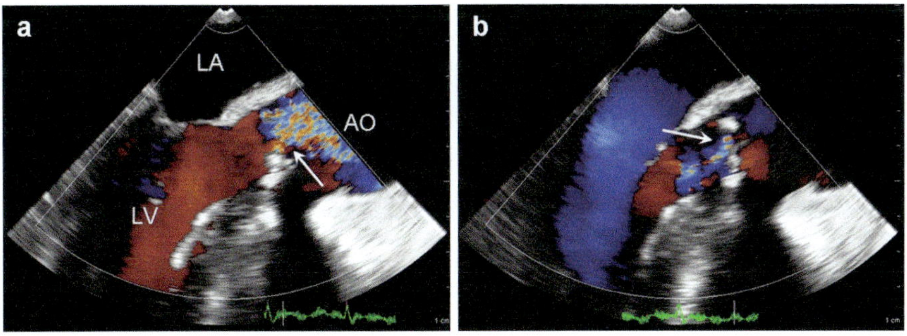

Fig. 5.85 Color Doppler showed turbulent left atrium outflow in systole (arrow, **a**) and mild to moderate regurgitation in diastole (arrow, **b**)

Periaortic hematoma can be resulted from microrupture of the aorta. Compared with intramural hematoma, which is bleeding into the wall of the aorta, periaortic hematoma arises from a microperforation of all three layers of the aorta. Moreover, forms of the hematoma appear like a tissue-density mass around the outside of the aortic root. The perforation likely occurs after stretching of the aortic wall from bulky calcium during balloon deployment of the transcatheter heart valve.

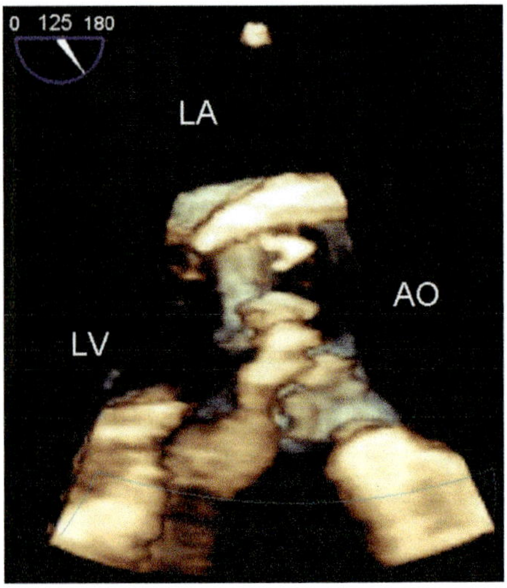

Fig. 5.86 Three dimensional long-axis view showed calcified aortic valve reduced cusp separation

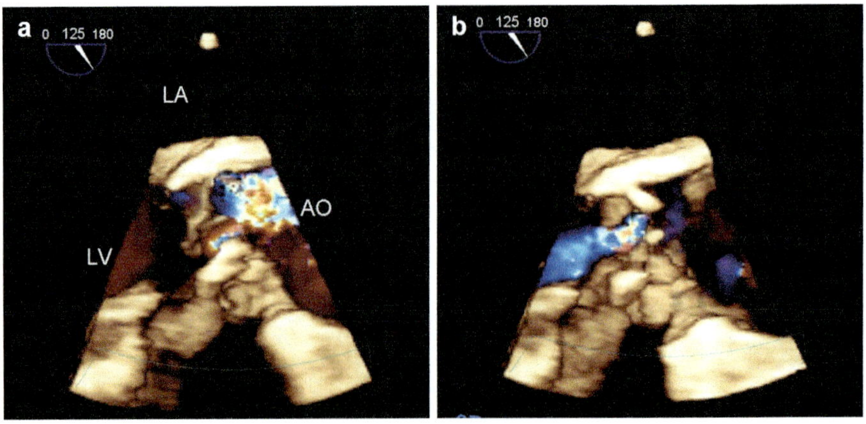

Fig. 5.87 Three dimensional color Doppler showed turbulent outflow across calcified aortic valve in systole (**a**) and mild to moderate aortic regurgitation in diastole (**b**)

This process performs to be self-limiting, with the microperforation sealing quickly once the balloon is deflated or the aorta is no longer stretched. Conservative managements of the periaortic hematoma, including administration of protamine, continued intubation with restricted activity, and meticulous blood pressure control, result in excellent outcomes. Failure to recognize this complication, nevertheless, may result in uncontrolled hypertension, leading to continued bleeding within the wall of the aorta and resulting in an intramural hematoma.

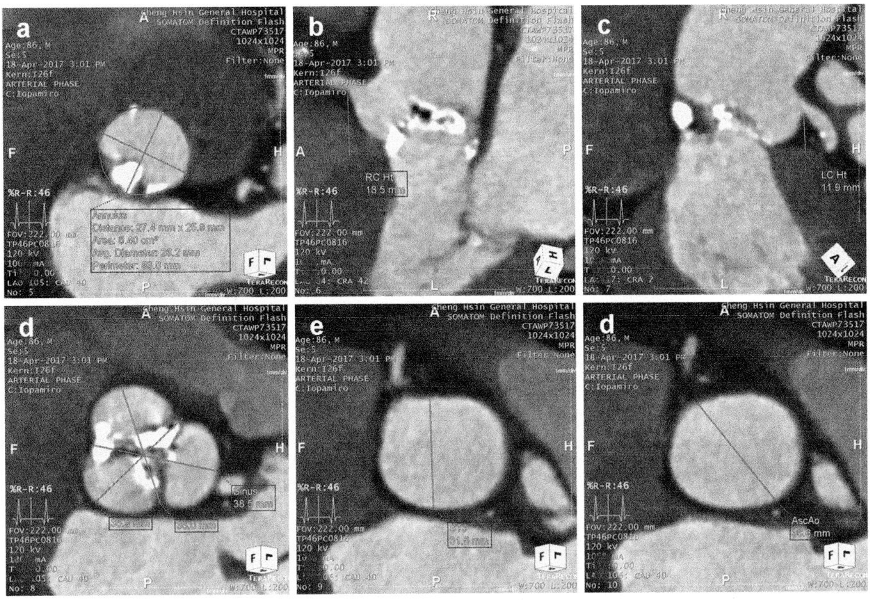

Fig. 5.88 Computed tomography of aortic root. (**a**) The maximum annular diameter is 27.4 mm, and the length perpendicular to it is 25.9 mm. The height of the right (**b**) and left coronary artery (**c**) from the basal annulus is 18.5 mm and 11.9 mm respectively. (**d**) Cross section revealed the maximum diameter of the left coronary sinus (38.5 cm), right coronary sinus (36.0 cm), and non-coronary sinus (35.9 cm). The diameter of sinotubular junction (**e**) and ascending aorta (**f**) is 31.5 and 36.6 mm individually

Fig. 5.89 During the transcatheter aortic valve implantation, the guiding wire (arrow heads) advanced cross the aortic valve

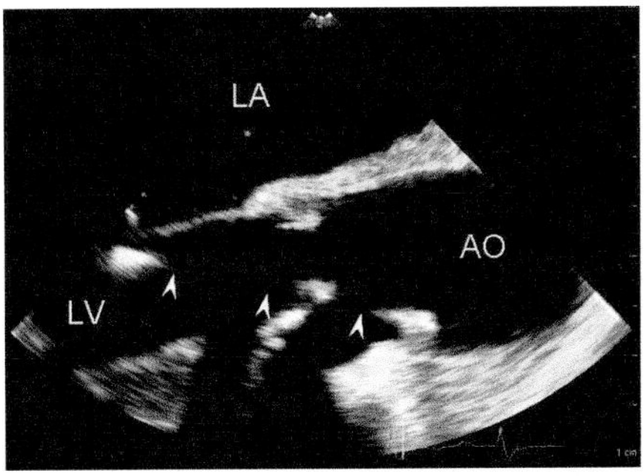

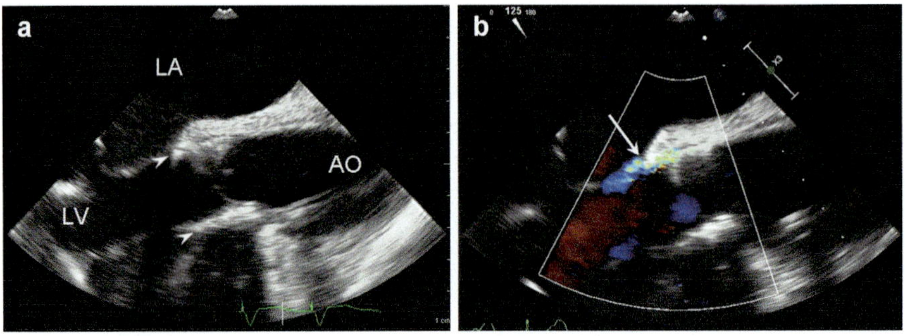

Fig. 5.90 When the SAPINE valve (29 mm, arrow heads, **a**) was first deployed, mild paravalvular leak (arrow, **b**) was present

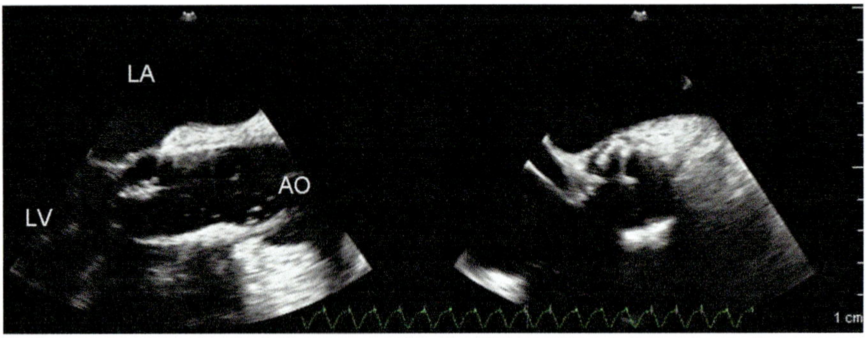

Fig. 5.91 To extend the SAPINE valve, the balloon catheter was inflated again. In x-plane view, air bubble filled the cavity within the prosthetic valve

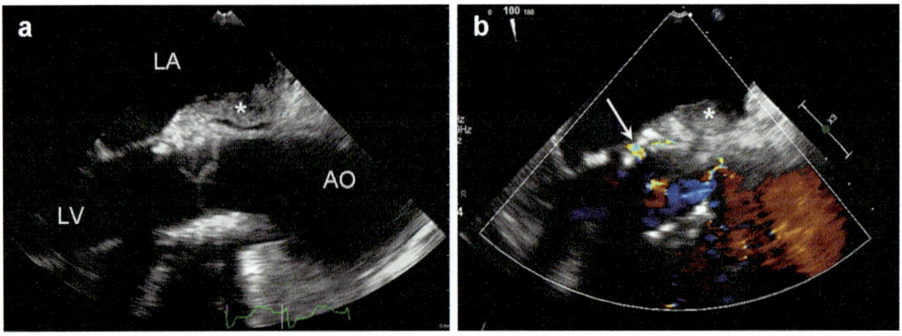

Fig. 5.92 After deployed again (**a**), the SAPINE valve presented normal function with trivial paravalvular leak (arrow, **b**). However, a hematoma (asterisk) was demonstrated around the outside of aortic root

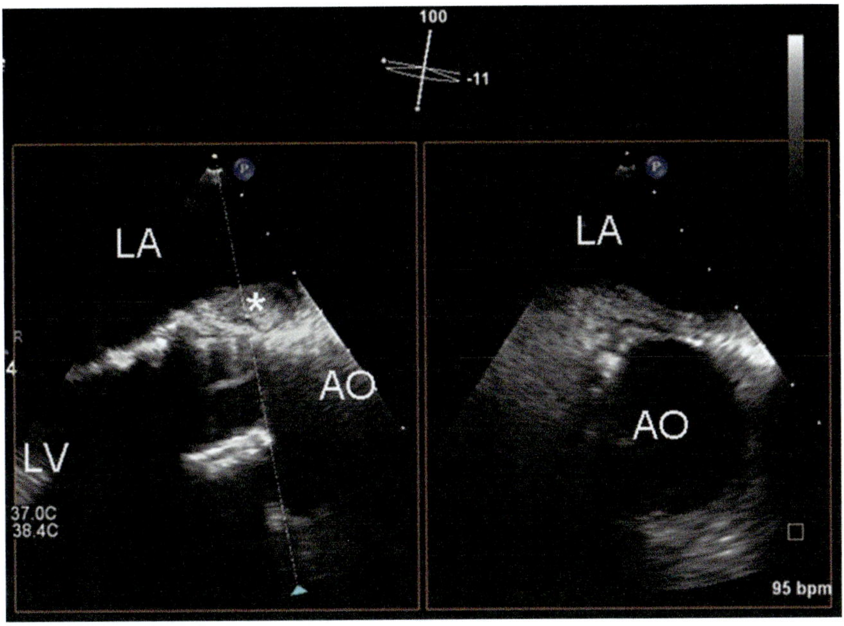

Fig. 5.93 In an x-plane view, a tissue-density hematoma (asterisk) was around the outside of the aortic root, which could be resulted from microrupture of the aorta

Fig. 5.94 In a three dimensional long-axis view, there was a hematoma (asterisk) around the outside of the aortic root

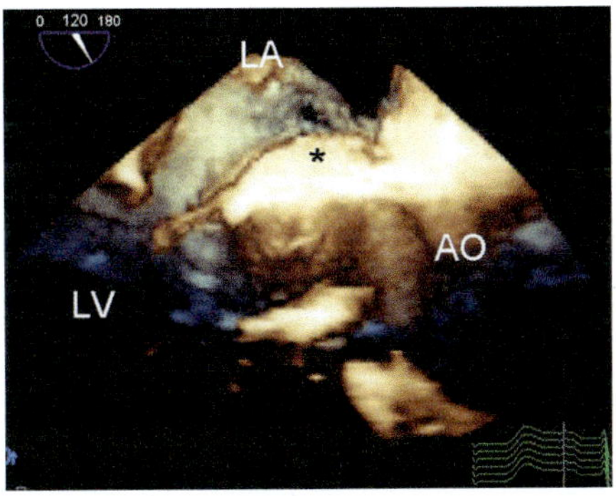

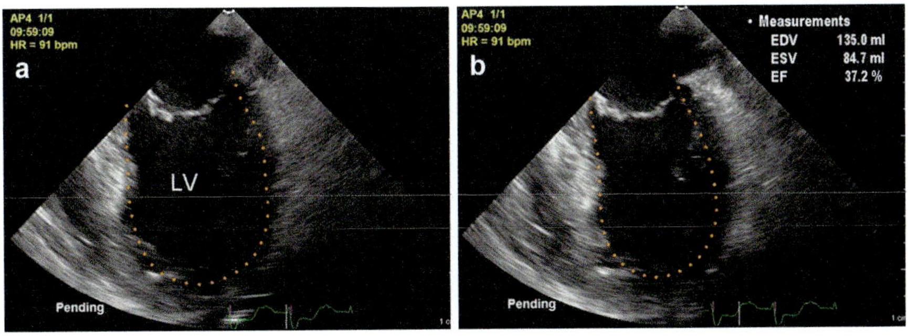

Fig. 5.95 Midesophageal four-chamber approach in diastole (**a**) and systole (**b**). Immediately after the SAPINE valve fully expanded, left ventricular dysfunction was revealed (*EDV* end diastolic volume, *ESV* end systolic volume, *EF* ejection fraction)

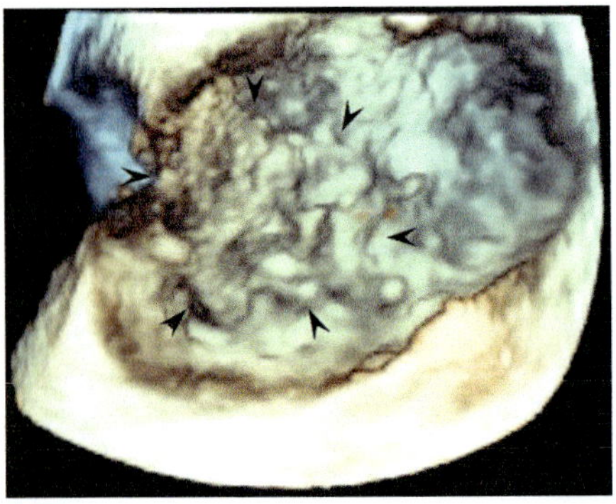

Fig. 5.96 During the procedure, there were some plaques seen in the descending aorta (within arrow heads)

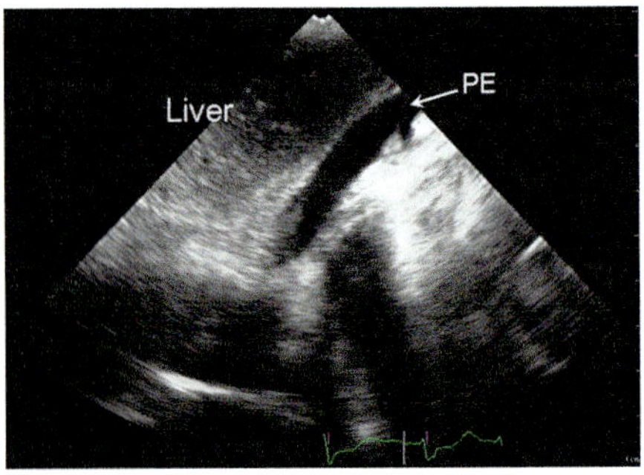

Fig. 5.97 After the procedure, pericardial effusion was also demonstrated, which could be the complication of aortic rupture

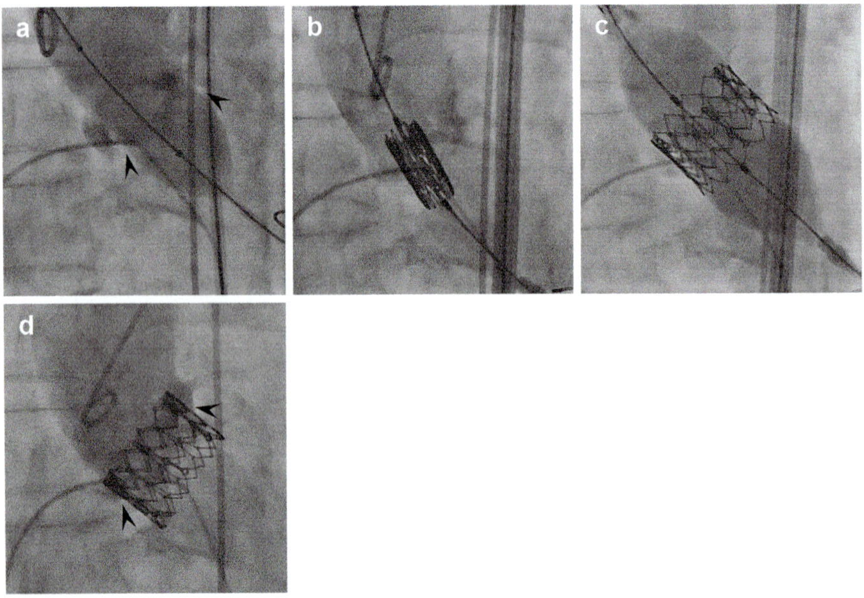

Fig. 5.98 Aortic root angiography during implantation of the SAPIEN valve. (**a**) The contrast injection showed the position of the cusps (arrow heads). (**b**) The SAPIEN valve was advanced onto the balloon and aligned between the aortic cusps. (**c**) The SAPINE valve was deployed by the balloon. (**d**) Position of the device was confirmed with one-half of it below the annular plane (arrow heads)

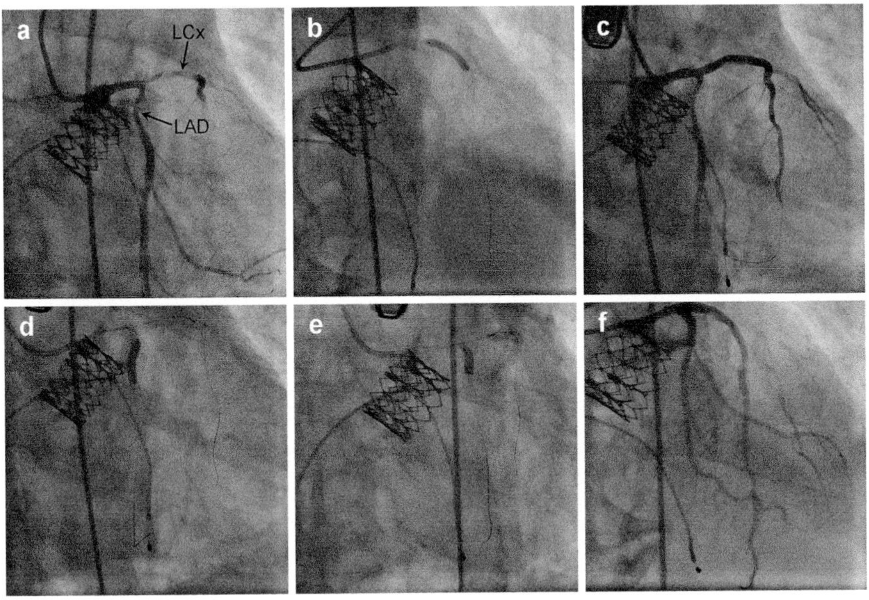

Fig. 5.99 Immediately after transcatheter aortic valve implantation, severe ST depression was noted by electrocardiogram. (**a**) Aortography showed impaired flow in left anterior descending artery (LAD) and haziness at proximal left circumflex (LCx). A dissection flap was noted in left main artery and proximal LCx. (**b**–**e**) Guiding wires advanced into the LAD and LCx. The arteries were dilated by balloons then stents were deployed. (**f**) Good angiography result with normal LAD and LCx flow was presented

5.10 Iatrogenic Ventricular Septal Defect and Following Rapid Tumor Invasion after Transcatheter Aortic Valve Implantation

An 86-year-old male patient had received a transcatheter aortic valve implantation for aortic stenosis. After the procedure, an iatrogenic linear tract at ventricular septum was revealed. To enclose the defect, an occluder implantation was indicated. However, the procedure was postponed because a mass was discovered in the right atrium and inferior vena cava by echocardiography.

Department of oncology was consulted for further treatment, where hepatocellular carcinoma at right lobe of liver (segment 6 and 7) involving right hepatic vein, IVC and extending to right atrium with metastatic lymphadenopathy and left adrenal gland metastases was confirmed. The patient received radiotherapy afterward.

Post-transcatheter aortic valve implantation ventricular septal defect most often results from a focal annular rupture that extends into the right ventricular outflow tract, but direct trauma to the septum from the transcatheter heart valve, like this patient, has also been described. Percutaneous closure should the first option to treat a post-transcatheter aortic valve implantation ventricular septal defect because patients who received transcatheter aortic valve implantation are frequently at high or prohibitive surgical risk. Consequently, open surgical procedure may not be feasible (Figs. 5.100, 5.101, 5.102, 5.103, 5.104, 5.105, 5.106, 5.107, 5.108, 5.109, 5.110, 5.111, 5.112, 5.113, 5.114, 5.115; Videos 5.100a, 5.100b, 5.101, 5.102, 5.103a, 5.103b, 5.104a, 5.104b, 5.105a, 5.105b, 5.106a, 5.106b, 5.107a, 5.107b, 5.108, 5.109a, 5.109b, 5.110, 5.111a, 5.111b, 5.112a, 5.112b, 5.113a, 5.113b, 5.114a, 5.114b, 5.115).

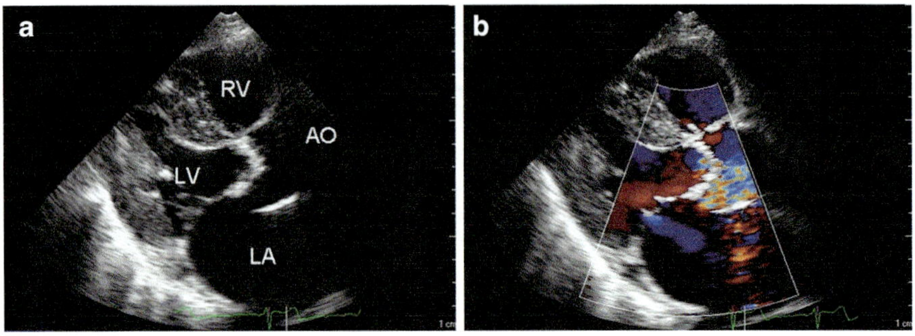

Fig. 5.100 Transthoracic parasternal long-axis view (**a**) with color Doppler (**b**) showed thickened aortic valve with restricted cusp mobility which reduced cusp separation caused turbulent left ventricular outflow

Fig. 5.101 Parasternal long-axis view showed thickened aortic valve with narrow aortic orifice

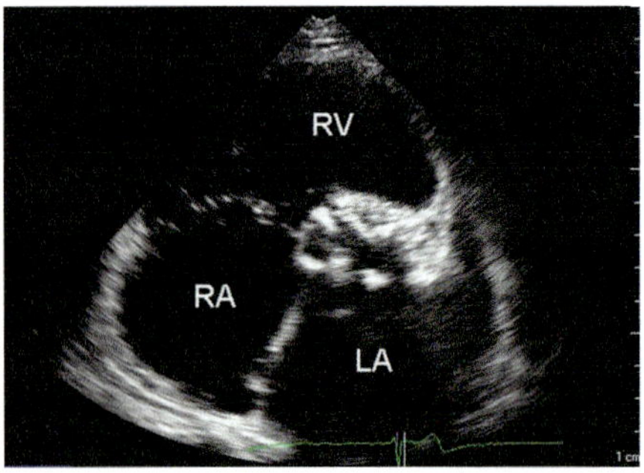

Fig. 5.102 Apical four-chamber view showed intact cardiac structure with normal function

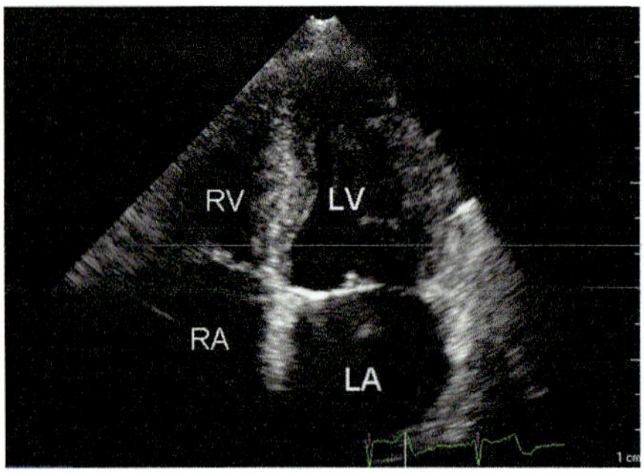

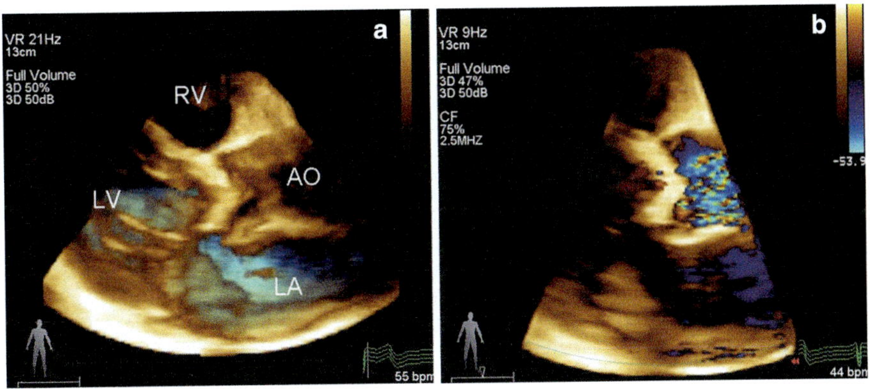

Fig. 5.103 Three dimensional parasternal long-axis view (**a**) with color Doppler (**b**) showed thickened aortic valve with restricted cusp mobility reduced cusp separation and caused turbulent left ventricular outflow

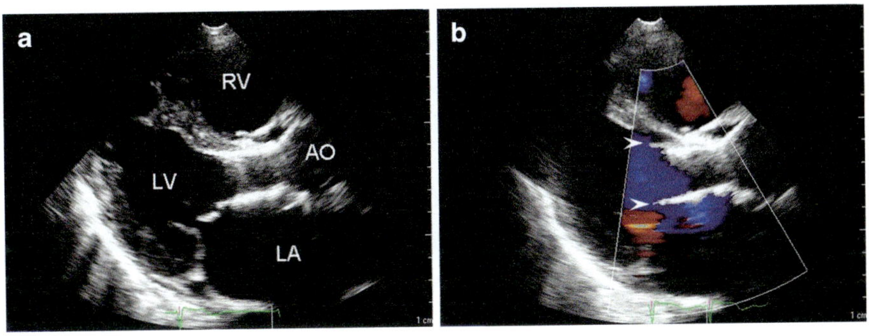

Fig. 5.104 After transcatheter aortic valve implantation, the CoreValve (29 mm, arrow heads) presented normal function (**a**) with trivial paravalvular leakage (**b**)

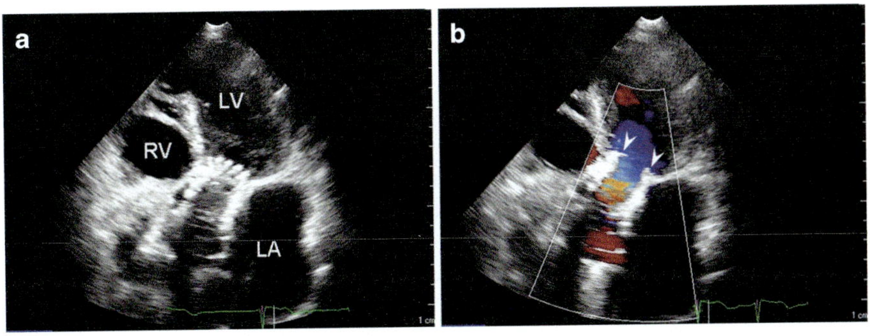

Fig. 5.105 In apical five-chamber view (**a**) with color Doppler (**b**), the CoreValve (arrow heads) presented normal function with trivial paravalvular leakage

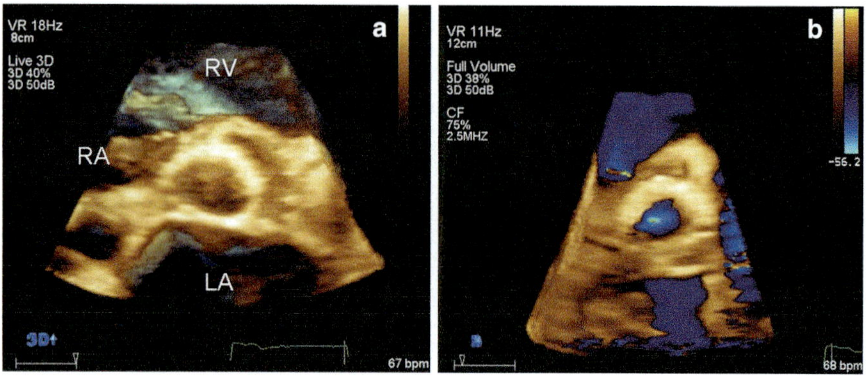

Fig. 5.106 In three dimensional parasternal short-axis view (**a**) with color Doppler (**b**), the CoreValve presented normal function with trivial paravalvular leakage

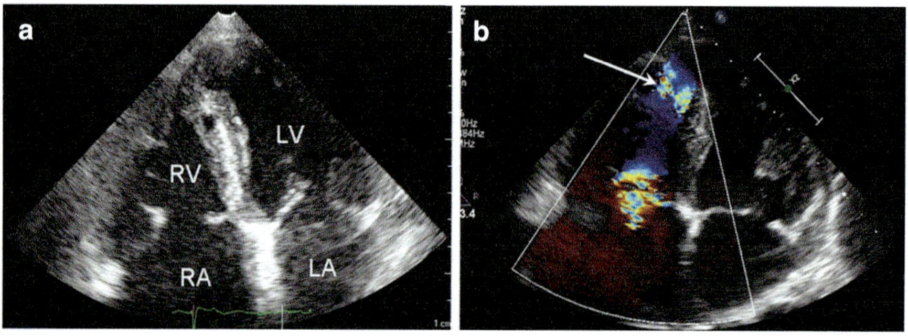

Fig. 5.107 In apical four-chamber view (**a**) with color Doppler (**b**), direct trauma of the ventricular septum was revealed. A linear tract near the apical ventricular septum with a left-to-right shunt (arrow) across it was demonstrated

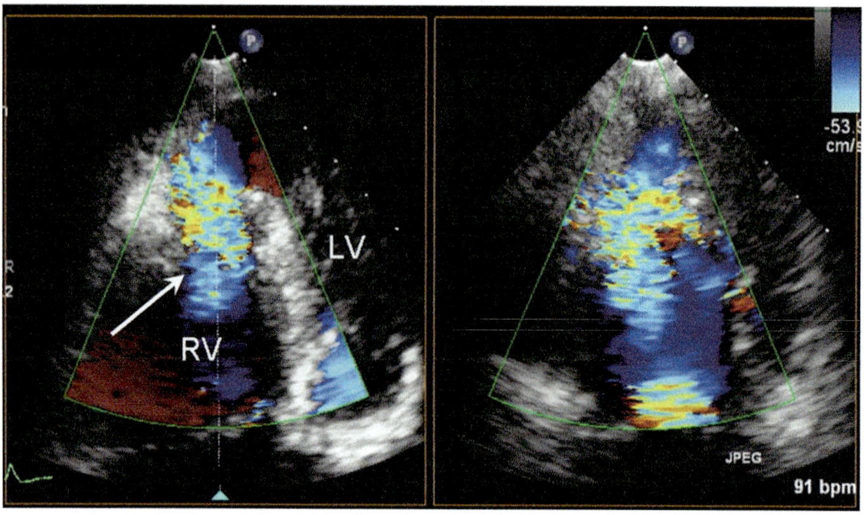

Fig. 5.108 In x-plane color Doppler, a linear tract near the apical ventricular septum with a left-to-right shunt (arrow) across it was demonstrated

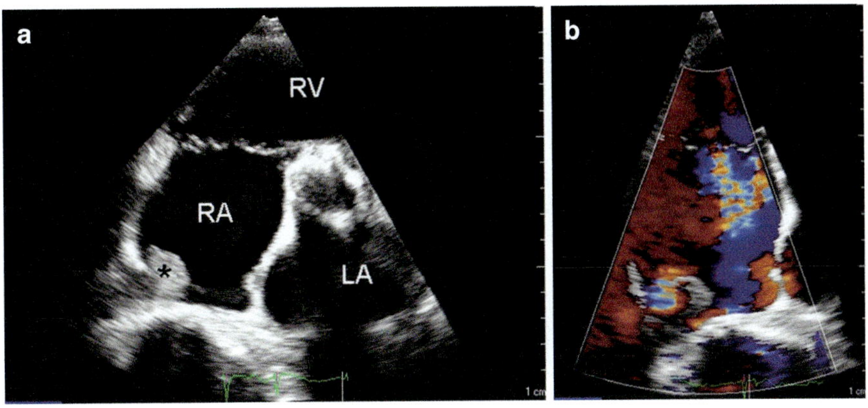

Fig. 5.109 Four-month following the transcatheter aortic valve implantation, transthoracic parasternal short-axis view showed a mass lesion (*) protruded into the right atrium (**a**) with flow occlusion (**b**)

Fig. 5.110 In subcostal four-chamber view, a mass lesion (*) protruded into the right atrium from inferior vena cava was demonstrated

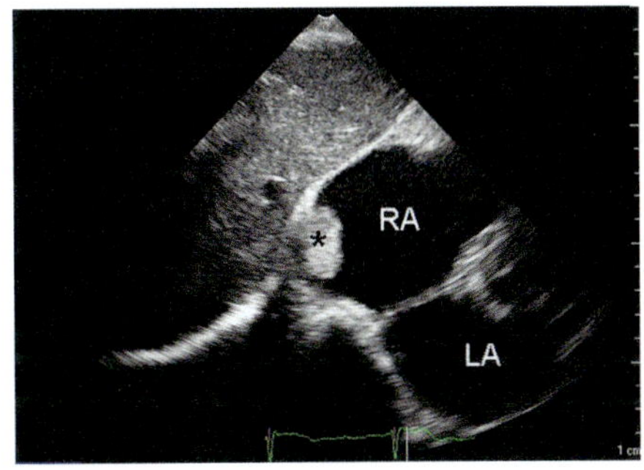

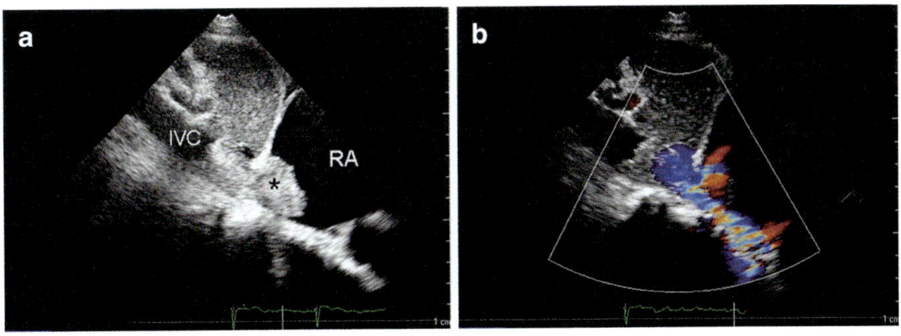

Fig. 5.111 Subcostal view of the inferior vena cava showed a mass lesion (*) extended into the right atrium from the vessel (**a**) with occlusion (**b**)

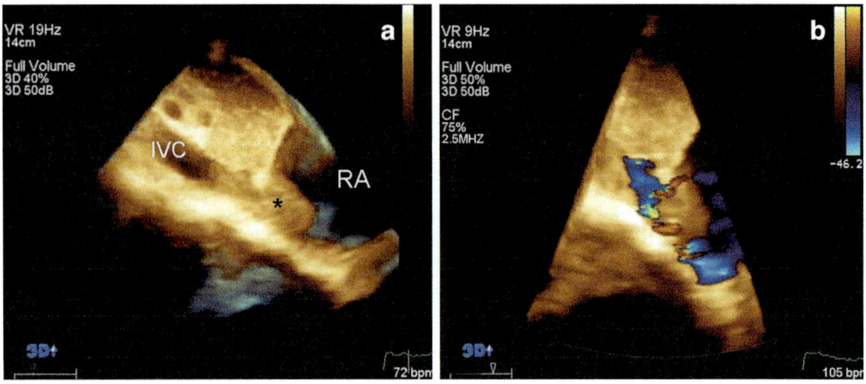

Fig. 5.112 In three dimensional subcostal view of the inferior vena cava, a mass lesion (*) extended into the right atrium from the vessel (**a**) with occlusion (**b**) was demonstrated

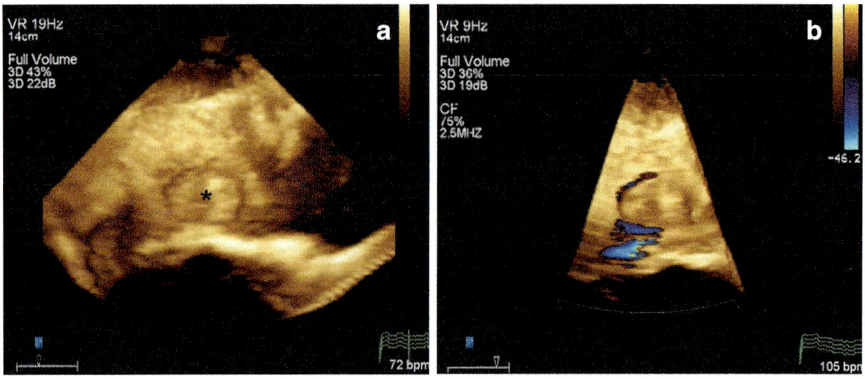

Fig. 5.113 In three dimensional subcostal view from the right atrium toward the inferior vena cava (**a**) with color Doppler (**b**), a mass lesion (*) extended into the right atrium and occluded the inflow

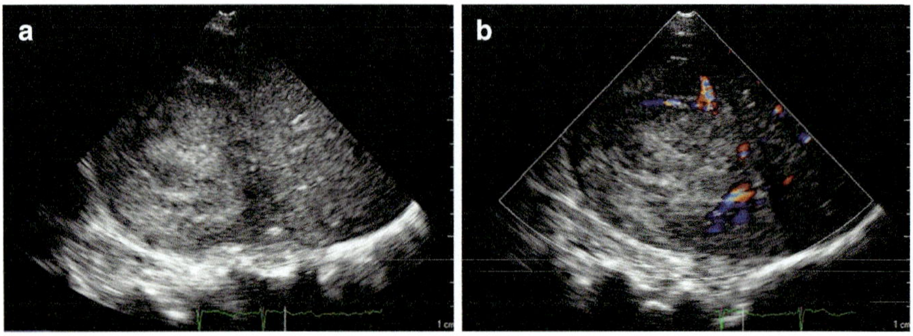

Fig. 5.114 In subcostal view of liver (**a**) with color Doppler (**b**), multiple hyperechoic masses (maximum was 11 mm × 9 mm) with blood supply was seen at right lobe liver

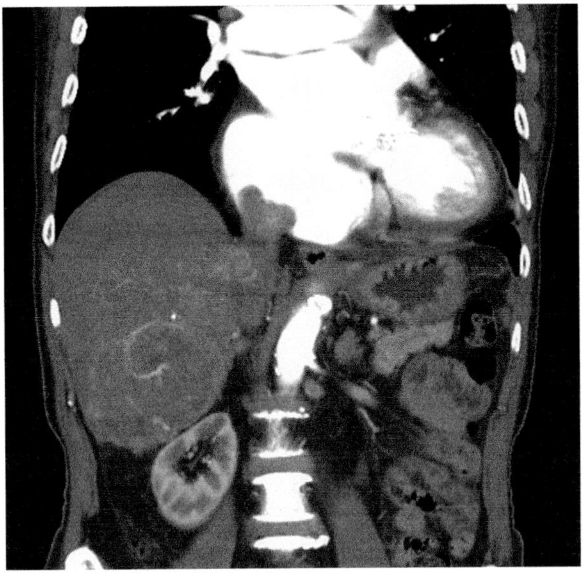

Fig. 5.115 Computed tomography showed multiple masses at right lobe of liver with extension to the right hepatic vein, inferior vena cava and the right atrium

5.11 Percutaneous Closure of Iatrogenic Left Ventricular Apical Pseudoaneurysm

A 76-year-old male patient had a previous surgical mitral valve replacement with porcine valve ten years ago. Recently, she suffered from progressive shortness of breath, dyspnea on exertion and pitting edema. Recurrent mitral regurgitation was revealed and an apical approached transcatheter mitral valve in valve replacement with SAPINE valve was done.

However, twenty two days following his operation, the patient developed mild dyspnea. A left ventricular apical pseudoaneurysm and right side pleural effusion were noted. Therefore, a left ventricular apex occluder implantation was scheduled (Figs. 5.116, 5.117, 5.118, 5.119, 5.120, 5.121, 5.122, 5.123, 5.124, 5.125; Videos 5.116, 5.117, 5.118a, 5.118b, 5.119, 5.120a, 5.120b, 5.120c, 5.120d, 5.121a, 5.121b, 5.122a, 5.122b, 5.123a, 5.123b, 5.124, 5.125).

The transapical approach for transcatheter mitral valve-in-valve implantation is a novel and promising alternative for patients who are not candidates for conventional redo surgical replacement. Complications include bleeding, stroke, mitral and aortic insufficiency, and hematoma. Pseudoaneurysms of the left ventricle are relatively infrequent. The risk of rupture of a left ventricular pseudoaneurysm is high while open surgical repair carries great mortality. As a result, percutaneous closure may offer a viable alternative to surgical intervention in this group.

Owing to the fact that transthoracic apical approach of echocardiogram is the closest view to evaluate the left ventricular apex, the implantation of apical false aneurysm occluder in this patient was monitored by it rather than a transesophageal one.

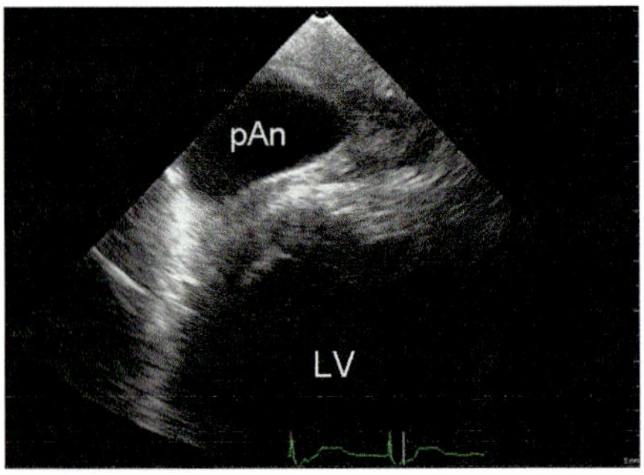

Fig. 5.116 In an apical approach of transthoracic echocardiogram, there was an echo lucent sac at the left ventricular apex, which was considered a pseudoaneurysm (pAn)

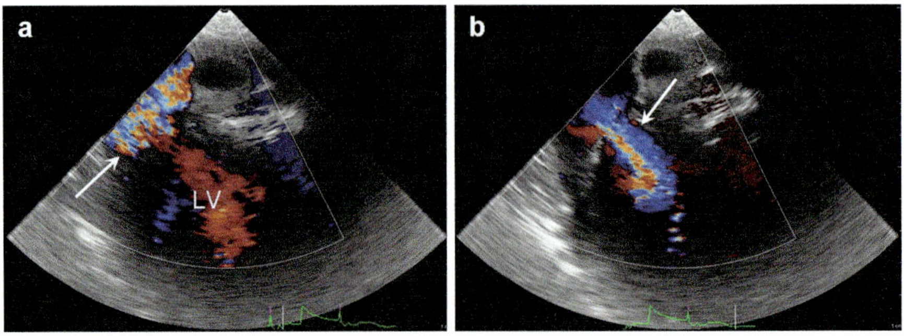

Fig. 5.117 Color Doppler demonstrated forward flow (arrow) into the pseudoaneurysm from the left ventricular cavity in systole (**a**) and retrograde flow into the cavity during diastole (**b**)

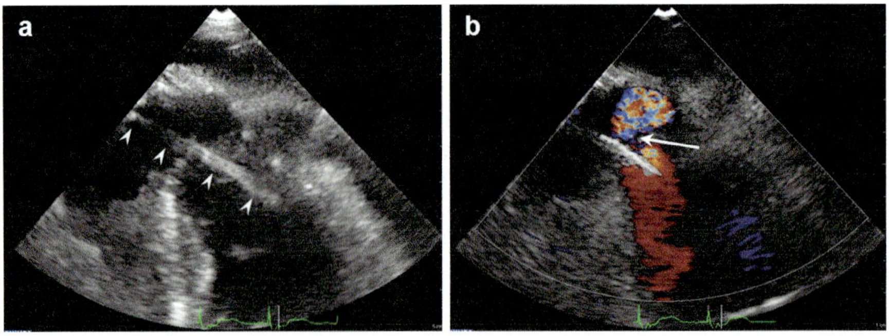

Fig. 5.118 During occluder implantation, a delivery cable (arrow heads, **a**) crossed the tear of left ventricular apex. (**b**) Forward flow (arrow) into the pseudoaneurysm in color Doppler demonstrated correct positioning of the occluder delivery system

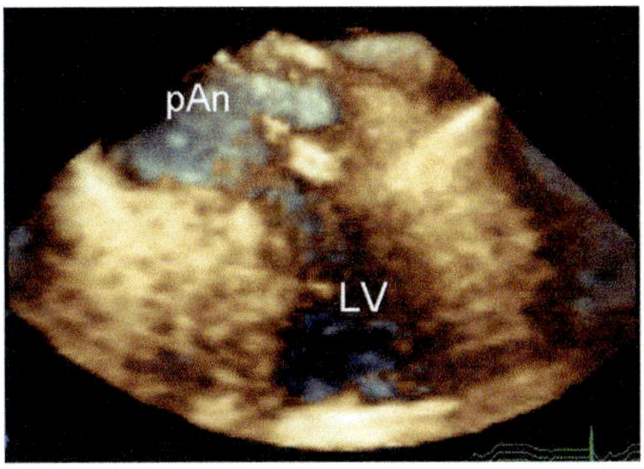

Fig. 5.119 In a three dimensional apical approach during the occluder implantation, the guiding catheter across the communication and advanced into the pseudoaneurysm

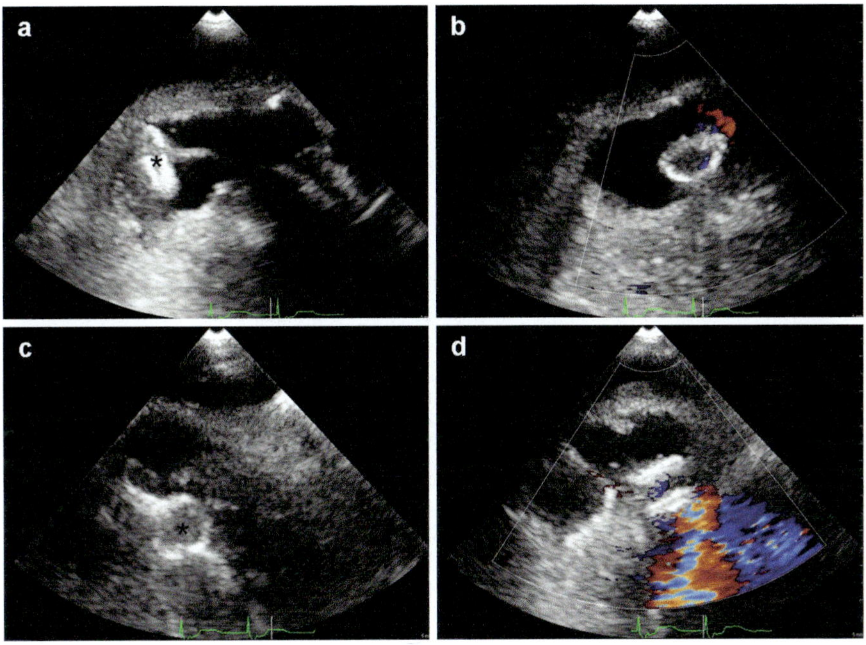

Fig. 5.120 During occluder implantation, the first disk of the occluder (asterisk, **a**) was deployed in the complex pouch. Than the delivery system was brought back (**b**).The remainder of the device was deployed in left ventricular cavity (asterisk, **c**). After the procedure, color Doppler showed mild residual flow across the occluder (**d**)

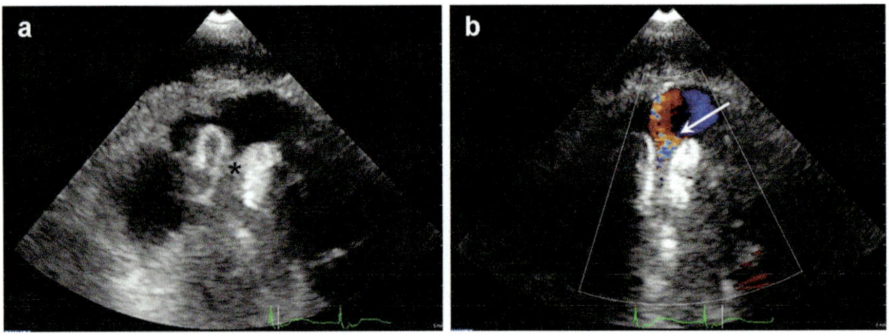

Fig. 5.121 In a modified apical approach after the occluder implantation, the device (asterisk, **a**) filled the tunnel of the tract. Color Doppler revealed mild residual flow (arrow, **b**) across the occluder into the pseudoaneurysm

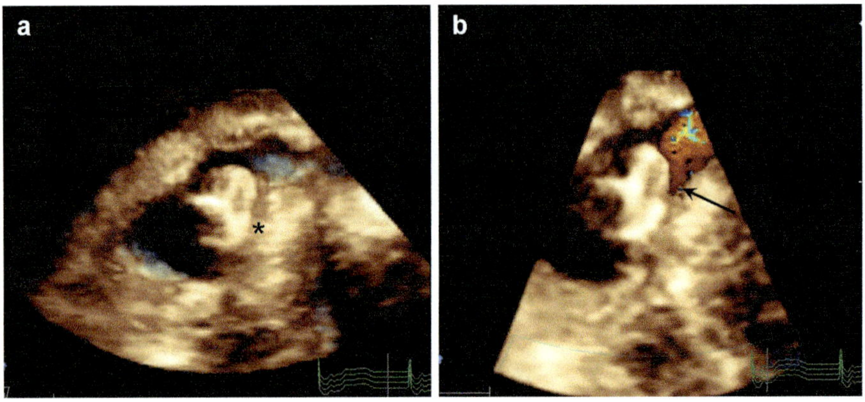

Fig. 5.122 Three dimensional modified apical approach after the occluder implantation showed the device (asterisk, **a**) filled the tunnel of the tract. Color Doppler revealed mild residual flow (arrow, **b**) across the occluder into the pseudoaneurysm

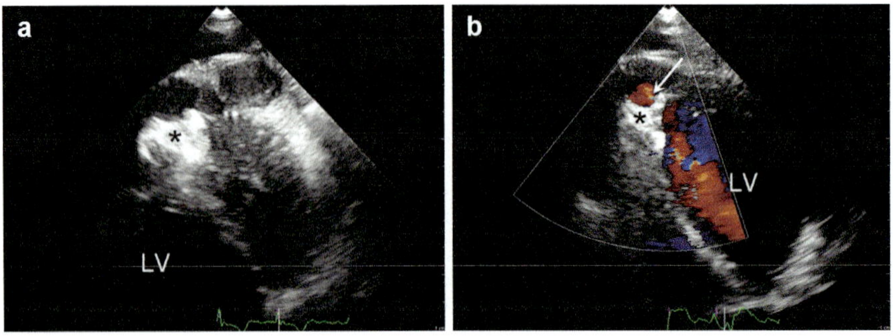

Fig. 5.123 On post-operative day 20, a modified apical approach showed the device (asterisk, **a**) remained in the correct position and thrombus formation in the cavity of the pseudoaneurysm. Color Doppler revealed the residual flow reduced form mild to minimal (arrow, **b**)

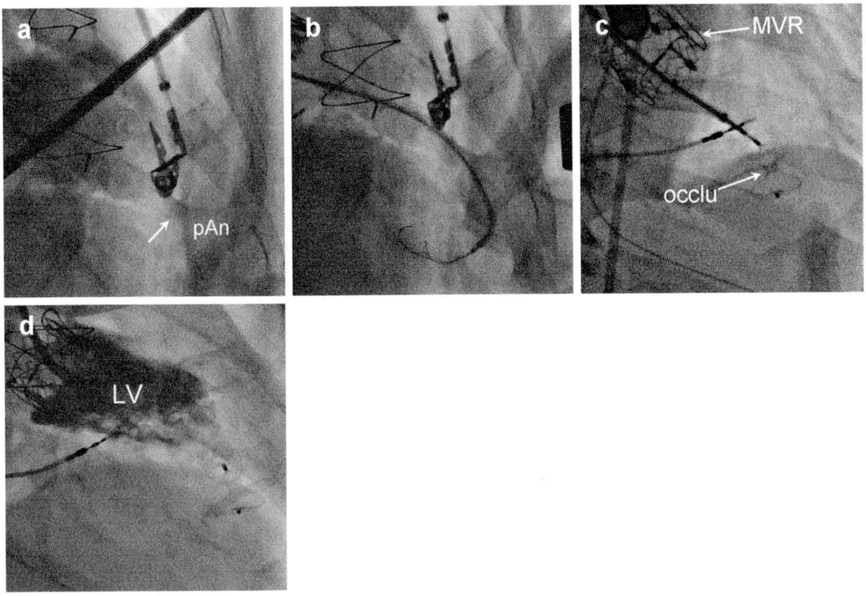

Fig. 5.124 Left-ventricular angiogram showed the tract (arrow, **a**) between left ventricular apex and the pseudoaneurysm (pAn). (**b**) The guiding catheter advanced into the pseudoaneurysm from the left ventricle. (**c**) The occluder (occlu) was delivered and both sides of the disks were deployed. (**d**) After the device was released, left-ventricular angiogram showed scarcely no residual flow across the occluder

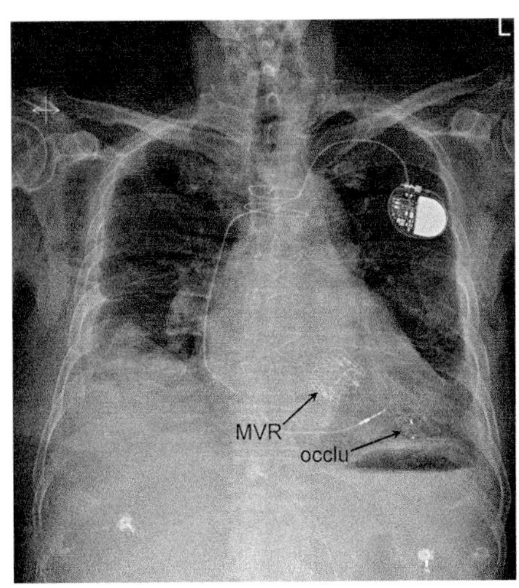

Fig. 5.125 Chest X ray showed the patient had received mitral valve replacement (MVR), SAPIEN valve and apex occluder (occlu) implantation

Suggested Readings

1. Abdelsalam E, Rodolfo R, Christopher F, et al. Persistent left ventricular false aneurysm after transapical insertion of an aortic valve. J Card Surg. 2011;26:51–3.
2. Ando T, Holmes AA, Taub CC, et al. Iatrogenic ventricular septal defect following transcatheter aortic valve replacement: a systematic review. Heart Lung Circ. 2016;25:968–74.
3. Darren M, Ali A, Pascal T, et al. Transcatheter heart valve failure: a systematic review. Eur Heart J. 2015;36:1306–27.
4. Dvir D, Leipsic J, Blanke P, et al. Coronary obstruction in transcatheter aortic valve-in-valve implantation: preprocedural evaluation, device selection, protection, and treatment. Circ Cardiovasc Interv. 2015;8:e002079.
5. Edgar T, Ronen G, Namal W, et al. Outcome of patients after transcatheter aortic valve embolization. J Am Coll Cardiol Intv. 2011;4:228–34.
6. Falipe F, Vedat T, Wilhelm R, et al. Successful post-dilation of a Lotus transcatheter aortic valve in case of prosthesis frame underexpansion due to leaflet calcification. JACC Cardiovasc Interv. 2015;8:866–8.
7. Généreux P, Head SJ, Hahn R, et al. Paravalvular leak after transcatheter aortic valve replacement: the new Achilles' heel? A comprehensive review of the literature. J Am Coll Cardiol. 2013;61:1125–36.
8. George DD, Jeffrey IW, Gennaro G, et al. Prosthetic heart valve thrombosis. JACC. 2016;68:2670–89.
9. Gian PU, Marco B, Angelo R, et al. The valve-in-valve technique for treatment of aortic bioprosthesis malposition: an analysis of incidence and 1-year clinical outcomes from the Italian CoreValve registry. JACC. 2011;2011:1062–8.
10. Hahn RT, Kodali S, Tuzcu EM, et al. Echocardiographic imaging of procedural complications during balloon-expandable transcatheter aortic valve replacement. JACC Cardiovasc Imaging. 2015;8:288–318.
11. Jan-Malte S, Nikos W, Georg N, et al. Next-generation transcatheter heart valves: current trials in Europe and the USA. Methodist Debakey Cardiovasc J. 2012;8(2):9–12.
12. John ML, Jason HR. Interventional procedures for adult structural heart disease. Philadelphia: Elsevier; 2014. Ch. 6, 7
13. John DC, John GW. Structural heart disease interventions. Philadelphia: Lippincott Williams & Wilkins; 2012. Ch. 18–20
14. Luu J, Ali O, Feldman TE, et al. Percutaneous closure of paravalvular leak after transcatheter aortic valve replacement. JACC Cardiovasc Interv. 2013;6(2):e6–8.
15. Martin BL, Nicolo P, Eugenia N, et al. Standardized endpoint definitions for transcatheter aortic valve implantation clinical trials: a consensus report from the Valve Academic Research Consortium. Eur Heart J. 2011;32:205–17.
16. Nathaniel BL, Nadira BH, Tamim MN, et al. Injuries to the aorta, aortic annulus, and left ventricle during transcatheter aortic valve replacement: management and outcomes. Circ Cardiovasc Interv. 2017;10:e004735.
17. Nicolas VM, Ramon RO, Ben R, et al. Transcatheter Lotus valve implantation in a degenerated Carpentier-Edwards bioprothesis. JACC Cardiovasc Interv. 2015;8:e27–8.
18. Schmidt T, Frerker C, Alessandrini H, et al. Redo TAVI: initial experience at two German centres. EuroIntervention. 2016;12(7):875–82.

Printed by Printforce, the Netherlands